CLINICAL DERMATOLOGY

For Ruth, Patricia and Arlene

Clinical Dermatology

J. A. A. HUNTER
BA MD FRCP (Edin)
Grant Professor of Dermatology
University of Edinburgh
The Royal Infirmary
Edinburgh

J. A. SAVIN
MA MD FRCP DIH
Consultant Dermatologist
The Royal Infirmary
Edinburgh

M. V. DAHL
BA MD
Professor of Dermatology
University of Minnesota
Minneapolis

SECOND EDITION

b

Blackwell
Science

© 1989, 1995 by
Blackwell Science Ltd
Editorial Offices:
Osney Mead, Oxford OX2 0EL
25 John Street, London WC1N 2BL
23 Ainslie Place, Edinburgh EH3 6AJ
238 Main Street, Cambridge
    Massachusetts 02142, USA
54 University Street, Carlton
    Victoria 3053, Australia

Other Editorial Offices:
Arnette Blackwell SA
    1, rue de Lille
    75007 Paris
    France

Blackwell Wissenschafts-Verlag GmbH
    Kurfürstendamm 57
    10707 Berlin
    Germany

    Feldgasse 13
    A-1238 Wien
    Austria

First published 1989
Reprinted 1990, 1992, 1994
Second edition 1995
Reprinted 1996

Set by Setrite Typesetters, Hong Kong
Printed and bound in Italy
by G. Canale & C. S.p.A., Turin

DISTRIBUTORS

    Marston Book Services Ltd
    PO Box 87
    Oxford OX2 0DT
    (*Orders*: Tel: 01865 791155
            Fax: 01865 791927
            Telex: 837515)

North America
    Blackwell Science, Inc.
    238 Main Street
    Cambridge, MA 02142
    (*Orders*: Tel: 800 215-1000
            617 876-7000
            Fax: 617 492-5263)

Australia
    Blackwell Science Pty Ltd
    54 University Street
    Carlton, Victoria 3053
    (*Orders*: Tel: 03 347-0300
            Fax: 03 349-3016)

A catalogue record for this title
is available from the British Library

ISBN 0-632-03714-8 (BSL)
ISBN 0-86542-841-7 (International Edition)

Library of Congress
Cataloging-in-Publication Data

Hunter, J.A.A.
    Clinical dermatology / J.A.A. Hunter,
J.A. Savin, M.V. Dahl. – 2nd ed.
        p.   cm.
    Includes index.
    ISBN 0-632-03714-8
    1. Skin – Diseases.   2. Dermatology.
I. Savin, John.   II. Dahl, Mark V.
III. Title.
    [DNLM: 1. Skin Diseases – diagnosis.
2. Skin Diseases – therapy.
WR 220 H945c 1994]
RL71.H934   1994
616.5 – dc20
DNLM/DLC
for Library of Congress

                                    94-16488
                                        CIP

Contents

Preface to the second edition

We were more than happy with the friendly reception given to the first edition of our book in 1989, and to its later reprintings. The favourable reviews reassured us that we were on the right lines. However, dermatology has forged ahead so rapidly since then that extensive updating and rewriting has become necessary more quickly than we expected. Every chapter has had to be revised: massive changes have been made in our sections on immunology, cytokines, fungal infections, and therapy. The new genetics is breeding in every chapter. We welcome you to our second edition.

Acknowledgement

We thank Dr A. McMillen, The Royal Infirmary, Edinburgh for providing Figs 15.30−15.33.

Preface to the first edition

Some 10% of those who go to their family doctors do so with skin problems. We have seen an improvement in the way these have been managed over the last few years, but the subject still baffles many medical students — on both sides of the Atlantic. They find it hard to get a grip on the soggy mass of facts served up by some textbooks. For them we have tried to create an easily-read text with enough detail to clarify the subject but not enough to obscure it.

There are many doctors too who are puzzled by dermatology, even after years in practice. They have still to learn how to look at the skin with a trained eye. Anyone who denies that clinical dermatology is a visual specialty can never have practised it. In this book we have marked out the route to diagnostic success with a simple scheme for recognizing primary skin lesions using many diagrams and coloured plates.

We hope that this book will help both groups — students and doctors, including some in general medicine and some starting to train as dermatologists — and of course their patients. We make no apologies for our emphasis on diagnosis and management, and accept that we cannot include every remedy. Here, we mention only those preparations we have found to be useful and, to avoid too many trade names, we have tabulated those used in the UK and the USA in a Formulary at the back of the book.

We have decided not to break up the text by quoting lists of references. For those who want to know more there are many large and excellent textbooks on the shelves of all medical libraries.

While every effort has been made to ensure that the doses mentioned here are correct, the authors and publishers cannot accept responsibility for any errors in dosage which may have inadvertently entered this book. The reader is advised to check dosages, adverse effects, drug interactions, and contraindications in the latest edition of the *British National Formulary* or *Drug Information* (American Society of Hospital Pharmacists).

Acknowledgements

The clinical photographs come from our departmental collections and we wish to thank all those who presented them. We are also most grateful to Moira Gray for typing and retyping the manuscript, to Mrs Angela McQuillin for preparing the diagrams and to the staff of Blackwell Scientific Publications for help and encouragement in preparing this book.

Introduction

The classification of skin diseases has never been easy. Early attempts, for example by Robert Willan (1757–1812) (Figure), the founder of modern dermatology, brought some order into a subject which was then in chaos, but have left us with an unfortunate legacy of cumbersome Latin names (e.g. lichen planus), based on a defunct botanical classification. These names still baffle many doctors who may already be in a state of panic when faced with a rash.

Another problem is that many have glimpsed dermatology only briefly during their medical training, as all too often the subject has been squeezed out of its place in the curriculum. The result is a growing number of doctors who quail before the skin and its reputed 2000 conditions, each with its own diverse presentations. They can see the eruptions clearly enough, but cannot describe or identify them. There are no machines to help them. Patients quickly spot their weakness and lose faith.

Our aim in this book has been to coax medical students and doctors through these difficulties. We have concentrated on common conditions, which make up the bulk of dermatology in developed countries, but mention some others, which may be rare, but which illustrate important general principles. We have tried to keep the terminology simple, and to cut out as many synonyms and eponyms as possible.

We believe that some understanding of the anatomy and physiology of the skin (Chapter 2) and of immunology (Chapter 3) is needed to follow the simple steps which lead to a sensible working diagnosis. This sequence starts with the identification of primary skin lesions (p. 36) and the patterns these can take up on the skin surface (p. 39). After this has been achieved investigations (pp. 39–43) will run along reasonable lines until a firm diagnosis is reached. Then, and only then, will the correct line of treatment snap into place.

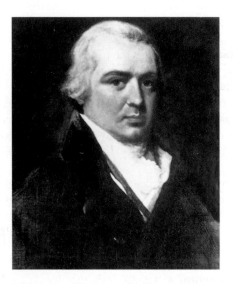

Robert Willan was able to use the Linnean system of botanical classification to divide skin diseases into eight orders.

But another cloud of mystery has settled here, over the subject of topical treatment. We attempt to blow this away in Chapter 24 with a few simple rules governing the selection of the right active ingredient (p. 277), and of the right vehicle in which it should be put up (p. 277). Correct choices here will be repaid by good results. Patients may be quick to complain if they are not doing well: equally they are delighted if their eruptions can be seen to melt rapidly away.

We admit, of course, that there are still problems in classification which will remain while the aetiology of so many skin diseases is still unknown. Nevertheless, whenever possible, we have grouped conditions which have the same cause, e.g. fungal infections (Chapter 15) and drug reactions (Chapter 23).

Failing this, some chapters are based on shared physiology, e.g. disorders of keratinization (Chapter 5) or on a shared anatomy, e.g. disorders of hair and nails (Chapter 8), of blood vessels (Chapter 13) or of the sweat glands (Chapter 14).

Finally, and most reluctantly, in some chapters we have been forced to group conditions which share certain physical characteristics, e.g. the bullous diseases (Chapter 11) and the papulosquamous disorders (Chapter 7): but this is unsound, and brings together some strange bedfellows. We are confident that modern research will reallocate their positions in the dormitory of dermatology.

CHAPTER 1

Skin disease in perspective

Dermatology may be defined as 'the study of skin and its diseases'. It is an immense subject, yet two-thirds of skin diseases are due to fewer than ten conditions. Perspective is important and an overview of the causes, prevalence and impact of skin disease is presented here.

Causes

The skin is the boundary between ourselves and what is around us. It reflects internal changes (Chapter 20) and reacts to changes in the environment. Usually it adapts easily, and returns to a normal state. Sometimes it fails to do so and a skin

disorder appears. Some of the internal and external factors which are important causes of skin disease are shown in Fig. 1.1. Often several will be operating at the same time: just as often no obvious cause for a skin abnormality can be found — and here lies much of the difficulty of dermatology.

Prevalence

No one who has worked in any branch of medicine will doubt the importance of diseases of the skin. A neurologist, for example, may know all about the Sturge—Weber syndrome, a gastroenterologist about the Peutz—Jeghers syndrome, and a cardiologist

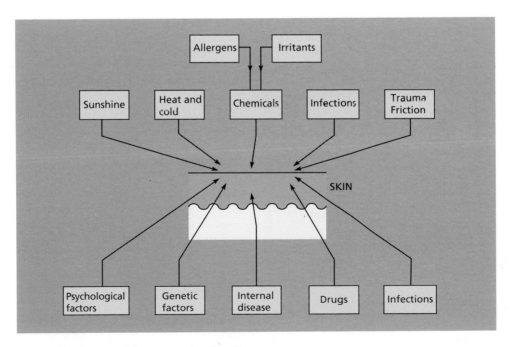

Fig. 1.1 Some internal and external factors causing skin diseases.

about the Leopard syndrome: but even in their own wards they will see far more of other common skin conditions such as drug eruptions, asteatotic eczema and scabies. They should know about these too.

In primary care, skin problems are even more important. They account for about 10% of all consultations in general practice in the UK; but this is only the tip of an iceberg of skin disease, the sunken part of which consists of problems which never get to doctors, being dealt with or ignored in the community.

How large is this problem? No one quite knows as those who are not keen to see their doctors seldom star in the medical literature. Nevertheless, a reasonable estimate of the iceberg of psoriasis in the UK is shown in Fig. 1.2. In the course of a single year most of those with psoriasis see no doctor, and only a few see a dermatologist.

Several large studies have confirmed that this is the case with other skin diseases too:

• 31.2% of a large representative sample of the US population were found to have significant skin disease which deserved medical attention. Scaled up, these figures would suggest that some 80 million of the US population have significant skin diseases.

• A community study of adults in the UK found 22.5% to have a skin disease needing medical attention: only one in five of these had seen a doctor within the preceding six months. Self-medication was far more common than any treatment prescribed by doctors.

Table 1.1 Some factors influencing the pattern of skin diseases in a community

High level of:	High incidence of:
Ultraviolet radiation	Skin malignancy in Caucasians
Heat and humidity	Fungal and bacterial infections
Industrialization	Contact dermatitis
Underdevelopment	Infestations
	Bacterial and fungal infections

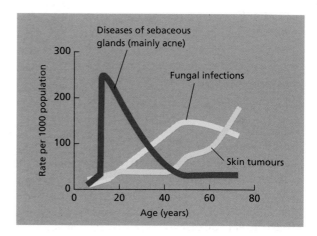

Fig. 1.3 The age-dependent prevalence of some skin conditions.

• Preparations used to treat skin disease can be found in about half of all homes in the UK: the ratio of non-prescribed to prescribed remedies is about six to one.

The pattern of skin disease in a community depends on many factors, both genetic and environmental. Some of these are listed in Table 1.1. In addition, within each community, different age groups suffer from different skin conditions. In the US for example, diseases of the sebaceous glands (mainly acne) peak at the age of about 18 and then decline, while the prevalence of skin tumours steadily mounts with age (Fig. 1.3).

Impact

Much of this book is taken up with ways in which skin diseases can do harm. Most fit into the five Ds shown in Fig. 1.4.

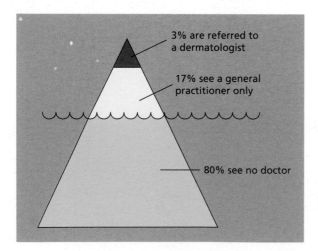

Fig. 1.2 The iceberg of psoriasis in the UK during a single year.

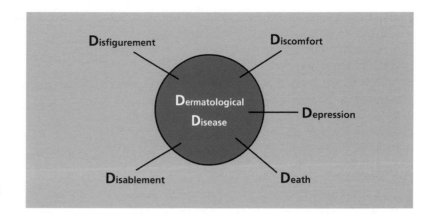

Fig. 1.4 The five Ds of dermatological disease.

Disfigurement

The range of possible reactions to disfiguring skin disease is described on p. 256. They vary from a leper complex, e.g. some patients with psoriasis (p. 51) to embarrassment, e.g. port-wine stains (Fig. 1.5) (p. 239) or androgenetic alopecia in both men and women (p. 75). Disorders of body image can lead those who have no skin disease to think that they have, or even to commit suicide in this mistaken belief (dermatological non-disease; p. 257).

Discomfort

Some people prefer pain to itch: skin diseases can offer both. Itchy skin disorders include eczema (p. 86), lichen planus (p. 67), scabies (p. 197) and dermatitis herpetiformis (p. 121). Pain is marked in e.g. shingles (p. 176), leg ulcers (p. 144) and glomus tumours (p. 240).

Disability

Skin conditions can ruin the quality of anyone's life. Each skin disease carries its own set of problems. At

Fig. 1.5 (a) This patient has a port-wine stain. (b) Her life is transformed by her clever use of modern camouflage cosmetics, which take her less than a minute to apply.

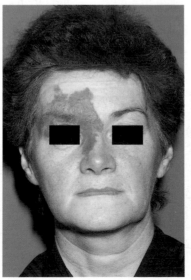

(a)

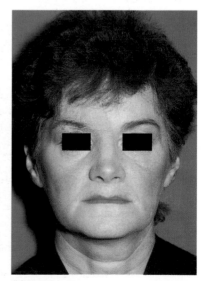

(b)

Table 1.2 The consequences of skin failure

Function	In skin failure	Treatment
Temperature control	Cannot sweat when too hot: cannot vasoconstrict when too cold. Hence temperature swings dangerously up and down	Controlled environmental temperature
Barrier function	Raw skin surfaces lose much fluid and electrolytes	Monitor and replace
	Heavy protein loss	High protein diet
	Bacterial pathogens multiply on damaged skin	Antibiotic
Cutaneous blood flow	Shunt through skin may lead to high output cardiac failure in those with poor cardiac reserve	Aggressively treat skin. Support vital signs
Others	Erythroderma may lead to malabsorption	Usually none needed
	Hair and nail loss later	Regrow spontaneously
	Nursing problems handling patients particularly with toxic epidermal necrolysis (p. 122) and pemphigus (p. 117)	Nurse as for burns

the most obvious level dermatitis of the hands can quickly destroy a manual worker's earning capacity as many hairdressers, nurses, cooks and mechanics know to their cost. In the USA for example, skin diseases account for almost half of all cases of occupational illness and cause more than 50 million days to be lost from work each year.

Disability and disfigurement may blend in a more subtle way, so that, for example, in times of unemployment even people with acne find it hard to get jobs. Psoriatics in the USA, already plagued by tactless hairdressers and messy treatments, have been shown to lose thousands of dollars in earnings by virtue of time taken off work. Even trivial psoriasis on the finger tips of blind people may have a huge effect on their lives by making it impossible to read Braille.

Depression

These physical, sensory and functional problems often lead to depression and anxiety, even in the most stable people.

Death

Death from skin disease is fortunately rare but does still occur, e.g. in pemphigus, toxic epidermal necrolysis and cutaneous malignancies.

However, the concept of skin failure is an important one. It may occur when any inflammatory skin disease becomes so widespread that it prevents normal functioning of the skin, with results as listed in Table 1.2.

LEARNING POINT
The words 'prevalence' and 'incidence' do not mean the same thing. Learn the difference and you join a small select band.
*1 The **prevalence** of a disease is the proportion of a defined population affected by it at a particular point in time.*
*2 The **incidence rate** is the proportion of a defined population developing the disease within a specified period of time.*

CHAPTER 2

The function and structure of the skin

The skin — the interface between humans and their environment — is the largest organ in the body. It weighs an average of 4 kg and covers an area of 2 m². A death from loss of skin, as in a burn, or in toxic epidermal necrolysis (p. 122), and the misery of unpleasant acne, remind us of its many important functions which range from the vital to the cosmetic (Table 2.1).

The skin has two layers. The outer is epithelial, the *epidermis*, which is firmly attached to, and supported by, connective tissue in the underlying *dermis*. Beneath the dermis is loose connective tissue, the *hypodermis*, which usually contains abundant fat (Fig. 2.1).

Epidermis

The epidermis is formed from many layers of closely packed cells, the most superficial of which are flattened and filled with keratins; it is therefore a stratified squamous epithelium. It adheres to the dermis partly by the interlocking of its downward projections (*epidermal ridges* or *pegs*) with upward projections of the dermis (*dermal papillae*) (Fig. 2.2).

The epidermis contains no blood vessels. It varies in thickness, from less than 0.1 mm on the eyelids to nearly 1 mm on the palms and soles. As dead surface squames are shed (accounting for some of the dust in our houses), the thickness is kept constant by cells dividing in the deepest (*basal* or *germinative*) layer. A generated cell moves, or is pushed by underlying mitotic activity, to the surface, passing through the *prickle* and *granular cell layers* before dying in the *horny layer*. The journey from the basal layer to the surface (epidermal turnover or transit time) takes about 60 days. During this time the cell's appearance changes. A vertical section through the epidermis summarizes the life history of a single epidermal cell (Fig. 2.3).

Table 2.1 Functions of the skin

Function	Structure/cell involved

Protection against:
  chemicals, particles
  ultraviolet radiation
  antigens, haptens
  microbes
	Horny layer
	Melanocytes
	Langerhans cells
	Langerhans cells
	Horny layer

Preservation of a balanced
  internal environment
Prevents loss of water,
  electrolytes and
  macromolecules
	Horny layer

Shock absorber
Strong, yet elastic and
  compliant
	Dermis and subcutaneous
	  fat covering

Temperature regulation	Blood vessels Eccrine sweat glands
Insulation	Subcutaneous fat
Sensation	Specialized nerve endings
Lubrication and waterproofing	Sebaceous glands
Protection and prising	Nails
Calorie reserve	Subcutaneous fat
Vitamin D synthesis	Keratinocytes
Body odour	Apocrine sweat glands
Psychosocial, display	Skin, lips, hair and nails

The *basal layer*, the deepest layer, rests on a basement membrane which attaches it to the dermis. It is a single layer of columnar cells, whose basal surfaces sprout many fine processes and hemidesmosomes, anchoring them the *lamina densa* of the basement membrane.

In normal skin some 30% of basal cells are preparing for division (growth fraction). Following mitosis, a cell enters the G_1 phase, synthesizes

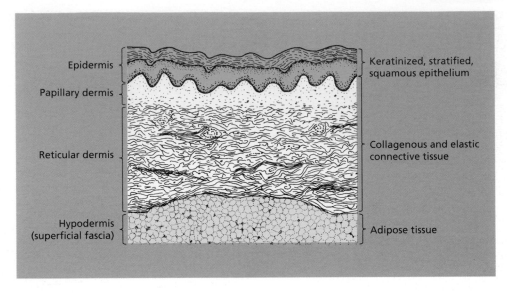

Fig. 2.1 Layers of the skin.

RNA and protein, and grows in size (Fig. 2.4). Later, something triggers the cell to divide. DNA is then synthesized (S phase) and chromosomal DNA is replicated. A short post-synthetic (G₂) phase of further growth occurs before mitosis (M). DNA synthesis continues through the S and G₂ phases, but not during mitosis. The G₁ phase is then repeated, and one of the daughter cells moves into the suprabasal layer. Having lost the capacity to divide, it then differentiates into a keratinocyte (Fig. 2.3) and synthesizes keratins. The cell cycle time in normal human skin is controversial; estimates of 50−200 hours reflect differing views on the duration of the G₁ phase.

Keratinocytes

The *spinous* or *prickle* cell layer is composed of such *keratinocytes*, which are firmly attached to each other by small interlocking cytoplasmic processes, abundant desmosomes and an intercellular cement of glycoproteins and lipoproteins. Under the light microscope, the desmosomes appear as 'prickles'. *Desmosomes* (Fig. 2.5a) are specialized attachment plaques which have been characterized biochemically. They contain desmoplakins. Cytoplasmic continuity between keratinocytes occurs at *gap junctions*, specialized areas on opposing cell walls. Tonofilaments are small fibres running from the

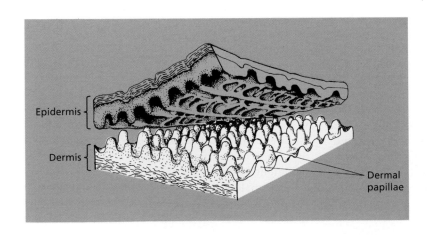

Fig. 2.2 The interlocking of epidermis and dermis.

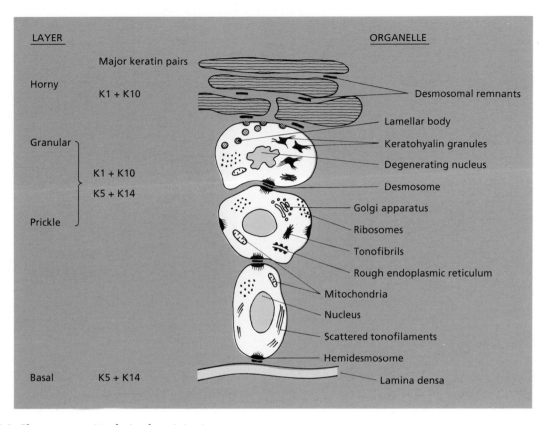

Fig. 2.3 Changes occurring during keratinization.

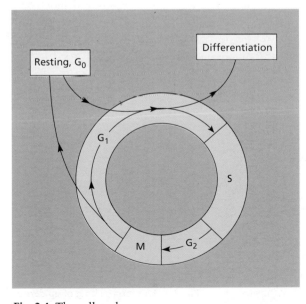

Fig. 2.4 The cell cycle.

cytoplasm to desmosomes. These are more numer-ous in cells of the spinous layer than in the basal layer, and are packed into bundles called *tonofibrils*. Many *lamellar granules* (membrane-coating granules, Odland bodies, keratinosomes) are seen in the super-ficial keratinocytes of this layer. They contain polysaccharides, free sterols, lipids and hydrolytic enzymes, and their contents are discharged into the intercellular space of the granular cell layer.

Differentiation continues in the *granular layer*, which normally has two or three layers of cells that are flatter than those in the spinous layer and have more tonofibrils. Granular layer cells contain lamel-lar granules and large, irregular basophilic granules of *keratohyalin* which merge with tonofibrils (Fig. 2.5). The keratohyalin granules contain profilaggrin, a histidine rich high molecular weight phosphoryl-ated protein, which is cleaved into filaggrin by speci-fic phosphatases as the granular cells move into

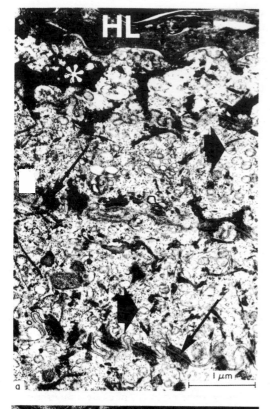

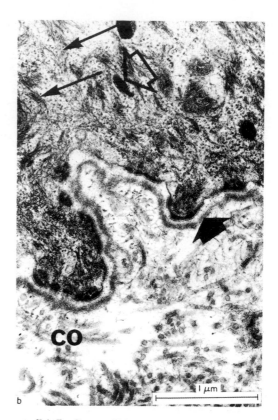

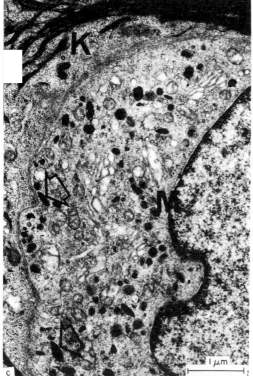

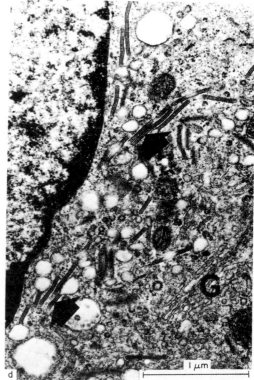

the horny layer. Hydrolytic and degrading enzymes found in the lysosomes of granular cells also destroy the cells' nuclei and intracytoplasmic organelles.

The *horny layer* (stratum corneum) is made of piled-up layers of flattened dead cells. Their cytoplasm is packed with keratin filaments embedded in a matrix derived from the keratohyalin granules. Horny cells normally have no nuclei or intracytoplasmic organelles. An insoluble envelope surrounds the horny cell and is formed by cross-linking of involucrin, synthesized high in the prickle cell layer. The envelope also contains loricrin, formed in the granular cell layer. Filaggrin, involucrin and loricrin can all be detected histochemically and are useful as markers of epidermal differentiation. Cells of the horny layer stick tightly together but flake off at the surface.

Keratinization

All cells have an internal skeleton made up of microfilaments (7 nm diameter; actin), microtubules (20–35 nm diameter; tubulin) and intermediate filaments (7–10 nm diameter). Keratins (from the Greek *keras* meaning horn) are the main intermediate filaments in epithelial cells and are comparable to vimentin in mesenchymal cells, neurofilaments in neurones and desmin in muscle cells. Keratins are no longer a biochemical curiosity as mutations in their genes cause epidermolysis bullosa simplex (p. 226) and bullous ichthyosiform erythroderma (p. 46).

The keratins are a family of more than 30 proteins, each produced by different genes. These separate into two gene families: one responsible for basic (Type I) and the other for acidic (Type II) keratins. The keratin polypeptide has a central helical portion with a non-helical N-terminal head and C-terminal tail. Individual keratins exist in pairs so that their double filament always consists of one Type I and one Type II keratin. Larger protofibrils are formed by the intertwining of adjacent filaments. The main keratins in the basal cell and prickle cells are keratins 5 and 14, but as differentiation occurs these are replaced by keratins 1 and 10 (Fig. 2.3). Two others (K6 and K16) are found in hyperproliferative states such as psoriasis.

During differentiation the keratin fibrils in the cells of the horny layer align, and aggregate, under the influence of filaggrin. Cysteine in keratins of the horny layer provides intra- and inter-chain disulphide links giving it the strength to withstand injury.

Cell cohesion

Firm cohesion in the spinous layer is ensured by 'stick and grip' mechanisms. The glycoprotein intercellular substance acts as a cement, sticking the cells together, and the intertwining of the small cytoplasmic processes of the prickle cells, together with their desmosomal attachments, accounts for the grip. The cytoskeleton of tonofibrils also rigidly maintains the cell shape. Lipids and sterol sulphates form electrochemical bonds, the rupture of which by steroid sulphatase, present in the horny layer, may account for the shedding of keratinized squames. One type of ichthyosis (p. 45) is characterized by a deficiency of steroid sulphatase; shedding then occurs in large scales.

The epidermal barrier

The horny layer prevents the loss of interstitial fluid from inside, and prevents the penetration of potentially harmful substances from outside. This *barrier function* is impaired when the horny layer is removed, experimentally by successive strippings with adhesive tape, or clinically by injury or skin disease. It is also decreased by excessive hydration or dehydration of the horny layer, and by detergents or lipid solvents.

The rate of penetration of a substance is proportional to its concentration difference across the layer. A rise in skin temperature aids penetration. The normal horny layer is slightly permeable to water but relatively impermeable to ions, such as

Fig. 2.5 (*Opposite*) Ultrastructure of the epidermis. (a) Horny and granular layer. HL, horny layers; white asterisk, keratohyalin granule; broad arrows, lamellar granules; fine arrows, desmosomes. (b) Dermo-epidermal junction. Fine arrows, tonofilaments; open arrow, melanosome; closed broad arrow, lamina densa; CO, collagen. (c) Part of melanocyte (M). Open arrows, melanosomes; K, part of keratinocyte. (d) Part of Langerhans cell. Broad arrows, Langerhans cell granules; G, Golgi apparatus.

sodium and potassium. Covalent substances (e.g. glucose and urea) also penetrate poorly, whilst some aliphatic alcohols pass through easily. In general the penetration of a solute dissolved in an organic liquid is that of the solvent.

Epidermal cell proliferation

Epidermopoiesis and its regulation

The thickness of the normal epidermis, and the number of cells in it, remain constant. This means that cell loss at the surface is balanced by cell production in the basal layer. Locally produced polypeptides (cytokines), growth factors and hormones may stimulate or inhibit epidermal proliferation; they interact in complex ways to ensure homeostasis. Cytokines and growth factors (Table 3.3) are produced by keratinocytes, Langerhans cells and lymphocytes within the skin. After binding to specific cell surface receptors, DNA synthesis is stimulated or inhibited via pathways of signal transduction, involving protein kinase C or inositol phosphate. Catecholamines, which do not penetrate the surface of cells, influence cell division via the cyclic AMP second messenger system. Steroid hormones bind to receptor proteins within the cytoplasm, pass to the nucleus and act at a transcriptional level.

Vitamin D synthesis

The steroid 7-dehydrocholesterol, found in keratinocytes, is converted by irradiation with sunlight to cholecalciferol. The vitamin becomes active after 25-hydroxylation in the kidney. Lack of sun and kidney disease may both cause vitamin D deficiency, and hence rickets.

Other cells in the epidermis

Keratinocytes make up about 85% of cells in the epidermis but three other types of cell are also found there: melanocytes, Langerhans cells and Merkel cells.

Melanocytes

Melanocytes are the only cells which can synthesize melanin. They migrate into the basal layer of the ectoderm from the neural crest. They are also found in hair bulbs, the retina and pia arachnoid. Each dendritic melanocyte associates with a number of keratinocytes, forming an 'epidermal melanin unit' (Fig. 2.6). The dendritic processes of melanocytes wind between the epidermal cells and end as discs in contact with them. Their cytoplasm contains discrete organelles, the *melanosomes*, containing varying amounts of the pigment melanin.

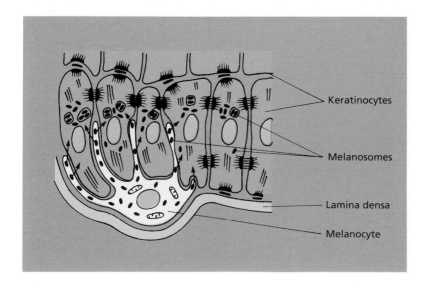

Fig. 2.6 The epidermal melanin unit. Arrows indicate transfer of melanosomes.

Melanogenesis

Melanocytes are the only cells in the epidermis to contain *tyrosinase* (dopa oxidase), the rate-limiting enzyme in melanogenesis. Tyrosinase, a copper-dependent enzyme, converts the substrate, tyrosine (derived from the essential amino acid phenylalanine), to melanin (Fig. 2.7). Dopa is formed by the oxidation of tyrosine, and further enzymic action leads to the formation of dopaquinone. Eumelanins, brown or black pigments are then formed by polymerization. Phaeomelanins and trichochromes, the pigments in red hair, are synthesized in the same way as eumelanin, except that cysteine reacts with dopaquinone. Phaeomelanins and eumelanins intermesh to form mixed melanin polymers (Fig. 2.7).

Eumelanins and phaeomelanins differ from neuromelanins, the pigments found in the substantia nigra and in cells of the chromaffin system (adrenal medulla, sympathetic ganglia, etc.), which are derived from tyrosine by the enzyme tyrosine hydroxylase.

Melanin is made within melanosomes. These tiny particles, about $0.1\,\mu m \times 0.7\,\mu m$, are shaped like either American footballs (eumelanosomes, containing eumelanin) or British soccer balls (phaeomelanosomes, containing phaeomelanin). Eventually, fully melanized organelles pass into the dendritic processes of the melanocyte and are then injected into neighbouring keratinocytes. Once there, melanosomes are distributed throughout the cytoplasm.

Negroids are black, not because they have more melanocytes, but because their melanocytes produce more and larger melanosomes, which are broken down less rapidly than those of Caucasoids. Melanins protect against ultraviolet radiation damage by absorbing and scattering the rays and by scavenging free radicals.

The control of melanogenesis

Melanogenesis is increased by a variety of stimuli, the most important of which is ultraviolet radiation. Tanning involves two distinct reactions.

The first, the immediate reaction, happens within

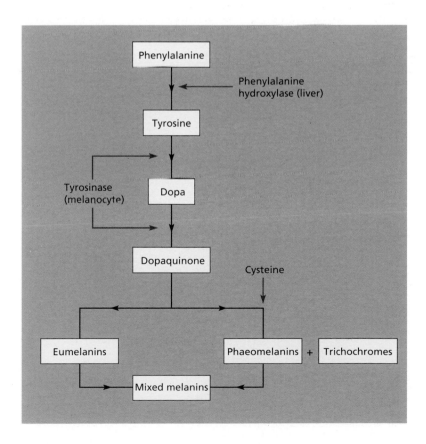

Fig. 2.7 Melanin synthetic pathway.

five minutes of exposure to long-wave ultraviolet (UVA: 320–400nm) and may be due to photo-oxidation of pre-formed melanin. This pigment-darkening reaction, which lasts about 15 minutes, is responsible for the well-known phenomenon of a 'false tan'.

The production of *new* pigment is delayed for some 24 hours after exposure to medium-wave ultra-violet (UVB: 290–320nm) and UVA. It depends on the proliferation of melanocytes, an increase in tyrosinase activity and melanosome production, and an increased transfer of new melanosomes to their surrounding keratinocytes.

A neat control mechanism involving glutathione has been postulated. Reduced glutathione in the epidermis, produced by the action of glutathione reductase on glutathione, inhibits tyrosinase. UVR and some inflammatory skin conditions may induce pigmentation by oxidizing glutathione and so blocking its inhibition of melanogenesis.

Melanocytes are also influenced by melanocyte stimulating hormone (MSH) peptides from the pituitary and other areas of the brain (Fig. 2.8). Their melanocyte stimulating activity is due to a common heptapeptide sequence. However, MSH peptides may play little part in the physiological control of pigmentation. Hypophysectomy will not cause black skin to lighten and only large doses of ACTH, in pathological states (Chapter 18), will increase skin pigmentation. It is now known that pro-opiomelanocortin and MSH peptides are also produced by both keratinocytes and melanocytes in the skin, so MSH may function in a paracrine or autocrine manner. In the skin α-MSH also acts as an anti-inflammatory agent by antagonizing the effects of IL-1 in inducing IL-2 receptors on lymphocytes (p. 22) and in inducing pyrexia.

Animal experiments indicate that oestrogens, progestogens, and possibly testosterone, may, in some circumstances, stimulate melanogenesis either

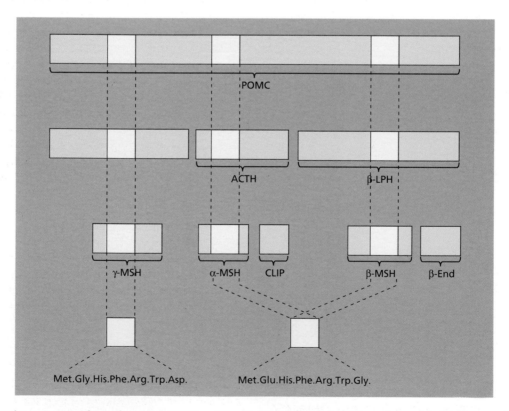

Fig. 2.8 Melanocyte stimulating hormone peptides. Abbreviations as in text. CLIP, corticotrophin-like intermediate lobe peptide; β-end, β-endorphin; POMC, pro-opiomelanocortin; βLPH, β-lipotrophin.

directly or by increasing the release of MSH peptides from the pituitary.

Genetics and skin pigmentation

Genetic differences determine the pigmentation of the different races. The Negroid in Britain, and the Caucasoid in Africa, remain respectively black and white. Nonetheless, there is some phenotypic variation in skin colour, for example tanning after sun exposure. Some genodermatoses with abnormal pigmentation are described in Chapter 22.

Langerhans cells

The Langerhans cell is a dendritic cell (Fig. 2.9), like the melanocyte, which also lacks desmosomes and tonofibrils but which has a lobulated nucleus. The specific granules within the cell look like sycamore seeds — plate-like structures with a rounded bleb protruding from their surface, which appear rod- or racquet-shaped on electron microscopy (see Fig. 2.5).

   Langerhans cells come from a mobile pool of precursors originating in the bone marrow. There are approximately 800 Langerhans cells per square mm in human skin and their dendritic processes fan out to form a striking network seen best in epidermal sheets (Fig. 2.10). Langerhans cells are alone among

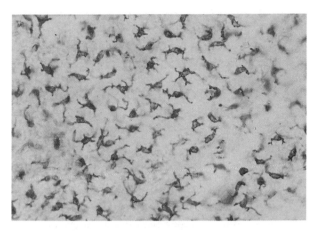

Fig. 2.10 ATPase positive Langerhans cells in an epidermal sheet: the network provides a reticulo-epithelial trap for contact allergens.

epidermal cells in possessing surface receptors for C3b and the Fc portions of IgG and IgE, and in bearing class II major histocompatibility complex antigens (HLA-DR, -DP and -DQ). Therefore they are best thought of as highly specialized macrophages.

   Langerhans cells play a key role in many immune reactions. They take up exogenous antigen, process it and present it to T lymphocytes either in the skin or in the local lymph nodes (p. 22). They probably play a part in immunosurveillance of viral and tumour antigens. In addition, ultraviolet radiation may induce skin tumours not only by causing mutations in the epidermal cells, but also by decreasing the number of epidermal Langerhans cells, so that cells bearing altered antigens are not recognized and destroyed by the immune system. Glucocorticoids, given topically or systemically, similarly reduce the density of epidermal Langerhans cells. The Langerhans cell is the principal cell in skin allografts to which the T lymphocytes of the host react during rejection; allograft survival might be prolonged by depletion of the Langerhans cells.

Merkel cells

Merkel cells are also found in normal epidermis and probably act as transducers for fine touch. These non-dendritic cells, lying in or near the basal layer, are the same size as keratinocytes and are concentrated in localized thickenings of the epidermis near

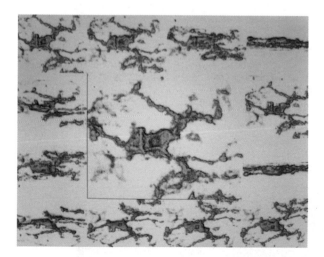

Fig. 2.9 Confocal scanning laser microscopy of a single epidermal Langerhans cell. The central panel shows a computerized reconstruction made up from serial slices. The images around the edge give a three-dimensional impression of the cell looked at from different angles.

hair follicles (hair discs). They contain membrane-bound spherical granules, 80–100 nm in diameter, which have a core of varying density, separated from the membrane by a clear halo. Sparse desmosomes connect these cells with neighbouring keratinocytes. Fine unmyelinated nerve endings are often associated with Merkel cells which express immuno-reactivity for various neuropeptides.

Epidermal appendages

The skin appendages are derived from epithelial germs during embryogenesis and, except for the nails, lie in the dermis. They include hair, nails, and the sweat and sebaceous glands.

The hair

The hair germ, a solid cylinder of cells, grows obliquely down into the dermis where it is met by a cluster of mesenchymal cells, bulging into the lower part of the hair germ to form the hair papilla. Eventually the papilla contains blood vessels bringing nutrients to the hair matrix. The sebaceous gland is an outgrowth at the side of the hair germ, establishing early the two parts of the pilosebaceous unit. The hair matrix, the germinative part of the follicle, is equivalent to the basal cells of the epidermis.

Melanocytes migrate into the matrix and are responsible for the different colours of hair (eumelanin: brown; phaeomelanin and trichochromes: red). Grey or white hair is due to low pigment production, and the filling of the cells in the hair medulla with minute air bubbles which reflect light. The anatomy of an adult hair follicle is shown in Fig. 2.11.

Hairs are classified into three main types:
1 *Lanugo hairs.* Fine long hairs covering the fetus, but shed about one month before birth.
2 *Vellus hairs.* Fine short unmedullated hairs covering much of the body surface. They replace the lanugo hairs just before birth.
3 *Terminal hairs.* Long, coarse medullated hairs seen, for example, in the scalp or pubic regions. Their growth is often influenced by circulating androgen levels.

Terminal hairs convert to vellus hairs in male-pattern alopecia and vellus hairs convert to terminal hairs in hirsutism (Chapter 8). The lips, glans penis, labia minora, palms and soles remain free of hair.

The hair cycle

Each follicle passes, independently of its neighbours, through regular cycles of growth and shedding. The three phases of follicular activity (Fig. 2.12) are known as:

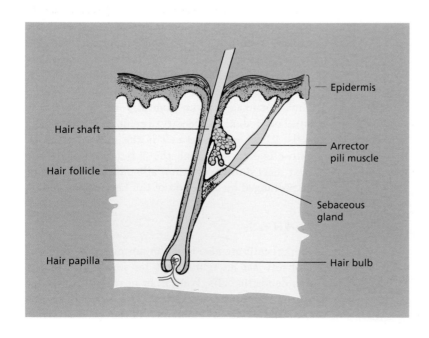

Fig. 2.11 Anatomy of the hair follicle.

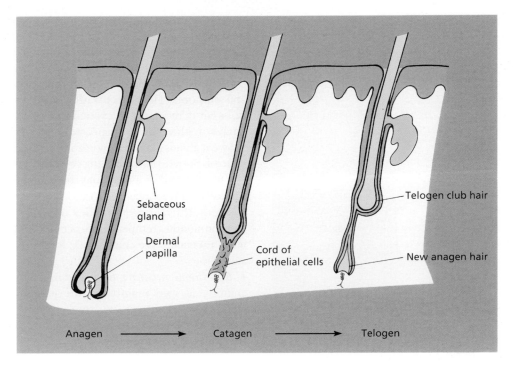

Sebaceous gland

Dermal papilla

Cord of epithelial cells

Telogen club hair

New anagen hair

Anagen ⟶ Catagen ⟶ Telogen

Fig. 2.12 The hair cycle.

1 *Anagen.* The active phase of hair production.
2 *Catagen.* A short phase of conversion from active growth to the resting phase. Growth stops, and the end of the hair becomes club-shaped.
3 *Telogen.* A resting phase at the end of which the club hair is shed.

The duration of each of these stages varies from region to region of the body. On the scalp, said to contain an average of 100 000 hairs, anagen lasts for up to five years, catagen for only a few days, and telogen for about three months. As many as 100 hairs may be shed from the normal scalp every day as a normal consequence of cycling. The proportion of hairs in the growing and resting stages can be estimated by looking at plucked hairs (a trichogram). On the scalp, about 85% are normally in anagen and 15% in telogen phase.

The cycle of alternating growth and rest is not synchronized in humans. There is no moulting period. However, some diseases (*see* Telogen effluvium, Chapter 8) and drugs may synchronize catagen so that large numbers of hairs are lost at the same time.

There are important racial differences in hair.

Asians tend to have straight hair, Negroids to have woolly hair and Europeans to have wavy hair. These differences are due to different cross-sectional shapes (round, flattened, etc.). Mongoloids have sparse facial and body hair when compared with Mediterranean people who also have more hair than northern Europeans.

The nail

The structure of the nail and nail bed is shown in Fig. 2.13. The hard keratin of the nail plate is formed in the nail matrix, which lies in an invagination of the epidermis (the nail fold) on the back of the terminal phalanx of each digit. The matrix runs from the proximal end of the floor of the nail fold to the distal margin of the lunule. From this area the nail plate grows forward over the nail bed, ending in a free margin at the tip of the digit. Longitudinal ridges and grooves on the under surface of the nail plate dovetail with similar ones on the upper surface of the nail bed. The nail bed is capable of producing small amounts of keratin which contribute to the nail and which are responsible for the 'false nail',

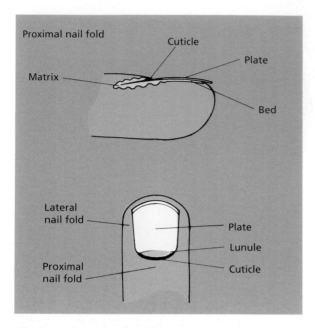

Fig. 2.13 The nail and nail bed.

formed when the nail matrix is obliterated by surgery or injury. The cuticle acts as a seal to protect the potential space of the nail fold from chemicals and from infection.

The rate at which nails grow varies from person to person: finger nails average between 0.5 and 1.2 mm per week, while toe nails grow more slowly. Nails grow faster in youth and in the summer. The nails provide strength and protection for the terminal phalanx. Their presence helps with fine touch and with the handling of small objects.

Eccrine sweat glands

Two to three million sweat glands are present all over the body, being most numerous on the palms, soles and axillae. The tightly coiled glands lie deep in the dermis, and the emerging duct passes to the surface by penetrating the epidermis in a corkscrew fashion. Sweat is formed in the coiled gland by active secretion, involving the sodium pump. Some damage occurs to the membrane of the secretory cells during sweating. Initially sweat is isotonic with plasma but, under normal conditions, it becomes hypotonic by the time it is discharged at the surface after the tubular resorption of electrolytes and water

under the influence of aldosterone and antidiuretic hormone.

In some ways the eccrine sweat duct is like a renal tubule. The pH of sweat is between 4.0 and 6.8, it contains sodium, potassium chloride, lactate, urea and ammonia. The concentration of sodium chloride in sweat is increased in cystic fibrosis, and sweat is analysed when this is suspected.

Sweat glands play an important role in temperature control, the skin surface being cooled by evaporation. Up to 10 litres of sweat may be excreted per day. Three stimuli induce sweating:
- *Thermal sweating* as a reflex response to a raised environmental temperature occurs all over the body, especially the chest, back, forehead, scalp and axillae.
- *Emotional sweating*, provoked mostly by fear and anxiety, is seen mainly on the palms, soles and axillae.
- *Gustatory sweating* is provoked by hot, spicy foods and affects the face.

The eccrine sweat glands are innervated by cholinergic fibres of the sympathetic nervous system. Sweating can therefore be induced by cholinergic, and blocked by anticholinergic, drugs. Central control of sweating resides in the pre-optic hypothalamic sweat centre.

Apocrine sweat glands

The apocrine glands in the adult are limited to the axillae, nipples, peri-umbilical area, perineum and genitalia. The coiled tubular glands (larger than those of eccrine glands) lie deep in the dermis, and during sweating the luminal part of their cells is lost (decapitation secretion). Apocrine sweat passes via the duct into the mid-portion of the hair follicle. The action of bacteria on apocrine sweat is responsible for body odour. The glands are innervated by adrenergic fibres of the sympathetic nervous system.

Sebaceous glands

Most sebaceous glands develop from hair germs, but a few free glands arise from the epidermis. The sebaceous glands associated with hair lie in the obtuse angle between the follicle and the epidermis. The gland itself is multilobed and contains cells full of lipid which, during secretion, are shed whole (holocrine secretion) so that sebum contains their remnants in a complex mixture of triglycerides, fatty acids, wax esters, squalene and cholesterol. Sebum is discharged into the upper part of the hair follicle (see Fig. 2.11). It lubricates and waterproofs the skin and protects it from drying; it is also mildly bacteriocidal and fungistatic. Free sebaceous glands may be found in the eyelid (meibomian glands), mucous membranes (Fordyce spots), nipple, peri-anal region and genitalia.

Sebaceous glands are stimulated by androgenic hormones, especially dihydrotestosterone. Human sebaceous glands contain 5α-reductase, 3β- and 17β-hydroxysteroid dehydrogenase, which convert weaker androgens to dihydrotestosterone. The sebaceous glands are stimulated by maternal androgens for a short time after birth, and then lie dormant until puberty when a surge of androgens stimulates a sudden increase in sebum excretion and sets the stage for acne (Chapter 14).

The dermo-epidermal junction

At the interface between the epidermis and dermis lies the basement membrane zone. With light microscopy it may be highlighted using a PAS stain, due to its abundance of neutral mucopolysaccharides. Electron microscopy (Fig. 2.14) shows that the *lamina densa* (rich in type IV collagen) is separated from the basal cells by an electron-lucent area, the *lamina lucida*. The plasma membrane of basal cells has *hemidesmosomes* (cf. desmosomes above). Fine *anchoring filaments* cross the lamina lucida and connect the lamina densa to the plasma membrane of the basal cells. *Anchoring fibrils* (of type VII collagen), dermal microfibril bundles, and single small collagen fibres (types I and III), extend from the papillary dermis to the deep part of the lamina densa. The lamina lucida contains at least four distinct macromolecules, laminin, the bullous pemphi-

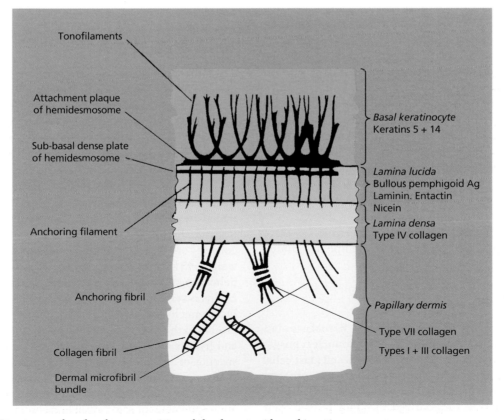

Fig. 2.14 Structure and molecular composition of the dermo-epidermal junction.

goid antigen, entactin and nicein. Laminin, a large non-collagen glycoprotein (molecular weight 800 kDa) produced by keratinocytes, aided by entactin, promotes adhesion between epithelial cells and type IV collagen, the main constituent of the lamina densa. The bullous pemphigoid antigen (molecular weight 230 kDa) is synthesized by basal cells and occurs in close association with the hemidesmosomes and laminin; its function is unknown but antibodies to it are found in the subepidermal blistering condition of pemphigoid (p. 119). Nicein may be a constituent of anchoring filaments.

The structures of the dermo-epidermal junction provide mechanical support, encouraging adhesion, growth, differentiation and migration of the overlying basal cells, and also act as a semipermeable filter which regulates the transfer of nutrients and cells from dermis to epidermis.

Dermis

The dermis lies between the epidermis and the subcutaneous fat. It supports the epidermis structurally and nutritionally. Its thickness varies, being greatest in the palms and soles and least in the eyelids and penis. In old age the dermis is thinned and loses its elasticity.

The dermis interdigitates with the epidermis (see Fig. 2.2) so that upward projections of the dermis, the dermal papillae, interlock with downward ridges of the epidermis, the rete pegs. This interdigitation is responsible for the ridges seen most readily on the finger tips (finger prints); it is important in the adhesion between epidermis and dermis, and increases the area of contact between them.

Like all connective tissues the dermis has three components: cells, fibres and amorphous ground substance.

Cells of the dermis

The main cells of the dermis are fibroblasts, but there are also small numbers of mononuclear phagocytes, lymphocytes, Langerhans cells and mast cells. Other blood cells, for example polymorphs, are seen during inflammation. The function of the resident dermal cells is summarized in Table 2.2 and their

Table 2.2 Functions of some resident dermal cells

Fibroblast	Synthesis of collagen, reticulin, elastin, fibronectin, glycosaminoglycans, collagenase
Mononuclear phagocyte	Mobile; phagocytose and destroy bacteria Secrete cytokines
Lymphocyte	Immunosurveillance
Langerhans cell	In transit between local lymph node and epidermis Antigen presentation
Mast cell	Stimulated by antigens, complement components, and other substances to release many mediators including histamine, heparin, prostaglandins, leukotrienes, tryptase and chemotactic factors for eosinophils and neutrophils

role in immunological reactions is discussed in Chapter 3.

Fibres of the dermis

The bulk of the dermis consists of interwoven fibres, principally of *collagen*, packed in bundles. Those in the papillary dermis are finer than those in the deeper, reticular dermis. When the skin is stretched, collagen, with its high tensile strength, prevents tearing, and the elastic fibres, intermingled with the collagen, return it to the unstretched state.

Collagen makes up 70–80% of the dry weight of the dermis. Its fibres are composed of thinner fibrils, which are in turn made up of microfibrils built from individual collagen molecules. These molecules consist of three polypeptide chains (molecular weight 95 kDa) forming a triple helix with a non-helical segment at both ends. The alignment of the chains is stabilized by covalent cross-links involving lysine and hydroxylysine. Collagen is an exceptional protein in that it contains a high proportion of proline and hydroxyproline and many glycine residues; the spacing of glycine as every third amino acid is a prerequisite for the formation of a triple helix. Defects in the enzymes needed for collagen synthesis are responsible for some skin diseases, including the

Table 2.3 Distribution of some types of collagen

Collagen type	Tissue distribution
I	Most connective tissues including tendon and bone
	Accounts for approximately 85% of skin collagen
II	Cartilage
III	Accounts for about 15% of skin collagen
	Blood vessels
IV	Skin (lamina densa) and basement membranes of other tissues
V	Ubiquitous including placenta
VII	Skin (anchoring fibrils)
	Fetal membranes

Ehlers–Danlos syndrome (Chapter 22) and conditions involving other systems including lathyrism (fragility of skin and other connective tissues) and osteogenesis imperfecta (fragility of bones).

There are many, genetically distinct, collagen proteins, all with triple helical molecules, and all rich in hydroxyproline and hydroxylysine. The distribution of some is summarized in Table 2.3.

Reticulin fibres are fine collagen fibres seen in fetal skin, and around the blood vessels and appendages of adult skin.

Elastic fibres account for about 2% of the dry weight of adult dermis. They have two distinct protein components: the amorphous elastin core and a surrounding 'elastic tissue microfibrillar component'. Elastin (molecular weight 72 kDa) is made up of polypeptides (rich in glycine, desmosine and valine) linked to the microfibrillar component through their desmosine residues. Defects in elastic tissue cause cutis laxa (sagging inelastic skin) and pseudoxanthoma elasticum (Chapter 22).

Ground substance of the dermis

The amorphous ground substance of the dermis consists largely of two glycosaminoglycans, hyaluronic acid and dermatan sulphate, with smaller amounts of heparan sulphate and chondroitin sulphate.

It has several important functions:

- It binds water, allowing nutrients, hormones and waste products to pass through the dermis.
- It is a lubricant between the collagen and elastic fibre networks during skin movement.
- It provides bulk, allowing the dermis to act as a shock absorber.

Muscles

Both smooth and striated muscle are found in the skin. The smooth arrector pili muscles are used by animals to raise their fur, and so to protect them from the cold. They are vestigial in humans, but may help to express sebum. Smooth muscle is also responsible for 'goose pimples' (bumps) from cold and nipple erection, and the dartos muscle raises the scrotum. Striated fibres, for example the platysma, and some of the muscles of facial expression, are also found in the dermis.

Blood vessels

Although skin consumes little oxygen, it has an abundant blood supply to regulate body temperature. The blood vessels lie in two main horizontal layers (Fig. 2.15). The deep plexus is just above the subcutaneous fat, and its arterioles supply the sweat glands and hair papillae. The superficial plexus is in the papillary dermis and arterioles from it become capillary loops in the dermal papillae. An arteriole from the deep dermis supplies an inverted cone of tissue, with its base at the epidermis.

The blood vessels in the skin play an important role in thermoregulation. Arteriovenous anastamoses at the level of the deep plexus may shunt blood to the venous plexus under sympathetic nervous control at the expense of the capillary loops reducing surface heat loss by convection.

Cutaneous lymphatics

An afferent lymphatic begins as a blind-ended capillary in the dermal papilla and passes to a superficial lymphatic plexus in the papillary dermis. There are also two deeper horizontal plexuses, and collecting lymphatics from the deeper one run with the veins in the superficial fascia.

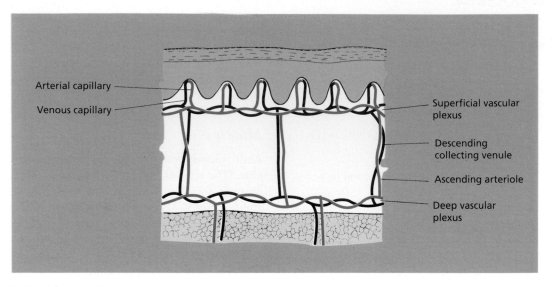

Fig. 2.15 Blood vessels of the skin.

Nerves

The skin is liberally supplied with about one million nerve fibres. Most end in the face and extremities. Their cell bodies lie in the dorsal root ganglia. Both myelinated and non-myelinated fibres are found, with the latter making up an increasing proportion peripherally. Most free sensory nerves end in the dermis; however, a few non-myelinated nerve endings penetrate into the epidermis. Some of these are associated with Merkel cells (p. 13). Free nerve endings detect potentially damaging stimuli of heat and pain (nocioceptors), while specialized end organs in the dermis, Paccinian and Meissner corpuscles, register deformation of the skin (mechanoreceptors) caused by pressure, vibration and touch. Autonomic nerves supply the blood vessels, sweat glands and arrector pili muscles.

Itching is an important feature of many skin diseases. It follows the stimulation of fine free nerve endings lying close to the dermo-epidermal junction. Areas with a high density of such endings (itch spots) are especially sensitive to itch-provoking stimuli. Impulses from these free endings pass centrally in two ways: quickly along myelinated A fibres, and more slowly along non-myelinated C fibres. As a result, itch has two components — a quick, localized, pricking sensation followed by a slow, burning, diffuse itching.

Many stimuli can induce itching (electrical, chemical and mechanical). In itchy skin diseases, pruritogenic chemicals such as histamine and proteolytic enzymes are liberated close to the dermo-epidermal junction. The detailed pharmacology of individual diseases is still poorly understood but prostaglandins potentiate chemically induced itching in inflammatory skin diseases.

LEARNING POINT
More and more diseases are being classified according to the abnormality of function and structure which they display rather than by their appearance.

CHAPTER 3

Immunology of the skin

The skin acts as a passive barrier to many chemicals and infectious agents: any that break through are dealt with by the immune system. This works in the skin just as it does in other tissues but the idea of the skin immune system (SIS) as a functionally independent immunological unit is helpful. It includes the skin with its blood vessels, and lymphatics with their local lymph nodes; it contains circulating lymphocytes and resident immune cells.

Immune reactions in the skin can be seen as obvious skin disease. This chapter outlines the intricate mechanisms involved in these reactions: the ways in which antigens are recognized by specialized skin cells, mainly Langerhans cells, and in which antibodies, lymphocytes, macrophages and polymorphs elicit inflammation. This may be interesting in theory but often it is difficult to see how this can help an individual reacting to an apparently harmless substance like nickel.

Table 3.1 Components of skin immune system (SIS)

Functional unit	Epidermis, dermis, blood vessels, lymphatics, and local lymph nodes
Cells	Keratinocytes
	Langerhans cells
	Lymphocytes
	L cells/null cells
	Monocytes/macrophages
	Granulocytes
	Mast cells
Molecules	Antigens and haptens
	Antibodies
	Complement
	Cytokines
	Adhesion molecules
	Histocompatibility antigens

Table 3.1 lists the main immunological components of skin. Each will be described in some detail.

The epidermal barrier

The most important function of the skin is to protect the body by preventing the loss of fluids and electrolytes, and the penetration of harmful substances (p. 5). The horny layer is a dry, mechanical barrier from which contaminating organisms and chemicals are continually being removed by washing and desquamation. It is only when these organisms breach the horny layer that the cellular components, described below, come into play. Their activity helps us when it deals with pathogens (e.g. molluscum contagiosum), but can damage us when it is an over-reaction to a chemical (e.g. nickel dermatitis), or is misdirected as in responses to one's own tissues (e.g. pemphigus) or to grafted foreign cells or tissues.

Cellular components of skin immune system

Keratinocytes (p. 6)

The prime role of these cells is to make keratins (p. 9) and to give structural support to the outermost epithelium of the body. In addition they produce large numbers of cytokines (see Table 3.3) and have immunological functions in their own right (see Fig. 3.4). Keratinocytes can be induced by γ-interferon to express HLA-DR. They can also produce α-melanocytes stimulating hormone (p. 12) which is immunosuppressive.

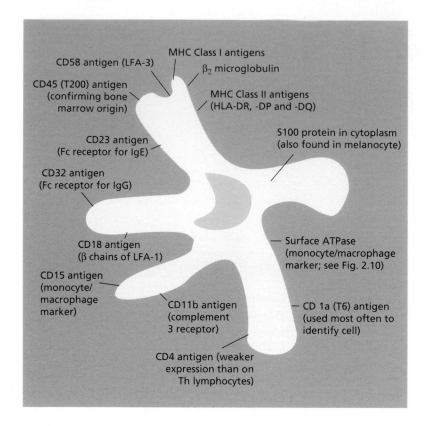

Fig. 3.1 Phenotype of human epidermal Langerhans cell.

Langerhans cells (p. 13)

These dendritic cells (Fig. 3.1) come from the bone marrow and circulate through the epidermis, the dermis, lymphatics (as 'veiled cells') and the T cell area of the lymph nodes where they are called 'dendritic' or 'interdigitating' cells. Some of their important phenotypic markers, many determined by specific monoclonal antibodies, are shown in Fig. 3.1.

The dendrites of Langerhans cells ramify between keratinocytes and interact with chemicals (often haptens) and organisms which have breached the epidermal barrier. The immune response begins with the activation of CD4$^+$ T cells by antigen presented by the Langerhans cell to them. The Langerhans cell takes up the offending antigen and digests it into small peptides. These then associate intracellularly with MHC class II proteins and the complex so formed moves to the cell surface where it is then recognized by the T cell receptor (TCR). Other surface molecules involved in T cell recognition and the adhesion between the T cell and antigen presenting cell are shown in Fig. 3.2.

When the Langerhans cell and naive CD4 T cell (so called because it has not met an antigen before) are apposed, the Langerhans cell releases IL-1 to trigger the T cell to release IL-2 (T cell growth factor) and to express receptors for IL-2 on the T cell surface (Fig. 3.3).

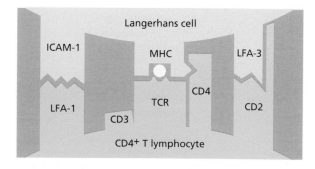

Fig. 3.2 Interactions between surface molecules on a CD4$^+$ T cell and a Langerhans cell.

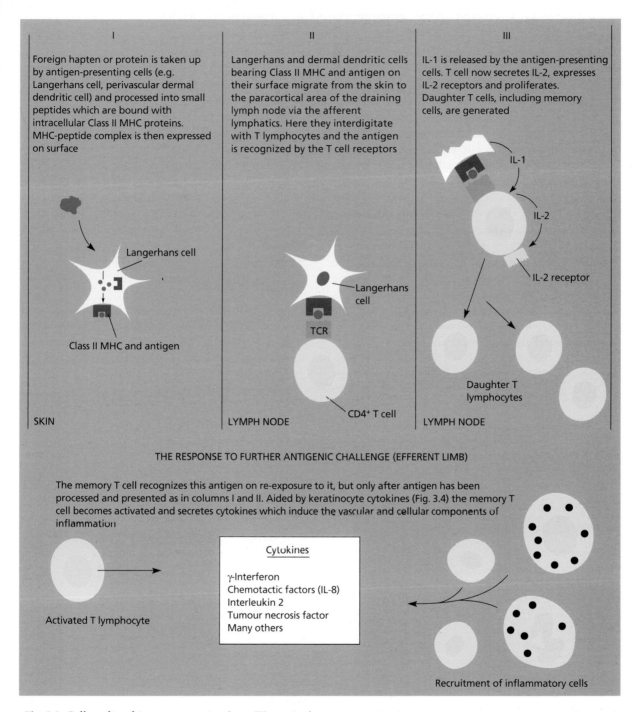

I

Foreign hapten or protein is taken up by antigen-presenting cells (e.g. Langerhans cell, perivascular dermal dendritic cell) and processed into small peptides which are bound with intracellular Class II MHC proteins. MHC-peptide complex is then expressed on surface

Langerhans cell

Class II MHC and antigen

SKIN

II

Langerhans and dermal dendritic cells bearing Class II MHC and antigen on their surface migrate from the skin to the paracortical area of the draining lymph node via the afferent lymphatics. Here they interdigitate with T lymphocytes and the antigen is recognized by the T cell receptors

Langerhans cell

TCR

CD4⁺ T cell

LYMPH NODE

III

IL-1 is released by the antigen-presenting cells. T cell now secretes IL-2, expresses IL-2 receptors and proliferates. Daughter T cells, including memory cells, are generated

IL-1

IL-2

IL-2 receptor

Daughter T lymphocytes

LYMPH NODE

THE RESPONSE TO FURTHER ANTIGENIC CHALLENGE (EFFERENT LIMB)

The memory T cell recognizes this antigen on re-exposure to it, but only after antigen has been processed and presented as in columns I and II. Aided by keratinocyte cytokines (Fig. 3.4) the memory T cell becomes activated and secretes cytokines which induce the vascular and cellular components of inflammation

Activated T lymphocyte

Cytokines

γ-Interferon
Chemotactic factors (IL-8)
Interleukin 2
Tumour necrosis factor
Many others

Recruitment of inflammatory cells

Fig. 3.3 Cell-mediated immune reaction (type IV reaction).

This process of induction (sensitization) takes place mainly in the lymph nodes and produces a clone of lymphocytes which are specifically sensi- tized to, and so will recognize, the particular antigen next time it is encountered. These lymphocytes leave the node and travel to the superior vena cava via the thoracic duct. They are then distributed throughout the entire circulation, though homing mechanisms (see adhesion molecules) ensure that some are relatively tissue specific (i.e. those from skin will return to skin). On return to the skin they play an important role in immunosurveillance against further incursions by the original antigen.

On further challenge with this antigen, an inflammatory response will occur in the skin. The antigen, once more processed and presented by the Langerhans cells, stimulates antigen-specific T cells to make lymphokines which bring other inflammatory cells into the area (Fig. 3.3). Neighbouring keratinocytes also secrete mediators including IL-1, IL-6 and G-CSF, which aid this response (Fig. 3.4).

These lymphokines recruit other, non-specific lymphocytes into the area and they too produce lymphokines. In immunological jargon this is augmentation by recruitment. It means that only a few of the lymphocytes, perhaps less than 5%, in an immunological inflammatory reaction of this sort can actually recognize the specific antigen which provoked it. The rest are uncommitted lymphocytes recruited to the site by the committed ones.

The lymphokines have a variety of other actions on lymphocytes, polymorphs and macrophages which are essential for the immune destruction of cells containing foreign antigen, tumours and transplanted tissue.

Keratinocytes are not only capable of enhancing T cell activation but can produce molecules (e.g. prostaglandin E, hydroxy-eicosatetraenoic acids [HETES], α-MSH and TGF-β) which inhibit activation (Fig. 3.4). These are produced by keratinocytes in normal (resting) epidermis and may help to prevent immune reactions being invoked in response to minor breaches of the barrier by harmless substances.

Dermal dendritic cells

These poorly characterized cells are found around the tiny blood vessels of the papillary dermis. They bear class II MHC antigens on their surface and, like Langerhans cells, probably function as antigen presenting cells.

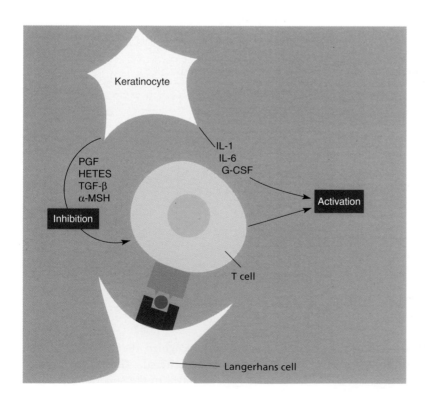

Fig. 3.4 Modulation of T cell activation by keratinocyte.

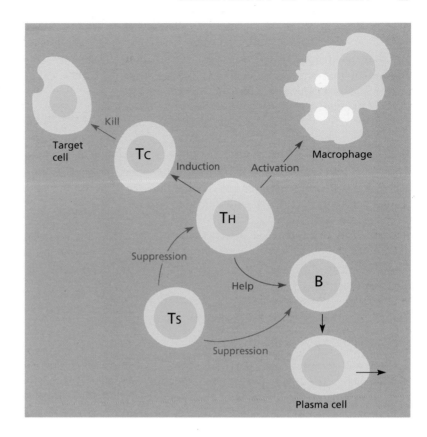

Fig. 3.5 Lymphocyte interactions.

Lymphocytes

The interactions and function of lymphocytes are shown in Fig. 3.5.

T cells

These lymphocytes develop and acquire their antigen receptors (TCR) in the thymus. They differentiate into subpopulations which are recognized by their different surface molecules (for CD terminology see below) and which are functionally distinct.

T helper (TH)/inducer cells

These help B cells to produce antibody and also induce cytotoxic T cells to recognize and kill virally infected cells and allogeneic grafts. TH cells recognize antigen in association with MHC class II molecules (see Fig. 3.2) and when triggered by antigen release cytokines which attract and activate other inflammatory cells.

Helper T cells are divided into TH_1 and TH_2 according to the main cytokines which they produce (Fig. 3.6). Those with specificity for antigens relevant in atopic dermatitis may have TH_2 cytokine profiles (p. 87).

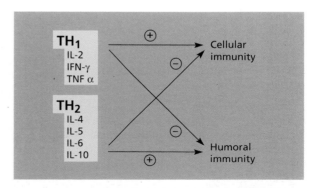

Fig. 3.6 T helper/inducer cells (both TH_1 and TH_2 produce IL-3 GM-CSF and TNF-α).

T delayed hypersensitivity (TD) cells

These are a subgroup of TH cells which are probably distinct in that when activated they bring macrophages and other inflammatory cells to the site of a delayed hypersensitivity reaction.

T cytotoxic (TC) cells

These lymphocytes are capable of destroying allogeneic and virally infected cells which they recognize via MHC class I molecules on their surface.

T suppressor (Ts) cells

These regulate the action of other T and B lymphocytes.

T cell receptor and T cell gene receptor rearrangements

Most T cell receptors are composed of an α and β chain, each with a variable (antigen binding) and constant domain, which are associated with the T3 cell surface molecule (see Fig. 3.2). Many different combinations of separate gene segments, termed V, D and J, code for the variable domains of the receptor. Analysis of rearrangements of the gene for the receptor is used to determine if a T cell infiltrate is most likely malignant or reactive. The identification of a specific band on analysis of DNA from the lesion which cannot be matched by the patient's DNA from other sites indicates monoclonal T cell proliferation, suggesting either malignancy or a T cell response to a single antigen.

B cells

These lymphocytes develop in fetal liver and later in the bone marrow. When mature they bear surface immunoglobulins which act as their antigen receptors. They reside in secondary lymphoid tissues where they respond to antigen stimuli by differentiating into plasma cells under the control of T cell cytokines.

CD (cluster of differentiation) antigens

Lymphocytes are now described according to their CD number which signifies surface protein recognized by monoclonal antibodies. Some CD numbers are the same as OKT (T) antigens (e.g. CD4 = T4, CD8 = T8).

L cells/null (non-T, non-B) cells

These leucocytes have properties between those of T and myelomonocytic cells. Most have receptors for FcIgG. This subpopulation contains NK and K cells.

NK (natural killer) cells

These are large granular leucocytes which can kill virally infected or tumour cells which have not previously been sensitized with antibody.

K (killer) cells

These are not a separate cell type, but rather Tc or NK or monocytic leucocytes which can kill target cells sensitized with antibody. In antibody-mediated cellular cytotoxicity, antibody binds to antigen on the surface of the target cell: the K cell binds to the antibody at its other (Fc) end by its Fc receptor and the target cell is then lysed (Fig. 3.7).

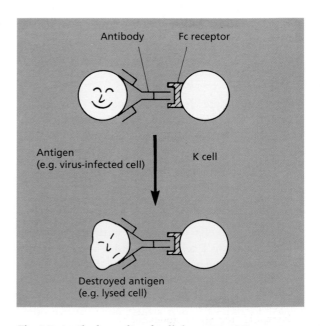

Fig. 3.7 Antibody-mediated cellular cytotoxicity.

Cells of the monocyte/macrophage system

Monocytes

These circulating cells of the reticulo-endothelial system constitute 5% of the total leucocytes. They migrate into the tissues, where they are called macrophages.

Macrophages

These large and long living phagocytic cells are found in connective tissue, spleen, lymph nodes and secondary lymphoid organs. They may function as antigen presenting cells.

Granulocytes (polymorphs)

These constitute the majority of blood leucocytes and are recognized by their multilobed nuclei and granular cytoplasm. Their histological staining separates them into:

Neutrophils

These account for more than 70% of circulating leucocytes. They are short lived phagocytes and spend less than 48 hours in the circulation before migrating into the tissues under influence of chemotactic stimuli (e.g. IL-8). They have receptors for Fc of Ig and C_3 which enable them to phagocytose opsonized particles.

Eosinophils

These comprise 2–5% of circulating leucocytes. Their granules contain a basic protein which on release damages pathogens, especially parasites. They are found where histamine is released and their granules also contain histaminase.

Basophils

These constitute less than 1% of blood leucocytes. They are functionally similar to mast cells.

Mast cells

They are present in most connective tissues and are found predominantly around blood vessels. Their numerous granules contain inflammatory mediators (see Fig. 3.8). In rodents (and probably in humans) there are two distinct populations of mast cells, connective tissue and mucosal, which differ in their composition of inflammatory mediators and proteolytic enzymes (Table 3.2).

Molecular components of the skin immune system

Antigens and haptens

Antigens are molecules which are recognized by the immune system outlined above and which provoke an immune reaction, usually in the form of a

Table 3.2 Comparison of connective tissue with mucosal mast cells

	Connective tissue mast cell (predominate in skin)	Mucosal mast cell
Histamine	+	+
Heparin	+	
Chondroitin sulphate		+
Tryptase	+	+
Chymase	+	
Stain with Alcian Blue (after formalin fixation)	Red	Blue
Degranulated by substance P and compound 48/80	+	−
Susceptible to sodium cromoglycate	+	−

humoral or cell-bound antibody response. Haptens, often chemicals of low molecular weight, are unable to provoke an immune reaction themselves unless they combine with a protein. They are important sensitizers in allergic contact dermatitis (p. 93).

Superantigens

Bacterial toxins, released by *Staphylococcus aureus*, are prototypic superantigens. Sensitization to such superantigens is not necessary to prime the immune response. Superantigens align with a variety of class II MHC molecules outside their antigen presentation groove and, without any cellular processing, may directly signal different classes of T cells within the large family carrying a Vβ type of T cell receptor. By these means superantigens are capable of inducing massive T cell proliferation and cytokine production leading to disorders such as the toxic shock syndrome (p. 165).

Antibodies (immunoglobulins)

Antibodies are a class of serum proteins, found in the gamma globulin fraction, whose production is induced by antigen. They bind specifically to the antigen which induced their formation.

Immunoglobulin G (**IgG**) is responsible for the majority of the secondary response to most antigens. It can cross the placenta and binds complement to activate the classical complement pathway (see Fig.

3.9). IgG can coat neutrophils and macrophages (by their FcIgG receptors) and acts as an opsonin by cross-bridging antigen. IgG can also sensitize target cells for destruction by K cells. **IgM** is the largest Ig molecule. It is responsible for much of the primary response. It cannot cross the placenta. Like IgG it may fix complement. **IgA** is the most common Ig in secretions. It occurs in humans mostly as monomers but also as dimers. It does not bind complement but may activate complement via the alternative pathway (see Fig. 3.9). **IgE** binds to Fc receptors on mast cells and basophils where it sensitizes them to the release of inflammatory mediators in type I immediate hypersensitivity reactions (see Fig. 3.8).

Complement

Complement is one of the serum enzyme systems comprising many separate proteins which may be activated by the classical or alternative pathway (see Fig. 3.9). Complement activation is important in mediating inflammation, opsonization and cell lysis (see Figs 3.9–3.11).

Cytokines

Cytokines are small proteins secreted by cells such as lymphocytes, macrophages and also keratinocytes (Table 3.3). They regulate the amplitude and duration of inflammation by acting locally on nearby cells

Table 3.3 Some cytokines

Interleukins (IL)	Colony stimulating factors (CSF)	Growth factors (GF)
IL-1α*	Granulocyte (G)-CSF*	Epidermal (E) GF*
IL-1β*	Macrophage (M)-CSF*	Transforming (T) GF-α*
IL-2	GM-CSF*	Transforming (T) GF-β*
IL-4		
IL-6*		Fibroblast (F) GF-a
IL-8*		Fibroblast (F) GF-b*
IL-10		Platelet derived (PD) GF*

Interferons (IFN)	Cytotoxins	
IFN-α	Tumour necrosis factor (TNF)-α	
IFN-β	Tumour necrosis factor (TNF)-β	
IFN-γ		

* May be produced by keratinocytes

(paracrine action), on those cells that secreted them (autocrine) and occasionally on distant target cells (endocrine) via the circulation. The term cytokine may be used to cover interleukins, interferons, colony stimulating factors, cytotoxins and growth factors. Interleukins are produced predominantly by leucocytes, have a known amino acid sequence and are active in inflammation or immunity.

There are many cytokines (Table 3.3) and each may act on more than one type of cell causing numerous different effects. Cytokines frequently have overlapping actions. In a given inflammatory reaction some cytokines act synergistically while others antagonize these effects. This network of potent chemicals, each acting alone and in concert, moves the inflammatory response along in a controlled way. Cytokines bind to specific cell surface receptors and produce a biological response by regulating the transcription of genes in the target cell via signal transduction pathways involving, for example, the protein kinase C or protein kinase A systems. This biological response reflects a balance between the production of the cytokine, the expression of its receptors on the target cells and the presence of inhibitors.

Adhesion molecules

Cellular adhesion molecules (CAMs) are surface glycoproteins which are expressed on many different types of cell; they are involved in cell–cell and cell–matrix adhesion and interactions. CAMs are fundamental in the interaction of lymphocytes with antigen presenting cells, keratinocytes and endothelial cells, and are important in lymphocyte trafficking in the skin during inflammation. CAMs have been classified into four families: cadherins, immunoglobulin superfamily, integrins and selectins. CAMs of special relevance in the skin are listed in Table 3.4.

Histocompatibility antigens

Like other cells in the body, those in the skin express surface antigens directed by genes of the major histocompatibility complex (HLA) on human chromosome 6. In particular, HLA A, B and C antigens (the class I antigens) are expressed on all nucleated cells including keratinocytes, Langerhans cells, and cells of the dermis. HLA-DR, -DP, -DQ and -DZ antigens (the class II antigens) are expressed

Table 3.4 Some cellular adhesion molecules which are important in the skin

Family	Nature	Example	Site	Ligand
Cadherins	Glycoproteins Adherence dependent on calcium	Desmoglein	Desmosomes in epidermis	Other cadherins
Immunoglobulin superfamily	Numerous molecules which are structurally similar to immunoglobulins	Intercellular adhesion molecule-1 (ICAM-1)	Endothelial cells Keratinocytes Langerhans cells	LFA-1
		Cluster of differentiation antigen 2 (CD2)	T lymphocytes Some NK cells	LFA-3
		Vascular cell adhesion molecule 1 (VCAM-1)	Endothelial cells	VLA-4
Integrins	Surface proteins comprising two non-covalently bound α and β chains	Very late activation proteins (β1-VLA)	T lymphocyte	VCAM
		Leucocyte function antigen 1 (LFA-1)	T lymphocyte	ICAM-1
		Macrophage activation antigen 1 (Mac-1)	Macrophages Monocytes Granulocytes	C3b component of complement
Selectins	Adhesion molecules with lectin-like domain which binds carbohydrate	E selectin (previously called ELAM-1)	Endothelial cells	SLe^x (CD15)

only on some cells. For example, they are poorly expressed on keratinocytes except during certain reactions (e.g. allergic contact dermatitis) or diseases (e.g. lichen planus). Helper T cells recognize antigens only in the presence of cells bearing class II antigens. Class II antigens are also important for certain cell–cell interactions. On the other hand, class I antigens mark target cells for cell-mediated cytotoxic reactions such as the rejection of skin allografts and the destruction of cells infected by viruses.

Types of reactions in the skin

There are four basic types of immunological reaction (Table 3.5).

Type I: immediate hypersensitivity reactions

These are characterized by vasodilatation and an outpouring of fluid from blood vessels. Such reac-

Table 3.5 Some immunological reactions in the skin

Type I
Immediate hypersensitivity reactions (mediated by IgE and mast cells)
  anaphylaxis
  wheal-flare reactions
  angioedema

Type II
Humoral cytotoxic reactions (mediated by IgG, IgM and complement)
  complement-mediated cytolysis
  antibody-mediated phagocytosis
  immunologically mediated hormone-like reactions

Type III
Immune complex diseases (mediated by IgG, IgM, IgA and complement)
Arthus reactions
Serum sickness
Vasculitis

Type IV
Cell-mediated reactions (mediated by lymphocytes and lymphokines)
  delayed hypersensitivity
  cell-mediated cytotoxicity
  antibody-dependent cellular cytotoxicity
  granulomatous reactions

tions can be mimicked by drugs or toxins, which act directly, but immunological reactions are mediated by antibodies, and are manifestations of allergy. IgE and IgG4 antibodies, produced by plasma cells in organs other than the skin, attach themselves to mast cells in the dermis. Mast cells contain inflammatory mediators, either in their granules or in their cytoplasm. The IgE antibody is attached to the mast cell by its Fc end, so that the antigen combining site dangles from the mast cell like a hand on an arm (Fig. 3.8). When specific antigen combines with the hand parts of the immunoglobulin (the antigen binding site or Fab end), the mast cell liberates its mediators into the surrounding tissue. Of these mediators, histamine (from the granules) and leukotrienes (from the cell membrane) induce vasodilatation, and endothelial cells retract allowing transudation into the extravascular space. The vasodilatation causes a pink colour and the transudation causes swelling. Urticaria and angioedema (p. 105) are examples of immediate hypersensitivity reactions occurring in the skin.

Antigen can be delivered to the skin from outside. A bee sting, for example, will induce swelling in everyone by direct pharmacological activity. However, some people, with IgE antibodies against antigens in the venom, swell even more at the site of the sting as the result of a specific immunological reaction. If they are extremely sensitive, they may develop wheezing, wheals, and anaphylactic shock (p. 272; Fig. 23.4), due to massive release of histamine into the circulation.

Antigens can also reach mast cells from inside the body. A person allergic to shellfish, for example, may develop urticaria within seconds, minutes, or hours of eating one. Antigenic material is absorbed from the gut, passes to tissue mast cells via the circulation, and elicits an urticarial reaction after binding to specific IgE on mast cells in the skin.

Type II: humoral cytotoxic reactions

In the main, these involve IgG and IgM antibodies which, like IgE, are produced by plasma cells and are present in the interstitial fluid of the skin. When they meet an antigen, they fix and activate complement through a series of enzymatic reactions which generate mediator and cytotoxic proteins (Fig. 3.9), e.g. if bacteria enter the skin, IgG and IgM

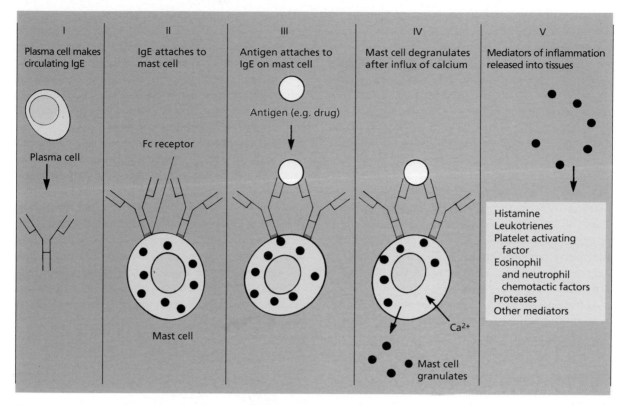

Fig. 3.8 Anaphylactic (type I) reaction.

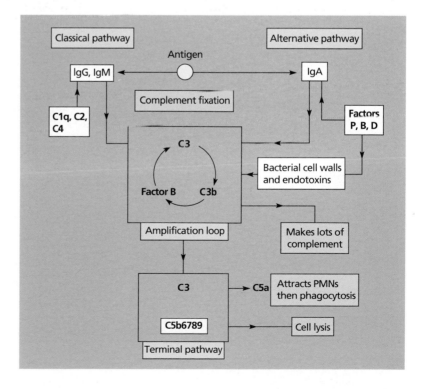

Fig. 3.9 Scheme of complement
activation.

antibodies bind to antigens on them. Complement is activated through the classical pathway and a number of mediators are generated. Amongst these are the chemotactic factor, C5a, which attracts polymorphs to the area of bacterial invasion, and the opsonin, C3b, which coats the bacteria so that they can be ingested and killed by the polymorphs when these arrive (Fig. 3.10). In certain circumstances, activation of complement can kill cells or organisms directly by the 'membrane attack complex' (C5b6789) in the terminal complement pathway (Fig. 3.9). Complement can also be activated by bacteria directly through the alternative pathway (Fig. 3.9). Antibody is not required. The bacterial cell wall causes more C3b to be produced by the alternative pathway factors B, D, and P (properdin). Aggregated IgA can also activate the alternative pathway.

Activation of either pathway produces C3b, the pivotal component of the complement system. Through the amplification loop, a single reaction can flood the area with C3b, C5a, and other amplification loop and terminal pathway components. Complement is the mediator of humoral reactions.

Humoral cytotoxic reactions are typical of defence against infectious agents such as bacteria. However, they also mediate certain autoimmune diseases such as pemphigoid (Chapter 13).

Occasionally antibodies bind to the surface of a cell and make it active without causing its death or activating complement. Instead, the cell is stimulated to produce a hormone-like substance which may mediate disease. Pemphigus (Chapter 13) is a blistering disease of skin in which this type of reaction is important. IgG antibodies react with an antigen on epidermal cells and induce them to release a proteolytic enzyme which dissolves the intercellular glue sticking the cells together. The keratinocytes fall apart from each other and the patient develops bullae and erosions.

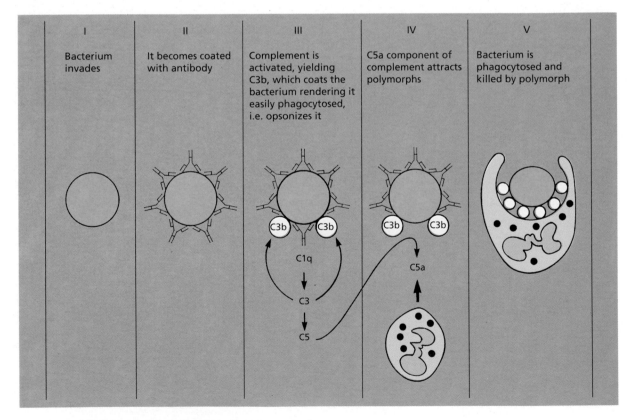

I	II	III	IV	V
Bacterium invades	It becomes coated with antibody	Complement is activated, yielding C3b, which coats the bacterium rendering it easily phagocytosed, i.e. opsonizes it	C5a component of complement attracts polymorphs	Bacterium is phagocytosed and killed by polymorph

Fig. 3.10 Antibody-mediated phagocytosis (type II reaction).

Type III: immune complex disease

Antigen may combine with antibodies near vital tissues so that the ensuing inflammatory response damages them. When an antigen is injected intradermally it combines with appropriate antibodies on the walls of blood vessels, complement is activated, and polymorphonuclear leucocytes are brought to the area (an Arthus reaction). Degranulation of polymorphs liberates lysosomal enzymes which damage the vessel walls.

Antigen–antibody complexes may also be formed in the circulation, move to the small vessels in the skin, and lodge there (Fig. 3.11). Complement will then be activated and inflammatory cells will injure the vessels as in the Arthus reaction. This causes oedema and the extravasation of red blood cells — the palpable purpura which characterizes vasculitis (Chapter 12).

Type IV: cell-mediated immunity

As its name implies, this is mediated by lymphocytes rather than by antibodies. Sensitized lymphocytes entering the skin interact with antigens processed by antigen-presenting cells, such as macrophages and Langerhans cells (Fig. 3.3). The lymphocytes are stimulated to enlarge, divide and to secrete cytokines which can injure tissues directly and kill cells or microbes.

Cell-mediated immune reactions are important in granulomatous reactions, delayed hypersensitivity reactions, and allergic contact dermatitis. They probably play a role in some photosensitive disorders, in protecting against cancer, and in mediating reactions to the bites of hostile or hungry insects.

Antigens coming from inside a cell, such as intracellular fungi or viruses, are presented to T cells by the class I MHC molecule (see above). Presentation

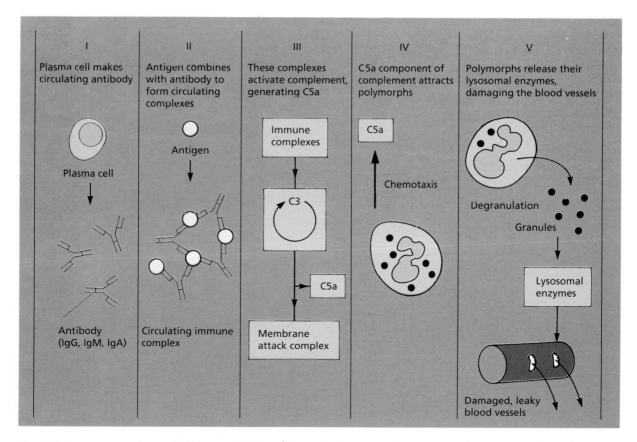

Fig. 3.11 Immune complex-mediated vasculitis (type III reaction).

in this manner makes the infected cell liable to destruction by lymphocytes. Cells can also kill other cells.

Granulomas are formed when cell-mediated immunity fails to eliminate antigen. Foreign body granulomas occur because a material remains undigested. Immunological granulomas require persistence of antigen, but the response is augmented by a cell-mediated immune reaction. Lymphokines, released by lymphocytes sensitized to the antigen, cause macrophages to differentiate into epithelioid cells and giant cells. These cells secrete other cytokines which influence inflammatory events. Immunological granulomas of the skin are characterized by Langhans giant cells (not to be confused with Langerhans cells; p. 13), epithelioid cells, and a surrounding mantle of lymphocytes.

Granulomatous reactions in the skin also arise when infectious organisms cannot be destroyed (e.g. in tuberculosis, leprosy, leishmaniasis), or when a chemical cannot be eliminated (e.g. zirconium or beryllium). Similar reactions are also seen in persisting inflammation of undetermined cause (e.g. in rosacea, granuloma annulare, sarcoidosis, and certain forms of panniculitis).

Immunodeficiency

The immune system defends the host against infectious agents which threaten it; hence immunodeficiency often leads to cutaneous infection.

Immunodeficiency should be considered in the following circumstances:
● Recurrent infections, particularly when severe, extensive or of several organs.
● Failure to respond to appropriate antibiotics.
● Infection with ordinary organisms in unusual sites, especially when resistant to treatment.
● Infections with opportunistic organisms in any site.
● Prolonged infection with weight loss, failure to thrive, severe diarrhoea, or graft-versus-host reaction.
● Atypical syndromes mimicking lupus erythematosus.

Many chronic infections of the skin are due to favourable local conditions rather than to immunodeficiency. For example, fungal infections of the toe webs become chronic because the skin there is moist and ideal for fungal growth. Recurrent infection in many organs, however, is the hallmark of an immunodeficient state.

LEARNING POINTS
1 Many skin reactions are good examples of immune mechanisms at work.
*2 However, do not blame the immune system as the prime cause of any disorder. If **Treponema pallidum** had not been discovered, syphilis might still be listed as an autoimmune disorder.*

CHAPTER 4

Diagnosis of skin disorders

The key to successful treatment is accurate diagnosis. This requires a careful history, a thorough physical examination, and the intelligent use of the laboratory.

Dermatology is different from other specialties because the diseases can easily be seen. Keen eyes, aided sometimes by a magnifying glass, are all that are needed for a complete examination of the skin. Often it is best to examine the patient briefly before obtaining a full history. A quick look will prompt the right questions.

History

The key points in the history are listed in Table 4.1 and should include a description of the events surrounding the onset of the skin lesions, and the progression of individual lesions and of the disease in general, including any responses to treatment. Many patients try a few salves before seeing a physician. Some try all the medications in their medicine cabinets, many of which can aggravate the problem. A careful inquiry into drugs taken for other conditions is often useful. Ask also about previous skin disorders, occupation, hobbies and disorders in the family.

Examination

To examine the skin properly, the lighting must be uniform and bright. The patient should undress. Do not be put off this too easily by the elderly, the stubborn, the shy, or the surroundings. Sometimes make-up must be washed off or wigs removed. There is nothing more embarrassing than missing the right diagnosis because clothing or make-up has obscured an important sign.

Table 4.1 Outline of dermatological history

History of present skin condition	*General health at present*
• Duration	• Ask about fever
• Site at onset, details of spread	
• Itch	
• Burning	
• Pain	
• Wet, dry, blisters	
• Exacerbating factors	
Past history of skin disorders	*Past general medical history*
	• Enquire specifically about asthma and hay fever
Family history of skin disorders	*Family history of other medical disorders*
• If positive — inherited versus infection/infestation	
Social and occupational history	
Should include details of:	
• Hobbies	
• Travels abroad	
• Relationship of rash to work and holidays	
• Alcohol intake	
Drugs used to treat present skin condition	*Drugs prescribed for other disorders* (including those taken before onset of skin disorder)
• Topical	
• Systemic	
• Physician prescribed	
• Patient initiated	

Distribution

Diagnosis in dermatology is based both on the distribution of lesions and on their morphology and configuration. For example, on inspection, an area of seborrhoeic dermatitis may look very like one of atopic dermatitis; but the key to diagnosis lies in the location of the rash. Seborrhoeic dermatitis affects the scalp, forehead, eyebrows, nasolabial folds, and central chest; atopic dermatitis typically affects the antecubital and popliteal fossae.

Determine if the skin disease is localized, universal, or symmetrical. Depending on the disease, or group of diseases, suggested by the morphology you may want to check special areas, like the feet in a patient with hand eczema, or the gluteal cleft in a patient you think might have psoriasis. Examine as much of the skin as possible. Look in the mouth and remember to check the hair and the nails (Chapter 8). Note negative as well as positive findings, for example the way the shielded areas are spared in a photosensitive dermatitis. Always keep your eyes open for incidental skin cancers which the patient may have ignored.

Morphology

After the distribution has been noted, next define the morphology of the primary lesions. Many skin diseases have a characteristic morphology, but scratch marks, ulceration, and other events may later change this appearance. The rule is to find an early or 'primary' lesion and to inspect it closely. What is its shape? What is its size? What is its colour? What are its margins like? What are the surface characteristics? What does it feel like?

Most types of primary lesion have one name if small, and a different one if large. The scheme is summarized in Table 4.2.

There are many reasons why you should describe skin diseases properly:
- Skin disorders are often grouped by their morphology. Once the morphology is clear, a differential diagnosis comes easily to mind.
- If you have to describe a condition accurately, you will have to look at it carefully.
- You can paint a verbal picture if you have to refer the patient for another opinion.
- You will sound like a physician and not a homoeopath.
- You will be able to understand the terminology of this book.

Terminology of lesions (Fig. 4.1)

Primary lesions

Erythema is redness due to vascular dilatation.

A *papule* is a small solid elevation of skin, less than 0.5 cm in diameter.

A *plaque* is an elevated area of skin greater than 2 cm in diameter but without substantial depth.

A *macule* is a small flat area of altered colour or texture.

Table 4.2 Terminology of primary lesions

	Small (less than 0.5 cm)	Large (greater than 0.5 cm)
Elevated solid lesions	Papule	Nodule (greater than 0.5 cm in both width and depth) Plaque (greater than 2 cm in width but without substantial depth)
Flat area of altered colour or texture	Macule	Large macule (patch)
Fluid-filled blister	Vesicle	Bulla
Pus-filled lesion	Pustule	Abscess
Extravasation of blood into skin	Petechia (pinhead size) Purpura (up to 2 mm in diameter)	Ecchymosis Haematoma
Accumulation of dermal oedema	Wheal (can be any size)	Angioedema

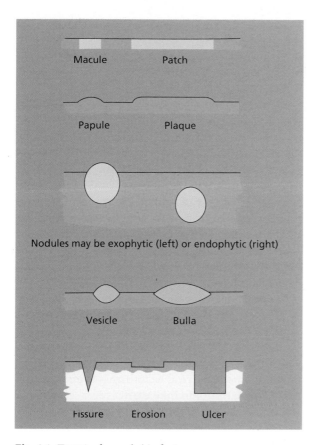

Fig. 4.1 Terminology of skin lesions.

A *vesicle* is a circumscribed elevation of skin, less than 0.5 cm in diameter, and containing fluid.

A *bulla* is a circumscribed elevation of skin over 0.5 cm in diameter and containing fluid.

A *pustule* is a visible accumulation of pus in the skin.

An *abscess* is a localized collection of pus in a cavity, more than 1 cm in diameter. Usually abscesses are nodules, and the term 'purulent bulla' is sometimes used to describe a pus-filled blister which is situated on top of the skin surface rather than in it.

A *wheal* is an elevated white compressible, evanescent area produced by dermal oedema. It is often surrounded by a red, axon-mediated flare. Although usually less than 2 cm in diameter, wheals may be huge.

Angioedema is a diffuse swelling of oedema which extends to the subcutaneous tissue.

A *nodule* is a solid mass in the skin, usually greater than 0.5 cm in diameter, in both width and depth, which can be observed as an elevation or can be palpated.

A *tumour* is harder to define, as the term is based more correctly on microscopic pathology than on clinical morphology. We keep it here as a convenient term to describe an enlargement of the tissues by normal or pathological material or cells that form a mass, usually more than 1 cm in diameter. Because the word 'tumour' scares patients, tumours are courteously called 'large nodules', especially if they are not malignant.

A *papilloma* is a nipple-like mass projecting from the skin.

Petechiae are pinhead-sized macules of blood in the skin.

The term *purpura* describes a larger macule or papule of blood in the skin. Such blood-filled lesions do not blanch if a glass lens is pushed against them (diascopy).

An *ecchymosis* is a larger extravasation of blood into the skin.

A *haematoma* is a swelling from gross bleeding.

A *burrow* is a linear or curvilinear papule, caused by a burrowing scabies mite.

A *comedo* is a plug of keratin and sebum wedged in a dilated pilosebaceous orifice. Open comedones are blackheads. The follicle opening of a closed comedo is nearly covered over by skin so that it looks like a pinhead-sized, ivory-coloured papule.

Telangiectasia is the visible dilatation of small cutaneous blood vessels.

Poikiloderma is a combination of atrophy, reticulate hyperpigmentation and telangiectasia.

Secondary lesions

These evolve from primary lesions.

A *scale* is a flake arising from the horny layer.

A *keratosis* is a horn-like thickening of the skin.

A *crust* may look like a scale, but is composed of dried blood or tissue fluid.

An *ulcer* is an area of skin from which the whole of the epidermis and at least the upper part of the dermis has been lost. Ulcers may extend into subcutaneous fat and heal with scarring.

An *erosion* is an area of skin denuded by a complete or partial loss of only the epidermis. Erosions heal without scarring.

An *excoriation* is an ulcer or erosion produced by scratching.

A *fissure* is a slit in the skin.

A *sinus* is a cavity or channel that permits the escape of pus or fluid.

A *scar* is a result of healing, where normal structures are permanently replaced by fibrous tissue.

Atrophy is a thinning of skin due to diminution of the epidermis, dermis or subcutaneous fat. When the epidermis is atrophic it may crinkle like cigarette paper, appear thin and translucent, and lose normal surface markings. Blood vessels may be easy to see in both epidermal and dermal atrophy.

Lichenification describes thickened skin with increased markings.

A *stria* is a streak-like, linear, atrophic, pink, purple or white lesion of the skin due to changes in the connective tissue.

Pigmentation, either more or less than surrounding skin, may develop after lesions heal.

Having identified the lesions as primary or secondary, adjectives can be used to describe them in terms of their:
- Colour (e.g. salmon-pink, lilac, violet).
- Sharpness of edge (e.g. well-defined, ill-defined).
- Surface contour (e.g. dome-shaped, umbilicated, spike-like) (Fig. 4.2).

- Geometric shape (e.g. nummular, oval, resembling the coast of Maine).
- Texture (e.g. rough, silky, smooth, hard).
- Smell (e.g. foul-smelling).
- Temperature (e.g. hot, warm).

Dermatologists also use a few special adjectives which warrant definition. *Nummular* means round or coin-like. *Annular* means ring-like. *Circinate* means circular. *Arcuate* means curved. *Discoid* means disc-like. *Gyrate* means wave-like. *Retiform* and *reticulate* mean net-like.

To describe a skin lesion, use the term for the primary lesion as the noun, and the adjectives mentioned above to define it. For example, the lesions of psoriasis may appear as 'salmon-pink, sharply demarcated, nummular plaques covered by large, silver, polygonal scales'.

Try not to use the terms 'lesion' or 'area'. Why say 'papular lesion' when you can say papule? It is almost as bad as the well worn 'skin rash'. By the way, there are very few diseases that are truly 'maculopapular'. The term is best avoided except to describe certain drug eruptions and viral exanthems. Even then, the terms 'scarlatiniform' (like scarlet fever — punctate, slightly elevated papules) or 'morbilliform' (like measles — a net-like, blotchy, slightly elevated, pink, exanthem) are more helpful.

Configuration

After unravelling the primary and secondary lesions, look for arrangements and configurations which are, for example, discrete, confluent, grouped, annular, arcuate, linear and dermatomal (Fig. 4.3). Note that while individual lesions may be annular, several individual lesions may arrange themselves into an annular configuration. Terms like annular, and other adjectives discussed under the morphology of individual lesions, may therefore apply to their groupings too. The Köbner or isomorphic phenomenon is the induction of skin lesions by, and at the site of, trauma such as scratch marks or operative incisions.

Special tools and techniques

A *magnifying lens* is a helpful aid to diagnosis because subtle changes in the skin become more apparent when enlarged.

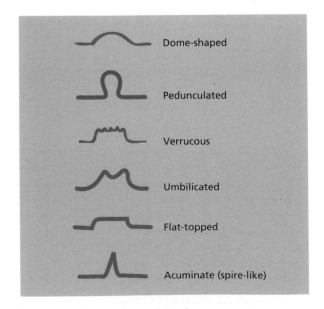

Dome-shaped

Pedunculated

Verrucous

Umbilicated

Flat-topped

Acuminate (spire-like)

Fig. 4.2 Surface contours of papules.

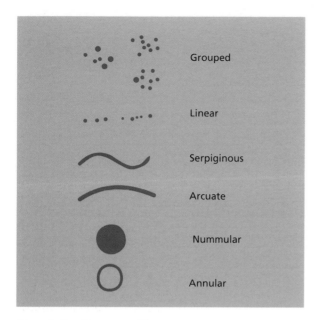

Fig. 4.3 Configuration of lesions.

A number of tests can be performed in the practice or office with results immediately available:

Potassium hydroxide preparations for fungal infections

If a fungal infection is suspected, scales or hair pluckings can be dissolved in an aqueous solution of 20% potassium hydroxide (KOH) containing 40% dimethyl sulphoxide (DMSO). The scale from the edge of a scaling lesion is vigorously scraped on to a glass slide with a No. 15 scalpel blade or the edge of a second glass slide. Other samples can include nail clippings, the roofs from tops of blisters, hair pluckings and the contents of pustules when a candidal infection is suspected. A drop or two of KOH solution is added before applying the coverslip. After 5–10 minutes, with the exception of nail clippings which take an hour or so to clear, the mount is examined under a microscope with the condenser lens lowered to increase contrast. With experience, fungal and candidal hyphae can be readily detected (Fig. 4.4). No heat is required if DMSO is included in the KOH solution.

Detection of scabies mite

The finding of burrows in an itchy patient is diag-

Skin lesions can also be examined using long-wave ultraviolet radiation emitted by a *Wood's light*. By demonstrating fluorescence, Wood's light may help in the diagnosis of fungus infections (Chapter 15), subtle disorders of pigmentation, erythrasma (p. 161), *Pseudomonas* infections, and pityriasis versicolor (p. 191).

In *diascopy*, a glass slide or clear plastic spoon is used to blanch vascular lesions and so to unmask their true colour. *Photography* helps to record the baseline appearance of a lesion or rash so that change at subsequent visits may be assessed objectively.

Assessment

Next try to put the disease into a general class. The titles of the chapters in this book are representative. Once classified, a differential diagnosis is usually forthcoming. Each diagnosis can then be considered on its merits, and laboratory tests may be used to confirm or refute diagnoses in the differential list. *At this stage you must make a working diagnosis or formulate a plan to do so!*

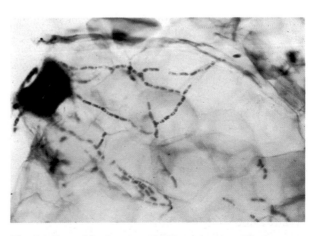

Fig. 4.4 Fungal hyphae in a KOH preparation. The polygonal shadows in the background are horny layer cells.

nostic of scabies. The retrieval of a mite from the skin will confirm the diagnosis and convince a sceptical patient of the infestation. The burrow should be examined under a magnifying glass; the acarus may be seen as a tiny black or grey dot at the most recent, least scaly end. It can be removed by a sterile needle and placed on a slide within a marked circle. Alternatively, if mites are not seen, questionable burrows are vigorously scraped with a No. 15 scalpel blade, moistened with liquid paraffin or vegetable oil, and the scrapings transferred to a slide. Patients never argue the toss when confronted by a magnified mobile mite.

Cytology (Tzanck smear)

Cytology can aid diagnosis of viral infections like herpes simplex and zoster, and bullous diseases such as pemphigus. A blister roof is removed and the cells from the base of the blister are scraped off with a No. 10 or 15 surgical blade. The cells are smeared on to a microscope slide, air-dried and fixed with methanol. They are then stained with Giemsa, toludine blue, or Wright's stain. Acantholytic cells (Chapter 11) are seen in pemphigus and multinucleus giant cells are diagnostic of herpes simplex or varicella zoster infections (Chapter 15).

Patch tests

Patch tests are invaluable in detecting allergens responsible for allergic contact dermatitis (Chapter 9). Either suspected antigens or a battery of antigens which are common culprits are tested (Fig. 4.5). Standard dilutions of the common antigens in appropriate bases are available commercially. The test materials are applied to the back under aluminium discs or patches; the occlusion encourages penetration of the allergen. The patches are left in place for 48 hours and then, after careful marking, are removed. The sites are inspected then and again at 96 hours. The test detects type IV delayed hypersensitivity reactions (Chapter 3). The readings are scored according to the reaction seen:

Not tested	NT
No reaction	0
Doubtful reaction (minimal erythema)	±

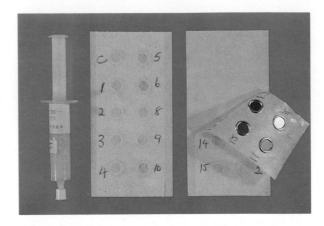

Fig. 4.5 Patch testing equipment. Syringe contains commercially prepared antigen, to be applied in aluminium cups.

Weak reaction (erythematous and maybe papular)	+
Strong reaction (erythematous and oedematous or vesicular)	++
Extreme reaction (erythematous and bullous)	+++
Irritant reaction	IR

A positive patch test does not prove that this substance is the cause of the current episode of contact dermatitis; the results must be interpreted in the light of the history and possible previous exposure to the allergen.

Patch testing requires attention to detail in applying the patches properly and skill and experience in interpreting the results.

Prick testing

Prick testing is much less helpful in dermatology. It detects immediate (type I) hypersensitivity (Chapter 3) and patients should not have taken systemic antihistamines for at least 48 hours prior to the test. Commercially prepared diluted antigens and a control are placed as single drops on marked areas of the forearm. The skin is gently pricked through the drops using separate sterile fine (e.g. Size 25 gauge, or smaller) needles. The drops are then removed with a tissue wipe. The prick should not cause bleeding. After 10 minutes the sites are inspected and the diameter of any wheal measured and recorded. Like patch testing, prick testing is not recommended for those without formal training in the procedure. Although the risk of anaphylaxis is small, resuscitation facilities including adrenaline and oxygen (p. 274) must be available. The relevance of positive results to the cause of the condition under investigation (usually urticaria or atopic dermatitis) is often debatable. Positive results should correlate with positive radio-allergosorbent tests (RAST; p. 89).

Skin biopsy

Skin biopsy is easily performed. There are two main types, punch and scalpel biopsy.

Punch biopsy

The skin is sampled with a small (3–4 mm diameter) tissue punch. Lignocaine (Lidocaine, USA) 1% is injected intradermally first, and a cylinder of skin is incised with the punch by rotating it back and forth. Skin is lifted up carefully with a needle or forceps and the base is cut off at the level of subcutaneous fat. The defect is cauterized or repaired with a single suture. The biopsy specimen must not be crushed with the forceps or critical histological patterns may be squashed.

The tissue can be sent to the pathologist with a summary of the history, a differential diagnosis, and the patient's age. Close liaison with the pathologist is essential, because the diagnosis may only become apparent with knowledge of *both* the clinical and histological features.

Scalpel biopsy

This provides more tissue than a punch biopsy. This technique can be used routinely, but is especially useful for biopsying disorders of the subcutaneous fat and for obtaining specimens with both normal and abnormal skin for comparison. After selecting the lesion for biopsy, an elliptical piece of skin is excised. The specimen should include the subcutaneous fat. Removing the specimen with forceps may cause crush artefact; this can be avoided by lifting the specimen with either a Gillies hook or a syringe needle. The wound is then sutured; firm compression for 5 minutes stops oozing. 3/0 non-

Table 4.3 Guidelines for skin biopsies

- Sample a fresh lesion
- Obtain specimen from near the lesion's edge
- Avoid sites where a scar would be conspicuous
- Avoid the upper trunk or jawline where keloids are more likely to form
- Avoid the legs, where healing is slow
- Avoid lesions over bony prominences, where infection is more likely
- Use the scalpel technique for diagnosing scalp disorders and diseases of the subcutaneous fat or vessels
- Do not crush the tissue
- Place in proper fixative
- If two lesions are sampled, be sure they do not get mixed up or mislabelled. Label specimen containers *before* biopsy is placed in them
- Make sure that patient's name, age and sex are clearly indicated on the pathology form
- Provide the pathologist with a legible summary of the history, the site of the biopsy, and a differential diagnosis
- Discuss the results with the pathologist

absorbable sutures are used for biopsies on the legs and back, 5/0 for the face, and 4/0 for elsewhere. Stitches are usually removed from the face in four days, from the anterior trunk and arms in seven days, and from the back and legs in ten days. Some guidelines for skin biopsies are listed in Table 4.3.

Laboratory tests

The laboratory is vital for the accurate diagnosis of many skin disorders. Tests include various assays of blood, serum and urine, bacterial, fungal and viral culture from skin and other specimens, immuno-fluorescent and immunohistological examinations (Figs 4.6 & 4.7), X-radiology, ultrasonography and other methods of image intensification. Specific details will be discussed as each disease is presented.

Treatment

This is the easiest part, but only if the diagnosis is correct. You can look up treatments, but you cannot look up diagnoses. Without a diagnosis, you will be asking 'what's a good treatment for scaling feet?' instead of 'what's good for tinea pedis?' (Would you ever ask yourself 'what's a good treatment for chest pain?') Once the diagnosis has been made, the

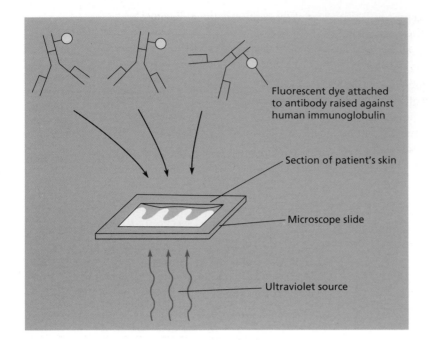

Fig. 4.6 Direct immunofluorescence detects antibodies in patient's skin. Here IgG antibodies are detected by staining with a fluorescent dye attached to antihuman IgG.

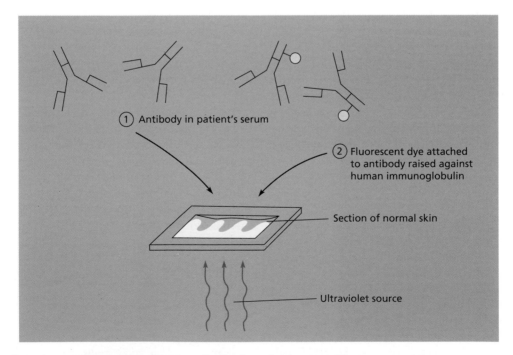

Fig. 4.7 Indirect immunofluorescence detects antibodies in patient's serum. There are two steps.
1 Antibodies in this serum are made to bind to antigens in a section of normal skin.
2 Antibody raised against human immunoglobulin, conjugated with a fluorescent dye can then be used to stain these bound antibodies (as in the direct immunofluorescence test).

treatment should take this into account, and also the age of the patient, the severity of the disorder, its extent, the disability it causes, the safety of the useful drugs, the cost of the drugs or treatments, and the likelihood of compliance with a treatment regimen. The patient's lifestyle should not be changed unless absolutely necessary.

Summary

Clinical dermatology is a visual specialty. You must see the disease and know what you see. Look closely and thoroughly. Take time. Examine the whole body. Locate primary lesions and check configuration and distribution. Ask appropriate questions, especially if the diagnosis is difficult. Classify the disorder and list the differential diagnosis. Use the history, examination, and laboratory tests to make a diagnosis if this cannot be made by clinical features alone. Then treat. Refer the patient to a dermatologist if:

- You cannot make a diagnosis.
- The disorder does not respond to treatment.
- The disorder is unusual or severe.
- You are just not sure.

LEARNING POINTS
1 A correct diagnosis is the key to correct treatment.
2 The term 'skin rash' is as bad as 'gastric stomach'.
3 Do not use long Latin descriptive names as a cloak for ignorance.
4 The history becomes more important when the diagnosis is difficult.
5 Undress patients and use a lens, even if it only gives you more time to think.
6 Remember the old adage that if you do not look in the mouth you will put your foot in it.

CHAPTER 5

Disorders of keratinization

The complex but orderly process of keratinization has been described on p. 9. In it, the living cells of the deeper epidermis are transformed into the dead cornified cells of the stratum corneum, from which they are shed in such a way that the surface of the normal skin does not seem scaly to the naked eye. In addition, shedding balances production, so that the thickness of the stratum corneum does not alter. If, however, the process of keratinization is abnormal, the stratum corneum may become thick or the surface of the skin may become dry and scaly. Such changes may be localized or generalized.

In this chapter we describe several skin disorders, mostly unrelated, which have as their basis a disorder of keratinization.

The ichthyoses

The word ichthyosis comes from the Greek word for a fish. It is applied to disorders which share, as their main feature, marked scaling in the absence of inflammation. Strictly speaking the scales lack the overlapping pattern of those of a fish, but the term is usefully descriptive and too well entrenched to be discarded. There are several types.

Ichthyosis vulgaris

Cause

Inherited as an autosomal dominant, this condition is common and affects about one person in 300.

Presentation

The dryness is usually mild and symptoms are few. The scales are small and branny, most obvious on the limbs and least obvious in the major flexures.

The skin creases of the palm may be accentuated. Keratosis pilaris (p. 44) is often present on the limbs.

Clinical course

The skin changes are usually not present at birth but develop over the first few years of life. Some patients improve in adult life, particularly during warm weather, but the condition seldom clears fully.

Complications

The already dry skin tends to chap in the winter and to be easily irritated by degreasing agents. This should be taken into account in the choice of a career. This type of ichthyosis is apt to appear in a stubborn combination with atopic eczema.

Differential diagnosis

It can usually be distinguished from less common types of ichthyosis on the basis of the pattern of inheritance and of the type and distribution of the scaling.

Investigations

None are usually needed.

Treatment

This is palliative. The dryness can be helped by the regular use of emollients which are best applied after a shower or bath. Emulsifying ointment, soft white paraffin, E45 and unguentum merck are all quite suitable (Formulary, p. 287) and the selection depends on the patient's preference. Many find proprietary bath oils and creams containing urea or lactic acid helpful also (Formulary, p. 287).

Sex-linked ichthyosis

Cause

This less common type of ichthyosis is inherited as a sex-linked recessive and therefore, in its complete form, is seen only in males, though some female carriers may show mild scaling. The condition affects some one in 6000 males in the UK and is associated with a deficiency of the enzyme steroid sulphatase which hydrolyses cholesterol sulphate. The responsible gene has been localized to the terminal part of the X chromosome at Xp 22.3 (see Chapter 22).

Presentation and course

In contrast to the delayed onset of the dominantly inherited ichthyosis vulgaris, scaling appears early, often soon after birth, and always by the first birthday. The scales are larger and browner (Fig. 5.1), and involve the major flexures as well as the skin generally. There is no association with atopy or keratosis pilaris. The condition persists throughout life.

Complications

Corneal opacities may appear in adult life.

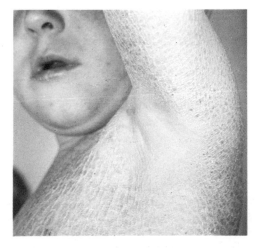

Fig. 5.1 Ichthyosis: large rather dark scales suggest the less common type inherited as a sex-linked recessive, though the sparing of the axilla may be against this.

Differential diagnosis

As for ichthyosis vulgaris. It is helpful to remember that only males are affected.

Investigations

None are usually needed. A few centres can measure steroid sulphatase in fibroblasts cultured from a skin biopsy.

Treatment

Oral aromatic retinoids are probably best avoided. Topical measures are as for ichthyosis vulgaris.

Collodion baby

This is a description and not a diagnosis. The bizarre skin charges are seen at birth. At first the stratum corneum is smooth and shiny, and the skin looks as though it has been covered with cellophane or collodion. Its tightness may cause ectropion and feeding difficulties. The shiny outer surface is shed within a few days leaving behind, most often, a lamellar ichthyosis, less often an X-linked ichthyosis, and occasionally a normal skin. Problems with temperature regulation and high water loss through the skin in the early days of life are best dealt with by the use of a high humidity incubator. Regular applications of a greasy emollient also limit fluid loss and make the skin supple. The much rarer 'Harlequin fetus' is covered with thick fissured hyperkeratosis. Ectropion is extreme and most affected infants die early.

Lamellar ichthyosis (LI) and non-bullous ichthyosiform erythroderma (NBIE)

Understandably, these rare conditions have often been confused in the past. Both may be inherited as an autosomal recessive, and in both the skin changes at birth are those of a collodion baby (see above). Later the two conditions can be distinguished by the finer scaling and more obvious redness of NBIE (Fig. 5.2). Both last for life and are sufficiently disfiguring for the long-term use of acitretin to be justifiable (Formulary, p. 305).

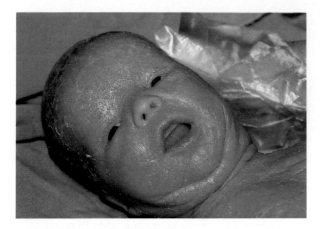

Fig. 5.2 Non-bullous ichthyosiform erythoderma in a neonate.

Epidermolytic hyperkeratosis
(bullous ichthyosiform erythroderma)

This rare condition is inherited as an autosomal dominant. Shortly after birth the baby's skin becomes generally red and shows numerous blisters. The redness fades over a few months, and the tendency to blister also lessens, but during childhood a gross brownish warty hyperkeratosis appears, sometimes in a roughly linear form and usually worst in the flexures. The histology is distinctive: a thickened granular cell layer contains large granules, and clefts may be seen in the upper epidermis. A few patients have localized areas of hyperkeratosis with the same histological features. Treatment is symptomatic and antibiotics may be needed if the blisters become infected. Acitretin (Formulary, p. 305) may be tried in severe cases.

Other ichthyosiform disorders

Sometimes ichthyotic skin changes are a minor part of a multisystem disease, but such associations are very rare. *Refsum's syndrome*, an autosomal recessive trait, is due to deficiency of a single enzyme concerned in the breakdown of phytanic acid, which accumulates in the tissues. The other features (retinal degeneration, peripheral neuropathy and ataxia) overshadow the minor dryness of the skin.

Rud's syndrome is an ichthyosiform erythroderma in association with mental retardation and epilepsy. In *Netherton's syndrome*, brittle hairs, with a

so-called 'bamboo deformity', are present with a curious gyrate and erythematous hyperkeratotic eruption (ichthyosis linearis circumflexa). Other conditions are identified by confusing acronyms. IBIDS stands for (I)chthyosis, (B)rittle hair, (I)mpaired intelligence, (D)ecreased fertility and (S)hort stature: the KID syndrome consists of (K)eratitis, (I)chthyosis and (D)eafness.

Acquired ichthyosis

It is unusual for ichthyosis to appear for the first time in adult life: if it does, an underlying disease should be suspected. The most frequent is Hodgkin's disease. Other recorded causes include other lymphomata, leprosy, sarcoidosis, malabsorption and a poor diet. The skin may also appear dry in hypothyroidism.

Other disorders of keratinization

Keratosis pilaris

Cause

This common condition is inherited as an autosomal dominant trait. The abnormality lies in the keratinization of hair follicles which become filled with horny plugs.

Presentation and course

The changes begin in childhood and tend to become less obvious in adult life. In the commonest type, the greyish horny follicular plugs are confined to the outer aspects of the thighs and upper arms, where the skin feels rough (Fig. 5.3). Less often the plugs affect the sides of the face and the eyebrows. There is an association with ichthyosis vulgaris.

Complications

Involvement of the cheeks may lead to an ugly pitted scarring. Rarely the follicles in the eyebrows may be damaged with subsequent loss of hair there.

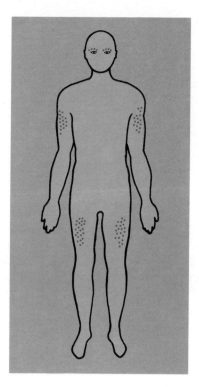

Fig. 5.3 The distribution of keratosis pilaris lesions.

Differential diagnosis

A rather similar pattern of widespread follicular keratosis (phrynoderma) can occur in severe vitamin deficiency. The lack is probably not just of vitamin A, as was once thought, but of several vitamins.

Investigations

None are needed.

Treatment

Keratolytics such as salicylic acid or urea in a cream base may be helpful though not curative (Formulary, p. 287).

Keratosis follicularis (Darier's disease)

Cause

This rare condition is inherited as an autosomal dominant trait. Fertility tends to be low and many cases represent new mutations. The basic defect is not fully understood but seems to involve tonofibrils and desmosomes. The abnormal gene has been mapped to the long arm of chromosome 12; a keratin gene seems a likely candidate.

Presentation

The first signs usually appear in the mid-teens, sometimes after over-exposure to sunlight. The characteristic lesions are small, pink and brownish papules with a greasy scale (Fig. 5.4b). These tend to coalesce into warty plaques in a 'seborrhoeic' distribution (Fig. 5.4a).

The severity of the condition varies greatly from person to person: early lesions are often seen on the sternal and interscapular areas, and behind the ears. In severe cases the skin may be widely affected, and the abnormalities remain for life, often causing much embarrassment and discomfort.

Other changes include lesions looking like plane warts on the backs of the hands, punctate keratoses or pits on the palms and soles, and a distinctive nail dystrophy in which white or pinkish lines or ridges run longitudinally to the free edge of the nail where they end in triangular nicks (Fig. 5.5).

Complications

Some patients are stunted and of poor intelligence. An impairment of delayed hypersensitivity may be the basis for a tendency to develop widespread herpes simplex and bacterial infections. Bacterial overgrowth is responsible for the unpleasant smell of some severely affected patients.

Differential diagnosis

The distribution of the lesions may be similar to that of seborrhoeic eczema, but discrete warty papules are not seen in this condition. The distribution differs from that of acanthosis nigricans (mainly flexural) and of keratosis pilaris (favours the outer upper arms and thighs).

Investigations

The diagnosis should be confirmed by a skin biopsy which will show characteristic clefts in the epidermis, and dyskeratotic cells.

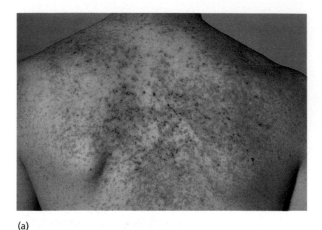

(a)

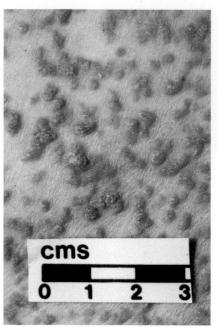

(b)

Fig. 5.4 (a) Extensive Darier's disease: in this case made worse by sun exposure. (b) The typical yellow-brown greasy papules of Darier's disease.

Treatment

Severe and disabling disease can be dramatically alleviated by long-term acitretin (Formulary, p. 305). Milder cases need only topical keratolytics, such as salicylic acid, and the control of local infection (Formulary, p. 290).

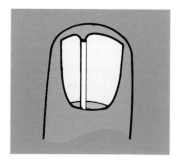

Fig. 5.5 The nail in Darier's disease. One or more longitudinal, pale or pink stripes run over the lunula to the free margin where they end in a triangular nick.

LEARNING POINTS

1 Life has been a living death for some patients with severe congenital disorders of keratinization. For them retinoids, used carefully, are the greatest advance in medicine.

2 The side effects of systemic retinoids preclude their use in minor disorders of keratinization.

Keratoderma of the palms and soles

Inherited types

Many genodermatoses share keratoderma of the palms and soles as their main feature. They cannot be described in detail here. The clinical patterns and modes of inheritance vary from family to family: punctate, striate, diffuse and mutilating varieties have been documented, sometimes in association with metabolic disorders such as tyrosinaemia, or with changes elsewhere.

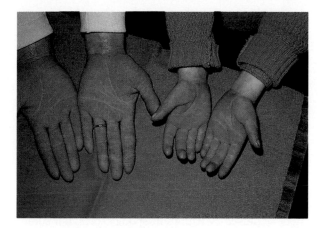

Fig. 5.6 Tylosis.

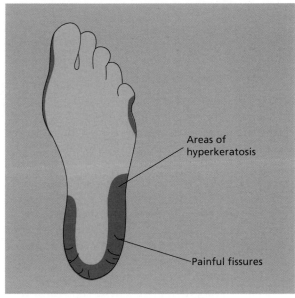

Fig. 5.7 Keratoderma climactericum — thickly keratotic skin, especially around the heels. Painful fissures are a problem.

The commonest pattern is a diffuse one, known also as tylosis (Fig. 5.6), which is inherited as an autosomal dominant trait. In a few families these changes have been associated with carcinoma of the oesophagus, but in most families this is not the case.

Treatment tends to be unsatisfactory but keratolytics such as salicylic acid and urea can be used in higher concentrations on the palms and soles than elsewhere (Formulary, p. 290).

Acquired types

It is not uncommon for normal people to have a few inconspicuous punctate keratoses on their palms, but it is no longer thought that these relate to internal malignancy.

Keratoderma of the palms and soles may be part of the picture of some generalized skin diseases such as pityriasis rubra pilaris (p. 69) and lichen planus (p. 67).

A distinctive pattern (*keratoderma climactericum*) is sometimes seen in middle-aged women at about the time of the menopause. It is most marked around the borders of the heels where painful fissures form and may interfere with walking (Fig. 5.7). Regular paring and the use of keratolytic ointments are often more helpful than attempts at hormone replacement, and the condition tends to settle over a few years. Acitretin in low doses may be worth a trial.

Knuckle pads

Cause

Sometimes these are familial; most often they are not. Trauma seems not to be important.

Presentation

Fibromatous and hyperkeratotic areas appear on the backs of many finger joints, usually beginning in late childhood and persisting thereafter. There may be an association with Dupuytren's contracture.

Differential diagnosis

Occupational callosities, granuloma annulare and viral warts should be considered.

Investigations

A biopsy may be helpful in the few cases of genuine clinical difficulty.

Treatment

None, including surgery, is satisfactory.

Callosities and corns

Both are responses to pressure. A callosity is a more diffuse type of thickening of the keratin layer which seems to be a protective response to widely applied repeated friction or pressure. Callosities are often occupational, for example they are seen on the hands of manual workers. Usually painless, they need no therapy.

Corns, on the other hand, have a central core of hard keratin which can hurt if forced inwards. They appear where there is high local pressure, often between bony prominences and shoes. Favourite areas include the backs of the toe joints, and the soles under prominent metatarsals. 'Soft corns' arise in the third or fourth toe clefts when the toes are squeezed together by tight shoes; such corns are often macerated.

The main differential is from hyperkeratotic warts, but these will show tiny bleeding points when pared down. A corn, however, has only its hard compacted avascular core surrounded by a more diffuse thickening of opalescent keratin.

The right treatment for corns is to eliminate the pressure which caused them, but patients may be slow to accept this. However, while regular paring may reduce the symptoms temporarily, well-fitting shoes are essential. Corns under the metatarsals may be helped by using soft spongy soles, but sometimes need orthopaedic alteration of weight bearing. Especial care is needed for corns on ischaemic or diabetic feet, which are at greater risk of infection and ulceration.

CHAPTER 6

Psoriasis

Psoriasis is a chronic, non-infectious, inflammatory disease of the skin, characterized by well-defined erythematous plaques bearing large, adherent, silvery scales. One to three per cent of most populations have psoriasis, which may be commonest in European and North American whites, uncommon in American blacks and almost non-existent in American Indians. It may start at any age but is rare under 10 years, and appears most often between 15 and 40. Its course is unpredictable but is usually chronic with exacerbations and remissions.

Cause and pathogenesis

The cause remains unknown. There is often a genetic predisposition, and the disease is sometimes triggered by an obvious factor. Some biochemical abnormalities are described below under separate headings but undoubtedly interact when establishing or perpetuating the inflammation. Theories about the pathogenesis of psoriasis tend to tag along behind fashions in cell biology; currently cytokines and adhesion molecules are in vogue.

Genetics

A child with one affected parent has a 16% chance of developing the disease, and this rises to 50% if both parents are affected. Genomic imprinting may explain why psoriatic fathers are more likely to pass on the disease to their children than are psoriatic mothers. If non-psoriatic parents have a child with psoriasis, the risk for subsequent children is about 10%. The disorder is concordant in 70% of monozygotic twins but only in 20% of dizygotic ones.

These figures are useful for counselling but do not spell out the precise mode of inheritance. Indeed the same family trees have been interpreted and reinterpreted by different experts as suggesting either an autosomal dominant inheritance with incomplete penetrance or a polygenic inheritance. Psoriasis is genetically heterogeneous.

Early onset psoriasis shows an obvious hereditary element with linkage to HLA-CW6. The risk of those with the HLA-CW6 genotype developing psoriasis is 20 times that of those without it. The hereditary element and the HLA associations are much weaker in late onset psoriasis.

Epidermal cell kinetics

In psoriasis there is increased epidermal proliferation due both to an excessive number of geminative cells entering the cell cycle, and perhaps to a decrease in cell cycle time. The growth fraction (p. 6) approaches 100% compared with 30% in normal skin. The epidermal turnover time (p. 5) is greatly shortened to 10 days as compared with 60 days in normal skin. This epidermal hyperproliferation accounts for many of the metabolic abnormalities associated with psoriasis. It is not confined to obvious plaques. similar but less marked changes occur also in apparently normal skin.

Altered epidermal maturation

During normal keratinization the profile of keratin types changes as a cell moves from the basal layer (K5 and K14) towards the surface (K1 and K10; p. 7). In psoriasis K6 and K16 are produced but their presence is secondary and non-specific, merely a result of increased epidermal proliferation.

Arachidonic acid metabolism (Fig. 6.1)

Arachidonic acid is bound to cell membranes and released from them by the activity of phospholipase

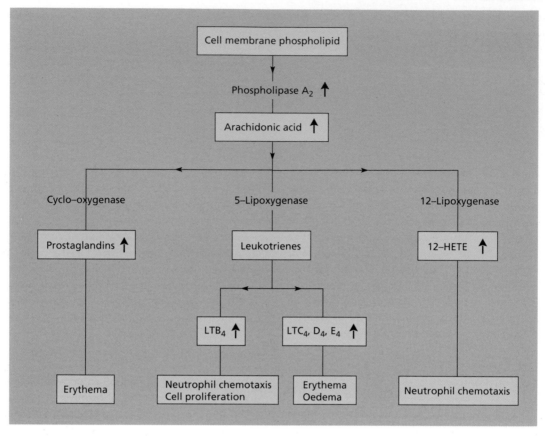

Fig. 6.1 Arachidonic acid and some of its metabolites in psoriasis. Broad arrows indicate those which are raised in lesional as compared with normal skin.

A$_2$. Levels of arachidonic acid, and of its metabolites prostaglandin E$_2$ (PGE$_2$), leukotriene B$_4$ (LTB$_4$), 12-hydroxy-eicosatetraenoic acid (12-HETE), and 15-HETE are elevated in the lesional skin of psoriasis. It is uncertain how these chemicals influence cell proliferation, though 12-HETE and other intermediates may inhibit adenylate cyclase and lower intracellular cyclic AMP (cAMP) (see below). LTB$_4$ attracts polymorphs strongly, and may be responsible for the micro-abscesses which are a feature of the histology (see below).

Cyclic nucleotides

There is evidence that cyclic guanosine monophosphate (cGMP) levels are increased in the lesions of psoriasis and therefore the ratio between cGMP and cAMP is increased. Beta-blockers, such as propa-

nolol, may worsen psoriasis by decreasing cAMP levels. Similarly, lithium exacerbates psoriasis and inhibits cAMP formation.

Polyamines

The biosynthesis of the polyamines putrescine, spermidine and spermine is intimately associated with cellular proliferation. Levels of the enzyme ornithine decarboxylase, catalysing the reaction ornithine to putrescine, are raised in the lesions of psoriasis, and the levels of the above polyamines are therefore elevated in lesional skin.

Proteinases and antiproteinases

Proteinases (e.g. plasminogen activator, cathepsins and certain complement components), and some proteinase inhibitors (e.g. α_1-antitrypsin and β_2-macroglobulin), regulate cell proliferation. Plasminogen activator is greatly increased in the lesions of psoriasis and parallels the mitotic rate; this increase may be due to deficiency of an inhibitor. Plasminogen activator is normally released following experimental injury, and in psoriasis its release could lead to the Köbner phenomenon (p. 38).

Calmodulin

The level of the specific calcium binding protein, calmodulin, is raised in lesions of psoriasis and falls with successful treatment. Interestingly, two drugs which help in psoriasis, dithranol and cyclosporin A, are calmodulin antagonists. The calcium–calmodulin complex, by influencing the activity of phospholipase A_2 (Fig. 6.1) and phosphodiesterase (catalyses cAMP to AMP), may also regulate cell proliferation abnormally in psoriasis.

Phosphatidyl inositol cycle

In psoriasis the activity of epidermal phospholipase C increases: this catalyses the conversion of phosphatidyl inositol in the cell membrane to inositol triphosphate (IP_3) and diacyglycerol (DG), both of which are involved in signal transduction. IP_3 induces intracellular calcium release which in turn activates calmodulin (see above). DG activates protein kinase C leading eventually to increased cell proliferation.

Inflammation

Psoriasis differs from the ichthyoses (p. 44) in its accumulation of inflammatory cells. This could be part of an immunological response to as yet unknown antigens. Certain interleukins and growth regulators are elevated, and adhesion molecules are expressed or upregulated in lesions of psoriasis. Immune events may well play a primary role in the pathogenesis of the disease and a hypothetical model might run as follows:

1 Keratinocytes are stimulated by various insults (e.g. trauma, infections, drugs, ultraviolet radiation) to release IL-1 and IL-8.
2 IL-1 upregulates the expression of intercellular adhesion molecule-1 (ICAM-1) and E selectin on vascular endothelium in the dermal papillae and ICAM-1 on keratinocytes. T helper lymphocytes accumulate in these papillary vessels because their lymphocyte function-associated antigen (LFA-1) sticks to adhesion molecules which are expressed on the vascular endothelium.
3 IL-8 from keratinocytes attracts T lymphocytes and neutrophils to migrate from papillary vessels into the epidermis where the T cells are held by adhesion of their LFA-1 with ICAM-1.
4 T cells accumulating in the epidermis are activated as a result of their interactions with Langerhans cells (possibly presenting unmasked retroviral or mycobacterial antigens or antigens shared by streptococci and keratinocytes) and keratinocytes. Activated T cells release IFN-γ, TNF-α and IL-2.
5 IFN-γ and TNF-α induce keratinocytes to express HLA-DR, to upregulate their ICAM-1 expression and to produce further IL-6, IL-8 and TGF-α. IL-2 ensures proliferation of the local T cells.
6 TGF-α acts as an autocrine mediator and attaches to epidermal growth factor (EGF) receptors inducing keratinocyte proliferation. IL-6 and TNF-α also have keratinocyte mitogenic properties.

Some see this chain of events as a type of wound healing which does not switch itself off.

Bacterial exotoxins produced by *Staphylococcus aurens* and certain streptococci may act as superantigens (p. 28) and promote marked T cell proliferation.

Cyclosporin (p. 64) which inhibits T helper cell function, improves psoriasis. This fits in with the idea that these lymphocytes are at the centre of the events underlying psoriasis. However, psoriasis is made worse by HIV infection: this paradox is hard to explain as the T helper lymphocyte is a major target for the HIV retrovirus.

The dermis

The dermis is abnormal in psoriasis. When psoriatic skin is grafted on to athymic mice, both epidermis and dermis must be present for the graft to sustain its psoriasis. The dermal capillary loops in psoriatic plaques are abnormally dilated and tortuous, and these changes come before epidermal hyperplasia in the development of a new plaque. Fibroblasts from psoriatics replicate more rapidly *in vitro* and produce more glycosaminoglycans than do those from non-psoriatics.

Precipitating factors

These include:

1 Trauma — in active psoriasis, lesions appear in skin damaged by scratches or surgical wounds (Köbner phenomenon) (Fig. 6.2).

2 Infection — beta-haemolytic streptococcal tonsillitis often triggers guttate psoriasis. AIDS often worsens it or precipitates explosive forms.

3 Hormonal — psoriasis frequently improves in pregnancy only to relapse post-partum. Hypocalcaemia secondary to hypoparathyroidism is a rare precipitating cause.

4 Sunlight — most psoriatics improve but 10% become worse.

5 Drugs — antimalarials, beta-blockers and lithium may worsen psoriasis. Psoriasis may 'rebound' after withdrawal of treatment with systemic steroids or potent topical steroids. The case against non-steroidal anti-inflammatory drugs remains not proven.

6 Cigarette smoking and alcohol — although the effects of confounding variables are difficult to unravel in epidemiological studies, there is growing

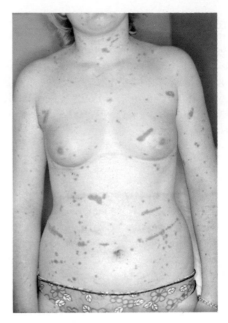

Fig. 6.2 Köbner phenomenon. Linear plaques of psoriasis, following scratching due to previous scabies.

evidence that both of these have an independent effect in precipitating or maintaining psoriasis.

7 Emotion — emotional upsets seem to cause some exacerbations.

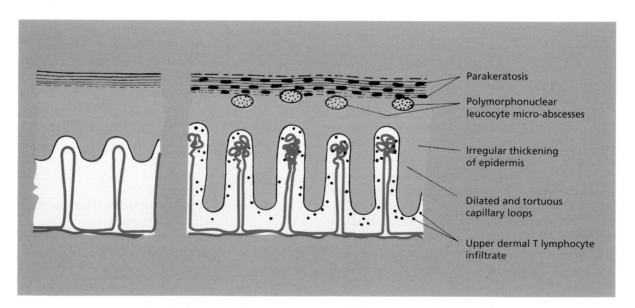

Fig. 6.3 Histology of psoriasis (right) compared with normal skin (left).

Histology (Fig. 6.3)

The main changes are:

1 Parakeratosis (nuclei retained in the horny layer).
2 Irregular thickening of the epidermis; but thinning over dermal papillae is apparent clinically when bleeding is caused by scratching and the removal of scales (Auspitz's sign).
3 Polymorphonuclear leucocyte micro-abscesses (described originally by Munro).
4 Dilated and tortuous capillary loops in the dermal papillae.
5 T lymphocyte infiltrate in upper dermis.

Presentation

Common patterns

Plaque pattern

This is the most common type. Lesions are well demarcated and range from a few millimetres to several centimetres in diameter (Figs 6.4 & 6.5). The lesions are pink or red with large, dry silvery-white

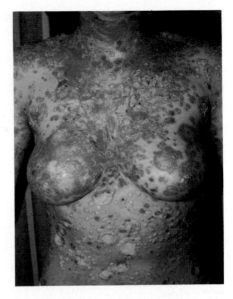

Fig. 6.5 Widespread plaques with coalescing lesions on chest.

scales (like candle grease). The elbows, knees, lower back, and scalp are sites of predilection (Fig. 6.6).

Guttate pattern

This is usually seen in children and adolescents and may be the first sign of the disease, often triggered by tonsillitis. Numerous small round red macules come up suddenly on the trunk and soon become scaly (Fig. 6.7). The rash often clears in a few months but plaque psoriasis may develop later.

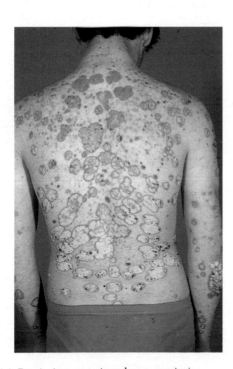

Fig. 6.4 Psoriasis: extensive plaque psoriasis.

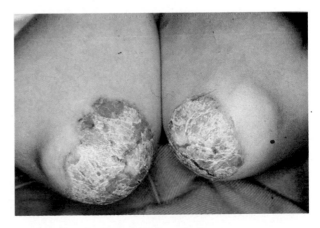

Fig. 6.6 Sharply defined plaques on elbows.

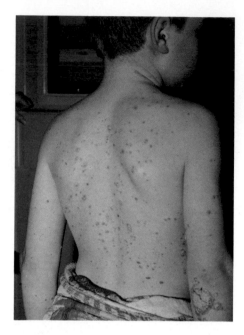

Fig. 6.7 Guttate lesions on trunk and plaques on elbow.

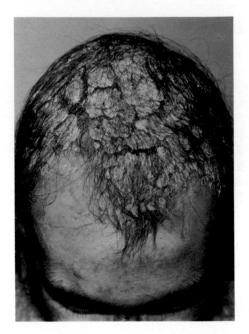

Fig. 6.8 Scalp psoriasis. The extent and associated marked hair loss are unusual.

Scalp

The scalp is often involved. Areas of scaling are interspersed with normal skin; their lumpiness is more easily felt than seen (Fig. 6.8). Frequently there is an overflow just beyond the scalp margin (Fig. 6.9). Significant hair loss is rare.

Nails

Involvement of the nails is common, with 'thimble pitting' (Fig. 6.10), onycholysis (separation of the nail from the nail bed) (Fig. 6.11) and sometimes subungual hyperkeratosis (Fig. 6.12).

Flexures

Psoriasis of the submammary, axillary and anogenital folds is not scaly though the glistening sharply demarcated red plaques (Fig. 6.13), often with fissuring in the depth of the fold, are still readily recognizable. Flexural psoriasis is commonest in women and in the elderly.

Palms

Palmar psoriasis may be hard to recognize as

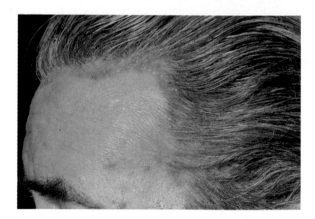

Fig. 6.9 Psoriasis of scalp margin.

its lesions are often poorly demarcated and barely erythematous.

Less common patterns

Napkin psoriasis

A psoriasiform spread outside the napkin (nappy/diaper) area may give the first clue to a psoriatic tendency in an infant (Fig. 6.14). Usually it clears

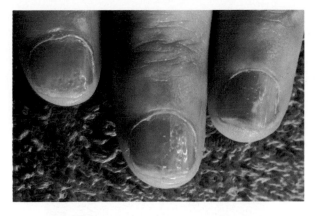

Fig. 6.10 Thimble-like pitting of nails with minor onycholysis.

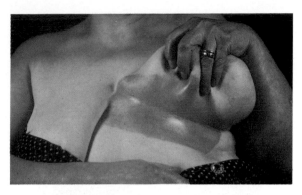

Fig. 6.13 Sharply defined glistening erythematous patch of flexural psoriasis.

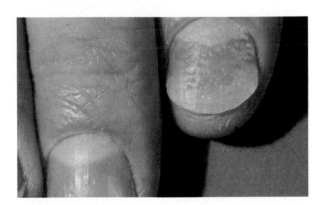

Fig. 6.11 Onycholysis and coarse pitting of little finger nail.

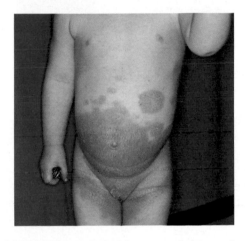

Fig. 6.14 Napkin psoriasis. Note constriction marks on thighs caused by polythene pants.

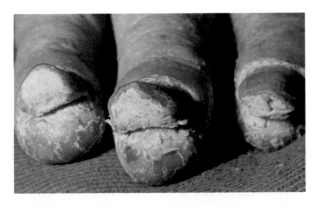

Fig. 6.12 Gross subungual hyperkeratosis.

quickly but there is an increased risk of ordinary psoriasis developing in later life.

Localized pustular psoriasis

This is a recalcitrant, often painful, condition which some regard as a separate entity. It affects the palms and soles which become studded with numerous sterile pustules, 3–10 mm in diameter, lying on an erythematous base. The pustules change to brown macules or scales (Fig. 6.15). Generalized pustular psoriasis is a rare but serious condition, with fever and recurrent episodes of pustulation within areas of erythema (Fig. 6.16).

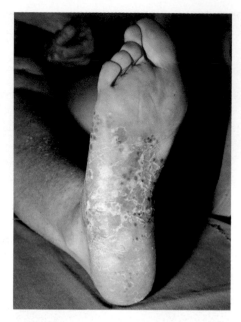

Fig. 6.15 Pustular psoriasis of right sole.

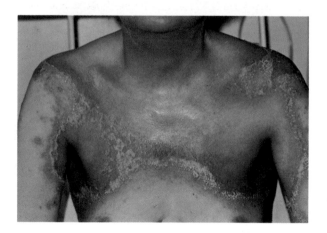

Fig. 6.16 Generalized pustular psoriasis. Clusters of superficial pustules at edge of spreading erythema.

Erythrodermic psoriasis

This is also rare and may be sparked off by the irritant effect of tar or dithranol, by a drug eruption or by the withdrawal of potent topical or systemic steroids. The skin becomes universally and uniformly red with variable scaling (Fig. 6.17). Malaise is accompanied by shivering and the skin feels hot and uncomfortable.

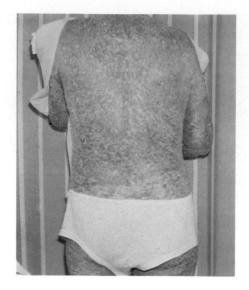

Fig. 6.17 Erythrodermic psoriasis.

Complications

Psoriatic arthropathy

Arthritis occurs in about 5% of psoriatics. Several patterns are recognized. Distal arthritis involves the terminal interphalangeal joints of the toes and fingers, especially those with marked nail changes (Fig. 6.12). Other patterns include involvement of a single large joint; one which mimics rheumatoid arthritis and may become mutilating (Figs 6.18 & 6.19); and one where the brunt is borne by the sacro-iliac joints and spine. Tests for rheumatoid factor are negative and nodules are absent. In patients with spondylitis and sacro-iliitis there is a strong correlation with the presence of HLA-B27.

Differential diagnosis

Discoid eczema (p. 100)

Lesions are less well defined and may be exudative or crusted, lack 'candle grease' scaling, and may be extremely itchy.

Seborrhoeic eczema (p. 98)

Scalp involvement is more diffuse and less lumpy.

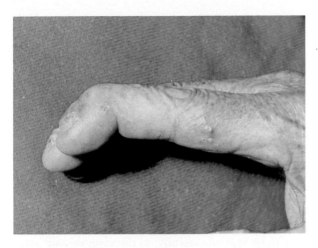

Fig. 6.18 Fixed flexion deformity of distal interphalangeal joints following arthropathy. Same patient as in Fig. 6.12.

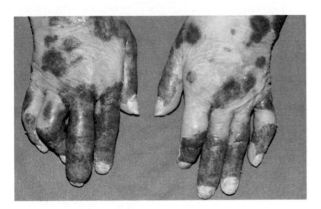

Fig. 6.19 Rheumatoid-like changes associated with severe psoriasis of hands and marked nail changes.

Flexural plaques are less well defined and more exudative. There may be signs of seborrhoeic eczema elsewhere, such as on the chest.

Pityriasis rosea (p. 66)

May be confused with guttate psoriasis but the lesions, which are oval rather than round, tend to run along rib lines. Scaling is of collarette type and a herald plaque may precede the rash.

Secondary syphilis (p. 167)

There is usually a history of a primary chancre. The scaly lesions are brownish and characteristically the palms and soles are involved. Oral changes, patchy alopecia and lymphadenopathy complete the picture.

Cutaneous T cell lymphoma (p. 242)

The lesions, which tend to persist, are not in typical locations and are often annular, arcuate or show bizarre outlines. Atrophy or poikiloderma may be present.

Tinea unguium (p. 184)

This is often confused with psoriasis but is more asymmetrical and there may be obvious tinea of neighbouring skin. Uninvolved nails are common. Pitting is not seen and nails tend to be crumbly and discoloured at their free edge.

Investigations

1 Biopsy is seldom necessary.
2 Throat swabbing for beta-haemolytic streptococci is needed in guttate psoriasis.
3 Skin scrapings and nail clippings may be required to exclude tinea.
4 Radiology and tests for rheumatoid factor are helpful in assessing arthritis.

Treatment

The need for this depends both on the patient's own perception of his or her disability, and on the doctor's objective assessment of how severe the skin disease is. The two do not always tally.

General measures

Instruction of the patient is of great importance. Explanations and reassurances must be geared to the patient's or the parent's intelligence. Patient information leaflets are helpful in reinforcing verbal advice. The doctor as well as the patient should keep the disease in perspective, and treatment must never be allowed to be more troublesome than the disease itself. At present there is no cure for psoriasis; all treatment is suppressive and aimed at either inducing a remission or making the condition more tolerable. Treatment for patients with chronic stable plaque psoriasis is relatively simple and may be safely administered by the family practitioner. Systemic treatment for severe psoriasis should be monitored by a dermatologist.

Physical and mental rest help to back up the specific management of acute episodes. Concomitant anxiety and depression should be treated on their own merits. See Table 6.1 for appropriate treatments.

Local treatment

Coal tar preparations

Crude coal tar and its distillation products have been used to treat psoriasis for many years. Their precise mode of action is uncertain but they do inhibit DNA synthesis.

Many preparations are available but it is wise to become familiar with a few. The less refined tars are smelly, messy and stain clothes, but are more effective than the cleaner refined preparations. Tar emulsions can also be added to the bath. Suitable

preparations are listed in the Formulary (p. 294). Surprisingly, no increase in skin cancer has been found in patients treated for prolonged periods with tar preparations; it has even been suggested that psoriatics are less likely than normal to develop skin cancer.

Dithranol

The use of dithranol (anthralin) has become popular in the last few decades. Like coal tar it inhibits DNA synthesis, but some of its benefits may be due to the formation of free radicals of oxygen.

Dithranol is more tricky to use than coal tar. It has to be applied carefully, to the plaques only, and, if left on for more than 30 minutes, covered with gauze dressings. As it is irritant, one should start with a weak (0.1%) preparation and then step up the strength at weekly intervals. Dithranol stronger than 1% is seldom necessary. Irritation of the surrounding skin can be lessened by the application of a protective bland paste, e.g. zinc paste.

Dithranol stains normal skin, but the purple-brown discoloration peels off after a few days. It

Table 6.1 Treatment options in psoriasis

Type of psoriasis	Treatment of choice	Alternative treatments
Stable plaque	Short-contact dithranol or Calcipotriol	Tar Topical steroids
Extensive stable plaque, (>30% surface area) recalcitrant to local therapy	UVB PUVA + etretinate	Methotrexate Cyclosporin A
Widespread small plaque	UVB	Tar
Guttate	Emollients while erupting; then UVB	Weak tar preparations Mild local steroids
Facial	Mild local steroids	
Flexural	Mild to moderately potent local steroids + antifungal	
Pustular psoriasis of hands and feet	Moderately potent or potent local steroids	Acitretin/etretinate (as available)
Acute erythrodermic, unstable or generalized pustular	Inpatient treatment with ichthammol paste, local steroids may be used initially with or without wet compresses	Acitretin/etretinate (as available) Methotrexate Cyclosporin A

also stains bathtubs, clothes, and anything else it touches. One popular regimen is to apply dithranol daily for five days in the week, and many patients clear within a month.

Short contact therapy, in which dithranol is applied for no longer than 30 minutes, is also effective. Initially a test patch of psoriasis is treated with a 0.1% dithranol cream, left on for 20 minutes and then washed off. If there is no undue reaction the application can be extended the next day and if tolerated the duration of application increased to 30 minutes. After the cream is washed off, a bland application such as soft white paraffin or emulsifying ointment is applied. Depending on response, the strength of the dithranol may be increased from 0.1% to 2% over two or three weeks. Suitable preparations are listed in the Formulary (p. 295).

As dithranol is so irritant it should not be applied to the face, the inner thighs, genital region or skin folds. Special care should be taken to avoid contact with the eyes. Recent research has shown that the application of triethanolamine after removal of dithranol reduces inflammation and staining due to dithranol without diminishing its therapeutic effect.

Calcipotriol (Calcipotriene, USA)

Ultraviolet radiation helps many patients with psoriasis (see below), perhaps by increasing the production of cholecalciferol in the skin (p. 295). Calcipotriol is an analogue of chlolecalciferol which does not cause hypercalcaemia and calciuria when used topically in the recommended dose. It has recently been introduced to treat mild to moderate psoriasis affecting less than 40% of the skin area. It is still not clear how it works but it does reduce epidermal proliferation and restores a normal horny layer. It also inhibits ornithine decarboxylase (p. 52).

Patients like calcipotriol as it is odourless, colourless and does not stain. Local and usually transient irritation may occur with the recommended twice daily application. One way of lessening this is to combine its use with that of a moderately potent steroid, the calcipotriol being applied in the evening and the steroid in the morning. Up to 100 g of calcipotriol may be used per week.

Our current practice, which may turn out to be unnecessary, is still to check the blood calcium and phosphate levels every six months.

Topical corticosteroids

Practice varies from centre to centre and from country to country. Many dermatologists, particularly in the USA, find topical corticosteroids helpful and use them as the mainstay of their long-term management of stable plaque psoriasis. Patients like them because they are clean and reduce scaling and redness.

In our view such usage is safe, but only under proper supervision by doctors well aware of problems such as dermal atrophy, tachyphylaxis, early relapses, the occasional precipitation of unstable psoriasis (Fig. 6.20), and rarely, in extensive cases, of adrenal suppression due to systemic absorption. A commitment by the prescriber to keep the patient under regular clinical review is especially important if the patient has to use more than 50 g/week of a moderately potent topical corticosteroid preparation. Combined tar–steroid preparations may also be helpful (Formulary, p. 291).

The regular use of topical corticosteroids is less controversial under the following circumstances:
1 In 'no choice' areas such as the face, ears, genitals and flexures where tar and dithranol are seldom tolerated (mildly potent steroid preparations should be used).

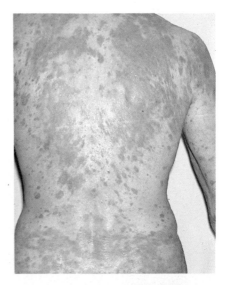

Fig. 6.20 Unstable psoriasis following long-term use of a potent topical steroid. There is no scaling and numerous small lesions are erupting around ill-defined plaques.

2 For patients who cannot use tar or dithranol because of allergic or irritant reactions (moderately potent preparations, except for 'no choice' areas where mildly potent ones should be used).
3 For unresponsive psoriasis on the scalp, palms and soles (moderately potent, potent and very potent [but only in the short term] preparations).
4 For patients with minor localized psoriasis (moderately potent or potent preparations).

Ultraviolet radiation

Most patients improve with natural sunlight and should be encouraged to sunbathe. During the winter, courses of artificial ultraviolet radiation (UVB) as an outpatient, or at home, may help (Fig. 6.21). Treatments, sufficient to produce a minimal erythema, should be given twice weekly for eight weeks. Goggles should be worn.

Combination therapy

Some of these treatments may be combined to clear chronic plaque psoriasis more quickly. For example, the Goeckerman regimen includes tar baths, crude coal tar and UVB therapy. The Ingram regimen combines tar baths, dithranol and UVB.

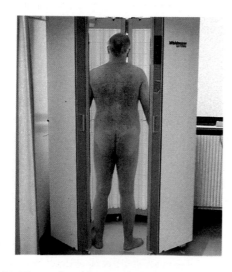

Fig. 6.21 Ultraviolet radiation therapy.

Special situations

Scalp psoriasis

This is often recalcitrant. Oily preparations containing 3% salicylic acid are useful (Formulary, p. 290). They should be rubbed into the scalp three times a week and washed out with a tar shampoo four to six hours later. If progress is slow they may be left on for one or two nights before shampooing. Salicylic acid and tar combinations are also effective.

Guttate psoriasis

A course of penicillin V or erythromycin is indicated for any associated streptococcal throat infection. Bland local treatment is often enough as the natural trend is towards remission. Suitable preparations include emulsifying ointment and zinc and ichthammol cream. Tar–steroid preparations are reasonable alternatives. A course of ultraviolet therapy (UVB) may be helpful after the eruptive phase is over.

Eruptive/unstable psoriasis

Bland treatment is needed and rest is important. Tar, dithranol and ultraviolet therapy are best avoided. Suitable preparations include emulsifying ointment and zinc and ichthammol cream.

Systemic treatment

A systemic approach should be considered if extensive psoriasis (>20% of the body surface) fails to improve with prolonged courses of tar or dithranol. As the potential side effects are great, local measures should be given a good trial first. The most commonly used systemic treatments are photochemotherapy with PUVA (*P*soralen + *U*ltra*V*iolet *A* treatment), retinoids, methotrexate, hydroxyurea, sulphasalazine and cyclosporin A.

Photochemotherapy; PUVA

In this ingenious therapy, a drug is photo-activated in the skin by ultraviolet radiation. An oral dose of 8-methoxypsoralen or 5-methoxypsoralen is followed by exposure to long wave ultraviolet radiation

(UVA: 320−400 nm). The psoralen reaches the skin and, in the presence of UVA, forms photo-adducts with DNA pyrimidine bases and cross-links between complementary DNA strands; this inhibits DNA synthesis and epidermal cell division.

The 8-methoxypsoralen (8-MOP) (crystalline formulation 0.6−0.8 mg/kg body weight or liquid formulation 0.3−0.4 mg/kg) or 5-methoxypsoralen (5-MOP) (1.2−1.6 mg/kg) is taken 1−2 hours before exposure to a bank of UVA tubes mounted in a cabinet similar to that seen in Fig. 6.21. Psoralens may also be administered in bath water for those unable to tolerate the oral regimen. The initial exposure is calculated either by determining the patient's minimal phototoxic dose (the least dose of UVA which after ingestion of 8-MOP produces a barely perceptible erythema 72 hours after testing) or by assessing skin colour and ability to tan. The usual starting dose is from 0.5 joules/cm^2 (skin type I: always burns and never tans) to 2.0 joules/cm^2 (skin type IV: never burns and always tans). Treatment is given two or three times a week with increasing doses of UVA, depending on erythema production and the therapeutic response. Protective goggles are worn during radiation and UVA opaque plastic glasses must be used after taking the tablets and for 24 hours after each treatment (see below). All phototherapy equipment should be serviced and calibrated regularly by adequately trained personnel. Accurate records of cumulative dosage and the number of treatments for each patient should be kept.

Clearance takes 5−10 weeks. Thereafter it is often possible to keep the skin clear by PUVA once a fortnight or every three weeks. However, as the side effects of PUVA relate to its cumulative dose (see below) maintenance therapy should not be used unless alternative treatments are deemed unsatisfactory. As far as possible PUVA therapy is avoided in younger patients.

Side effects

Erythema is the most common but is minimized by careful dosimetry. A quarter of patients itch during and immediately after radiation; fewer feel nauseated after taking 8-MOP. 5-Methoxypsoralen, not yet available in the USA, is worth trying if these effects become intolerable. Long-term side effects include premature ageing of the skin (with mottled pigmentation, scattered lentigines, wrinkles and atrophy), cutaneous malignancies (after a cumulative dose greater than 1000 joules), and theoretically cataract formation. The use of UVA blocking glasses (see above) for 24 hours after each treatment should protect against the latter. The long-term side effects relate to the total amount of UVA received over the years; this must be recorded and kept as low as possible without denying treatment when it is clearly needed.

Retinoids

Etretinate and acitretin (20−50 mg daily) (Formulary, p. 305), are analogues of vitamin A, and are amongst the few drugs helpful in pustular psoriasis. They are used to thin down thick hyperkeratotic plaques. Minor side effects are frequent and dose-related. They include dry lips, mouth, vagina and eyes, peeling of the skin, pruritus, thinning of the hair, and unpleasant paronychia. All settle on stopping or reducing the dose of the drug, but the use of emollients and artificial tears is often recommended.

Etretinate and acitretin may be used on their own for long periods but regular blood tests are needed to exclude abnormal liver function and elevation of serum lipids (mainly triglycerides but also cholesterol). Yearly X-rays should help to detect ossification of ligaments especially the paraspinal ones (DISH syndrome − disseminated interstitial skeletal hyperostosis). Children, and those with persistently abnormal liver function tests or hyperlipidaemia, should not be treated.

The most important side effect is *teratogenicity* and retinoids should not normally be prescribed to women of child-bearing age. If they have to be given, for unavoidable clinical reasons, effective oral contraceptive measures must be taken and these, in view of the long half-life of the drugs or their metabolite, should continue for *two years after treatment has ceased*. Blood donation should be avoided for at least one year after the last dose.

Retinoids and PUVA act synergistically and are often used together in the so-called Re−PUVA regimen. This clears plaque psoriasis quicker than PUVA alone, and needs a smaller cumulative dose of UVA. The standard precautions for both PUVA and retinoid treatment should, of course, still be observed.

Methotrexate

This folic acid antagonist (Formulary, p. 304) inhibits DNA synthesis during the S phase of mitosis. After an initial trial dose of 2.5 mg, in an adult of average weight the drug is given orally once a week and the dose increased gradually to a maintenance dose of 7.5−15 mg/week. This often controls even aggressive psoriasis. The drug is eliminated largely by the kidneys and so the dose must be reduced if renal function is poor. Aspirin and sulphonamides displace the drug from binding with plasma albumin, and frusemide (furosemide, USA) may decrease its renal clearance: note must therefore be taken of concurrent drug therapy (Formulary, p. 304) and the dose reduced accordingly. Minor and temporary side effects such as nausea and malaise are common in the 48 hours after administration. The most serious drawback to this treatment is hepatic fibrosis, the risk of which is greatly increased in those who drink excessive alcohol. Unfortunately routine liver function tests and scans cannot predict this reliably, and a liver biopsy is advised to exclude active liver disease. Exceptions are made for patients over 70 years old and when only short-term treatment with methotrexate is anticipated. Liver biopsy before treatment or early in the course of therapy should be repeated after every cumulative dose of 1.5−2 g. Blood checks to exclude marrow suppression, and to monitor renal and liver function, should also be performed; these are carried out weekly at the start of treatment but the interval may be slowly increased to monthly or every other month depending on when stable maintenance therapy is established. This drug is also teratogenic and should not be given to females in their reproductive years. Oligospermia has been noted in men and their fertility may be lowered; however, a child fathered by a man on methotrexate can be expected to be normal.

Cyclosporin

Cyclosporin inhibits cell mediated immune reactions. It blocks resting lymphocytes in the G0 or early G1 phase of the cell cycle and inhibits lymphokine release, especially that of IL-2. It also has a direct antiproliferative effect on epidermis.

Cyclosporin is effective in severe psoriasis, but patients requiring it should be under the care of specialists. The initial daily dose is 3−4 mg/kg/day and not more than 5 mg/kg/day. With improvement the dose can often be reduced but there are worries over long-term treatment which may include hypertension, kidney damage, and persistent viral warts with a risk of skin cancer. Blood pressure and renal function should be assessed carefully *before* starting. The serum creatinine should be measured every other week for the first three months of therapy, and then, if it remains stable, measurements need to be repeated only monthly (>2.5 mg/kg/day) or every other month (<2.5 mg/kg/day) depending on the dose. This should be reduced if the serum creatinine concentration rises to 30% above the baseline level on two occasions within two weeks. If these changes do not reverse themselves when the dose has been reduced for one month, then the drug should be stopped.

Hypertension is a common side effect of cyclosporin A: nearly 50% of patients develop a systolic blood pressure over 160 mmHg and/or a diastolic blood pressure over 95 mmHg. Usually these rises are mild or moderate and respond to concomitant treatment with the calcium channel blocker, nifedipine. If this cannot be tolerated, an angiotensin converting enzyme inhibitor should be used under specialist supervision. Diuretics, which may worsen renal function, and beta-blockers, which may themselves worsen psoriasis, should probably be avoided.

Cyclosporin interacts with a number of drugs (Formulary, p. 303) which should be avoided. Treatment with cyclosporin should not continue for longer than one year without careful assessment and close monitoring.

Other systemic drugs

Antimetabolites such as azathioprine and hydroxyurea help psoriasis, but less than methotrexate; they tend to damage the marrow rather than the liver. Regular blood monitoring is again essential. Sulphasalazine occasionally helps psoriasis.

LEARNING POINTS

1 The treatment must not be worse than the disease.

2 Do not aggravate eruptive psoriasis.

3 Never use systemic steroids.

4 Avoid the long-term use of potent or very potent topical corticosteroids.

5 Never promise a permanent cure, but be encouraging.

6 Great advances have been made over the last 20 years in the treatment of severe psoriasis, but patients taking modern systemic agents require careful monitoring.

CHAPTER 7

Other papulosquamous disorders

Psoriasis is not the only skin disease that is sharply marginated and scaly. The differential diagnosis of the most common papulosquamous diseases is given in Table 7.1. Eczema may also be raised and scaly, but is usually poorly marginated and fissures, crusts, or lichenifies (Chapter 11). Psoriasis is discussed in Chapter 6.

Pityriasis rosea

Cause

The cause of pityriasis rosea is not known. An infectious agent has been suspected but not proven; the disorder seems not to be contagious.

Presentation

Most patients develop one plaque (the herald plaque) before the others. It is larger (2–5 cm in diameter) than later lesions, and is rounder, redder, and more scaly. After several days many smaller plaques appear, mainly on the trunk, but some also occur on the neck and extremities (Fig. 7.1). An individual

Table 7.1 The papulosquamous diseases

Psoriasis
Pityriasis rosea
Lichen planus
Pityriasis rubra pilaris
Parapsoriasis
Mycosis fungoides
Pityriasis lichenoides
Discoid lupus erythematosus
Tinea
Nummular eczema
Seborrhoeic dermatitis
Secondary syphilis
Drug eruptions

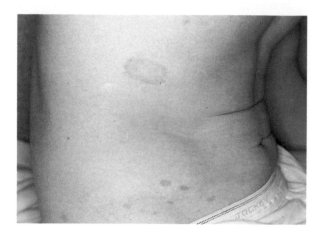

Fig. 7.1 The herald plaque of pityriasis rosea is usually on the trunk and is larger than the other lesions. Its annular configuration is shown well here.

plaque is oval, salmon pink, and shows a delicate scaling, adherent peripherally (a collarette) (Figs 7.2 & 7.3). The configuration of such plaques is often characteristic. Their longitudinal axes run down and out from the spine, along the lines of the ribs. Purpuric lesions are rare.

Course

The herald plaque precedes the generalized eruption by several days. Subsequent lesions enlarge over the first week or two. Itching is slight or moderate. The eruption lasts between two and ten weeks and then resolves spontaneously, sometimes leaving hyperpigmented patches which fade more slowly.

Differential diagnosis

Although the herald plaque is often mistaken for ringworm, the two disorders most likely to be misdiagnosed early in the general eruption are guttate

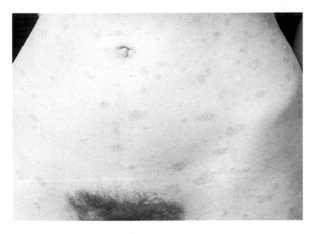

Fig. 7.2 The numerous small oval patches of pityriasis rosea showing collarettes of scales attached just inside the periphery of the lesions. The long axes of the lesion lie transversely here.

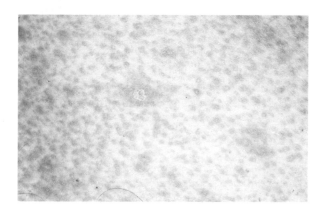

Fig. 7.3 Close-up of unusually severe pityriasis rosea: numerous erythematous follicular papules are seen as well as the standard oval plaques.

psoriasis and secondary syphilis. Tinea corporis and pityriasis versicolor can be distinguished by the microscopical examination of scales (p. 39) and secondary syphilis by its other features (mouth lesions, palmar lesions, condyloma lata, lymphadenopathy, alopecia) and by serology. Gold and captopril are the drugs most likely to cause a pityriasis rosea-like drug reaction, but barbiturates, penicillamine, and other drugs may also do so.

Investigations

Because secondary syphilis can mimic pityriasis rosea so closely, testing for syphilis is usually wise.

Treatment

No treatment is curative and active treatment is seldom needed. A moderately potent topical steroid or calamine lotion may help the itching. One per cent salicylic acid in soft white paraffin or emulsifying ointment reduces scaling. Sunlight or artificial UVB often relieves pruritus and may hasten resolution.

LEARNING POINTS
1 Check serology for syphilis if in doubt about the diagnosis.
2 Revise the diagnosis if rash persists for longer than three months.

Lichen planus

Cause

The cause of lichen planus is unknown, but chronic graft-versus-host disease can cause an eruption like lichen planus, as can certain drugs (see below).

Presentation

Typical lesions are violaceous or lilac-coloured, intensely itchy, flat-topped papules which arise usually on the extremities, particularly on the volar aspects of the wrists and legs (Fig. 7.4). One must look closely to see a white streaky pattern on the surface of these papules (Wickham's striae). White asymptomatic lacy lines, dots and occasionally small white plaques are also found in the mouth, particularly inside the cheeks, in about 50% of patients (Fig. 7.5). Variants of the classical pattern are rare and often difficult to diagnose (Table 7.2). Curiously,

Table 7.2 Variants of lichen planus

Annular
Atrophic
Bullous
Follicular
Hypertrophic
Ulcerative

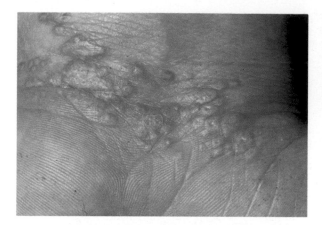

Fig. 7.4 Shiny flat-topped papules of lichen planus. Note Wickham's striae.

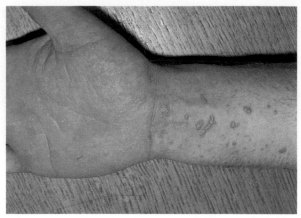

Fig. 7.6 Lichen planus. Note Köbner phenomenon on the wrist and pseudovesicular appearance on the palm.

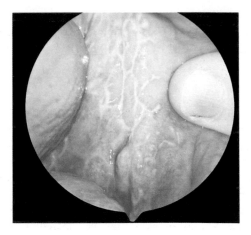

Fig. 7.5 Classic white lacy network lying on the buccal mucosa.

although the skin plaques are usually itchy, patients rub rather than scratch, so that excoriations are uncommon. As in psoriasis, the Köbner phenomenon may occur (Fig. 7.6). The nails are usually normal, but may be affected by changes ranging from fine longitudinal grooves to destruction of the entire nail fold and bed (p. 84).

Course

Individual lesions may last for many months and the eruption as a whole tends to last about one year. As the lesions resolve they become darker, flatter, and leave discrete brown or grey macules. About one in six patients will have a recurrence.

Complications

Essentially none, but nail or hair loss may be permanent. The ulcerative form of lichen planus in the mouth has led to squamous cell carcinoma. Ulceration, usually over bony prominences, may be disabling, especially if it is on the soles.

Differential diagnosis

Lichen planus should be differentiated from the other papulosquamous diseases listed in Table 7.1. Lichenoid drug reactions can mimic lichen planus. Gold and other heavy metals have often been implicated. Other drug causes include antimalarials, β-blockers, non-steroidal anti-inflammatory drugs, para-aminobenzoic acid, thiazide diuretics, and penicillamine. Contact with chemicals used to develop colour film may also produce similar lesions. It may be hard to tell lichen planus from generalized discoid lupus erythematosus if only a few large lesions are present or if the eruption is on the palms, soles, or scalp. Wickham's striae or oral lesions favour the diagnosis of lichen planus.

Investigations

The diagnosis is usually obvious clinically. The histology is also characteristic (Fig. 7.7), so a biopsy will confirm the diagnosis if this is needed.

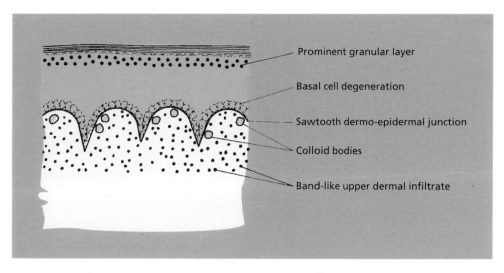

Fig. 7.7 Histology of lichen planus.

Treatment

Treatment can be difficult. If drugs are suspected as the cause, they should be stopped and unrelated ones substituted. Potent topical steroids will sometimes relieve symptoms and flatten the plaques. Systemic steroid courses work too, but are recommended only in special situations (e.g. unusually extensive involvement, nail destruction, or painful and erosive oral lichen planus). Treatment with PUVA (p. 62) may help reduce pruritus and help to clear up the skin lesions. Etretinate (Formulary, p. 305) has also helped some patients with stubborn lichen planus. Antihistamines may blunt the itch. Mucous membrane lesions are usually asymptomatic and do not require treatment.

LEARNING POINTS
1 A good diagnostic tip is to look for light reflected from shiny papules.
2 Always look in the mouth.
3 If you can recognize lichen planus you have pulled ahead of 75% of your colleagues.

Pityriasis rubra pilaris

Cause

This is unknown. A defect in vitamin A metab-olism was once postulated but has been disproved. The familial type has an autosomal dominant inheritance.

Presentation

The familial type develops gradually in childhood and persists throughout life. The more common acquired type begins in adult life with redness and scaling of the face and scalp. Later, red or pink areas grow quickly and merge, so that patients with pityriasis rubra pilaris are often erythrodermic. Small islands of skin may be 'spared' from this general erythema, but even here the follicles may be red and plugged with keratin (Fig. 7.8). Similarly, the generalized plaques, although otherwise rather like psoriasis, may also show follicular plugging.

Course

The palms and soles become thick, smooth, and yellow. They often fissure rather than bend. The acquired form of pityriasis rubra pilaris generally lasts for 6–18 months, but may recur. Even when the plaques have gone, the skin may retain a rough, scaly texture with persistent, small, scattered, follicular plugs.

Complications

There are usually no complications. However,

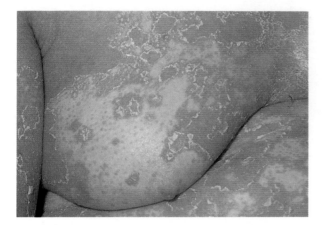

Fig. 7.8 Pityriasis rubra pilaris. Note the red plugged follicles, even in the 'spared' areas.

widespread erythroderma may cause patients to tolerate cold poorly.

Differential diagnosis

Psoriasis is the hardest disorder to tell from pityriasis rubra pilaris, but lacks its slightly orange colour. The thickening of the palms and soles, the follicular erythema in islands of uninvolved skin, and the follicular plugging within plaques, especially over the knuckles, are other features which help to separate them.

Investigations

A biopsy may help to distinguish psoriasis from pityriasis rubra pilaris, but the two disorders share many histological features.

Treatment

The disorder responds slowly to systemic retinoids such as acitretin (etretinate, USA; in the adult, 20–30 mg/day for six to eight months (p. 305)). Oral methotrexate in low doses, once a week may also help (p. 304). Topical steroids and keratolytics (e.g. 2% salicylic acid in soft white paraffin) reduce inflammation and scaling, but usually do not suppress the disorder completely. Systemic steroids are not indicated.

Parapsoriasis and premycotic eruption

Parapsoriasis is a contentious term which some would drop. We still find it useful clinically for lesions which look a little like psoriasis but which persist despite anti-psoriasis treatment.

Cause

The cause is unknown.

Presentation

Pink scaly plaques appear typically on the buttocks, breasts, abdomen or flexural skin (Fig. 7.9). Some distinguish benign parapsoriasis from a premycotic eruption (a forerunner of the cutaneous T cell lymphoma, mycosis fungoides, Fig. 7.10) though both may appear similar early in their development. The distinguishing features listed in Table 7.3 are helpful but not invariable. Both conditions are stubborn in their response to treatment. Itching is variable.

Complications

Patients with suspected premycotic eruptions should

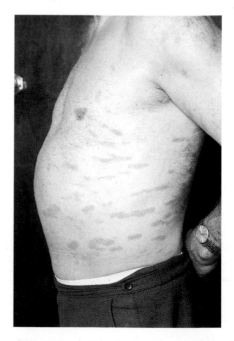

Fig. 7.9 Parapsoriasis. The benign type with finger-like lesions on the sides of the trunk.

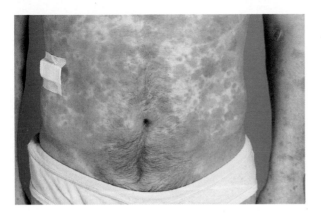

Fig. 7.10 A bizarre eruption: its persistence and variable colour suggested a premycotic eruption. Biopsy confirmed this.

Table 7.3 Distinguishing features of parapsoriasis and premycotic eruption

Parapsoriasis (benign type)	Premycotic eruption
Smaller plaques	Larger
Yellowish	Not yellow
Sometimes digitate	Asymmetrical with bizarre outline
No atrophy	Atrophy ± poikiloderma
Responds to UVB	Responds better to PUVA
Remains benign though rarely clears	Some progress to cutaneous T cell lymphoma

be followed up carefully even though the development of cutaneous T cell lymphoma may not occur for years. If poikiloderma (atrophy, telangiectasia and reticulate pigmentation) or induration develops, the diagnosis of cutaneous T cell lymphoma becomes likely.

Differential diagnosis

This includes psoriasis, tinea and nummular (discoid) eczema. In contrast to psoriasis and pityriasis rosea the lesions of parapsoriasis are characteristically asymmetrical. Topical steroids may cause atrophy and confusion.

Investigations

Several biopsies should be taken if a premycotic eruption is suspected, if possible from thick or atrophic, untreated areas. These may suggest early mycosis fungoides, with bizzare mononuclear cells both in the dermis and in microscopic abscesses within the epidermis. Electron microscopy may show abnormal lymphocytes with convoluted nuclei in the dermis or epidermis, though the finding of these cells, especially in the dermis, is non-specific. DNA probes can determine monoclonality of the T cells within the lymphoid infiltrate of mycosis fungoides based on rearrangements of the T cell receptor genes. The use of these probes and immunophenotyping help to differentiate benign parapsoriasis from premycotic eruptions.

Treatment

Treatment is controversial. Less aggressive treatments are used for benign parapsoriasis. Usually moderately potent steroids or ultraviolet radiation bring some resolution, but lesions tend to recur when these are stopped. For premycotic eruptions treatment with PUVA (p. 62) or topical nitrogen mustard is advocated by some, but it is not clear if this slows down or prevents the development of a subsequent cutaneous T cell lymphoma.

Pityriasis lichenoides

Pityriasis lichenoides is uncommon; it occurs in two forms. The numerous small circular scaly macules and papules of the chronic type are commonly confused with guttate psoriasis (p. 55). However, their scaling is distinctive in that single, silver-grey scales surmount the lesions (mica scales). The acute type is characterized by papules which become necrotic and leave scars like those of chickenpox. More often than not there are a few lesions of the chronic type in the acute variant and vice versa. UVB radiation may reduce the number of lesions and spontaneous resolution occurs eventually.

Other papulosquamous diseases

Discoid lupus erythematosus is typically papulosquamous; this is discussed with subacute cutaneous lupus erythematosus in Chapter 12. Fungus infections are nummular and scaly and can appear papulosquamous or eczematous; these are covered in Chapter 15. Seborrhoeic and nummular (discoid) eczema are discussed in Chapter 9. Secondary syphilis is discussed in Chapter 15.

Erythroderma/exfoliative dermatitis

Sometimes the whole skin becomes red and scaly. The disorders which can cause this are listed in Table 7.4. The best clue to the underlying cause is a history of a previous skin disease. Most often the histology is non-specific. Erythroderma is the term used when the skin is red with little or no scaling, whereas exfoliative dermatitis is preferred when scaling predominates.

Most patients have lymphadenopathy, and many have hepatomegaly as well. Temperature regulation is impaired and heat loss through the skin usually makes the patient feel chilly and shiver. Oedema, high output cardiac failure, tachycardia, anaemia, failure to sweat, and dehydration may occur. Treatment is symptomatic and that of the underlying condition.

Table 7.4 Causes of erythroderma/exfoliative dermatitis

Psoriasis
Pityriasis rubra pilaris
Ichthyosiform erythroderma
Pemphigus erythematosus
Contact, atopic, or seborrhoeic eczema
Reiter's syndrome
Lymphoma (including the Sézary syndrome)
Drug eruptions

LEARNING POINTS
The dangers of erythroderma are:
1 Poor temperature regulation.
2 High-output cardiac failure.
3 Protein deficiency.

CHAPTER 8

The hair and nails

The hair

To have too much hair is as bad as not having enough. These twin torments make sense only when seen against the background of the activity of normal hair follicles (Fig. 8.1).

Anatomy and physiology

The structure of a typical hair follicle has been described on p. 14.

Alopecia

The term means nothing more than loss of hair and this may have many causes and patterns. It is convenient for the clinician to subdivide alopecia into localized and diffuse types. In addition it is important to decide whether or not the hair follicles have been replaced by scar tissue: if they have, regrowth cannot occur. The presence of any disease of the skin itself should also be noted.

Localized alopecia

Some of the commonest causes are listed in Table 8.1; only a few can be dealt with in detail.

Alopecia areata

Cause

An immunological basis is suspected because of its association with thyroid disease, vitiligo and atopy. Histologically, T lymphocytes cluster like a swarm of bees around affected hair bulbs, having been attracted and made to divide by cytokines from the dermal papilla. The condition runs in some families. A few cases seem to follow emotional trauma. It affects some 2% of new patients seen at skin clinics.

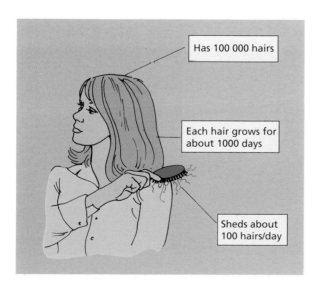

Fig. 8.1 An average scalp.

Has 100 000 hairs

Each hair grows for about 1000 days

Sheds about 100 hairs/day

Table 8.1 Some causes of localized alopecia

Non-scarring	Scarring
Alopecia areata	Burns, radiodermatitis
Androgenetic	Aplasia cutis
Hair-pulling habit	Result of kerion, carbuncle
Traction alopecia	Cicatricial basal cell carcinoma
	Lichen planus, lupus erythematosus
Scalp ringworm (human)	Necrobiosis, sarcoid, pseudopelade

Presentation

The typical patch is uninflamed, with no scaling, but with easily seen empty hair follicles (Fig. 8.2). Pathognomonic 'exclamation-mark' hairs may be seen around the edge of enlarging areas; they are broken off about 4 mm from the scalp, and are narrower and less pigmented proximally (Figs 8.3 & 8.4). Patches are most common in the scalp and beard but other areas, especially eyelashes and eyebrows, can be affected too. An uncommon diffuse

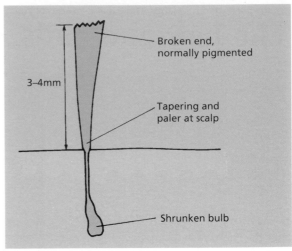

Fig. 8.4 An exclamation-mark hair.

pattern is recognized, with exclamation-mark hairs scattered widely over a diffusely thinned scalp. A few patients show fine pitting or wrinkling of the nails.

Course

The outcome is unpredictable. In a first attack, regrowth is usual within a few months. New hairs appear in the centre of patches as fine pale down and gradually regain their normal thickness and colour (Fig. 8.5), though the new hair may remain white in

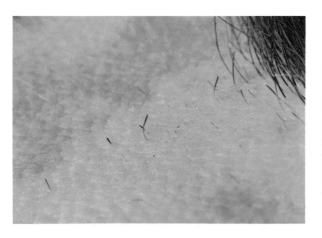

Fig. 8.2 The characteristic uninflamed patches of alopecia areata. Already some early regrowth of pale hair can be seen.

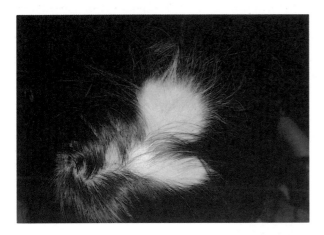

Fig. 8.3 Exclamation-mark hairs: pathognomonic of alopecia areata.

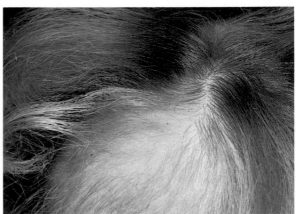

Fig. 8.5 Encouraging regrowth within a patch of alopecia areata.

older patients. Subsequent episodes tend to have more patches and regrowth is slower. Hair loss in some areas may co-exist with regrowth in others. A minority of patients lose all the hair from their heads (alopecia totalis) or from the whole skin surface (alopecia universalis).

Regrowth is tiresomely erratic but the following suggest a poor prognosis:
1 Onset before puberty.
2 Association with atopy or Down's syndrome.
3 Unusually widespread alopecia.
4 Involvement of the scalp margin (ophiasiform).

Differential diagnosis

Patches are not scaly, in contrast to ringworm, and are usually uninflamed, in contrast to lupus erythematosus and lichen planus. In the hair-pulling habit of children, and in traction alopecia, broken hairs may be seen but true exclamation-mark hairs are absent. Secondary syphilis can cause a 'moth-eaten' patchy hair loss also.

Investigations

None are usually needed. Syphilis can be excluded with serological tests if necessary. Organ-specific auto-antibody screens provide interesting information but do not affect management.

Treatment

A patient with a first or minor attack can be reassured about the prospects for regrowth. Tranquillizers may be helpful at the start. Avoid giving systemic steroids but intralesional triamcinolone leads to localized tufts of regrowth while not affecting the overall outcome. This may be useful to re-establish eyebrows or to stimulate hope. Spirit-based steroid lotions are often used but with limited success. Ultraviolet radiation or even PUVA therapy may help extensive cases: hair fall often returns when treatment stops. Contact sensitizers (e.g. diphencyprone) seem promising, but are still only being used in a few centres under trial conditions. Wigs are necessary for extensive cases.

Androgenetic alopecia (male-pattern baldness)

Cause

Although clearly familial, the exact mode of inheritance has not yet been clarified. Male-pattern baldness is androgen-dependent; in females, androgenetic alopecia, with circulating levels of androgen within normal limits, is seen only in those who are strongly predisposed genetically.

Presentation

The common pattern (Fig. 8.6), in which hair is lost first from the temples and then from the crown, is too well known to need further description. However, hair loss in women may be much more diffuse, particularly over the crown (Fig. 8.7). In bald areas, terminal hairs are replaced by finer vellus hairs.

Clinical course

Hair loss is relentless, tending to follow the family pattern with some losing hair quickly and others more slowly. The diffuse pattern seen in women tends to progress slowly.

Complications

Even minor hair loss may lead to great anxiety and monosymptomatic hypochondriasis (p. 257).

Differential diagnosis

The diagnosis is usually obvious in men, but other causes of diffuse hair loss have to be considered in women (p. 78).

Investigations

None are usually needed. In women virilization may have to be excluded.

Treatment

There is no effective treatment. Scalp surgery, hair transplants, and wigs are welcomed by some. Topical application of minoxidil lotions may slow hair loss and even stimulate new growth of hair in a minority

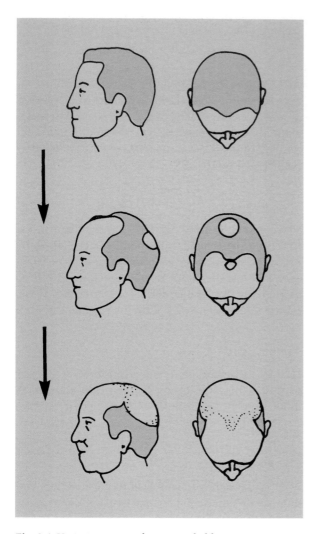

Fig. 8.6 Variations on male-pattern baldness.

of cases (Formulary, p. 296). Small and recently acquired patches respond best. When minoxidil treatment stops, the new hairs will fall out.

LEARNING POINTS
1 Minoxidil lotion helps only if the areas of hair loss are small and recent. Treatment must go on for ever.
2 Warn your patient about costly but useless hair clinics.

Trichotillomania

This is dealt with on p. 260.

Traction alopecia (Fig. 8.8)

Cause

Hair can be pulled out by several procedures intended to beautify, including hot-combing to straighten kinky hair, styling hair tightly as with a pony tail, and rolling hair excessively or too tightly.

Presentation

The changes are usually seen in girls and young women, particularly those whose hair has always tended to be thin anyway. The bald areas show short broken hairs, folliculitis, and sometimes scarring.

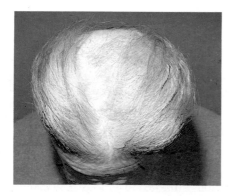

Fig. 8.7 Androgenetic alopecia most marked on the crown.

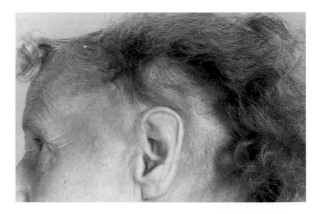

Fig. 8.8 Traction alopecia. The rollers she thought would help to disguise her diffuse hair loss made it worse at the scalp margins.

The pattern of hair loss is determined by the cosmetic procedure in use, hair being lost where there is maximal tug. The term 'marginal' alopecia is applied to one common pattern in which hair loss is mainly around the edge of the scalp — at the sides or at the front (Fig. 8.8).

Clinical course

Patients are often slow to accept that they are responsible for the hair loss themselves, and notoriously slow to alter their cosmetic practices. Even if they do, regrowth is often disappointingly incomplete.

Differential diagnosis

The pattern of hair loss provides the main clue to the diagnosis, and if the possibility of traction alopecia is kept in mind there is usually no difficulty. The absence of exclamation-mark hairs distinguishes it from alopecia areata, and of scaling from tinca capitis.

Treatment

Patients have to stop doing whatever is causing their hair loss. Rollers which tug can be replaced by those which only heat.

Patchy hair loss due to skin disease

Scalp ringworm

Inflammation, often with pustulation, is a feature of infections derived from animals, and the resultant scarring can be severe. The classical scalp ringworm derived from human sources causes areas of scaling with broken hairs. The subject is covered in more detail on p. 186.

Psoriasis

The rough removal of adherent scales can also remove hairs, but regrowth is the rule

Scarring alopecia

Hair follicles can be damaged in many ways. If the follicular openings can no longer be seen with a lens, regrowth of hair cannot be expected.

Sometimes the cause is obvious: a severe burn, trauma, a carbuncle, or an episode of inflammatory scalp ringworm. Discoid lupus erythematosus (p. 128), lichen planus (p. 67) and localized scleroderma (p. 133) can also lead to scarring alopecia. The term 'pseudopelade' is applied to a slowly progressive, non-inflamed type of scarring which leads to irregular areas of hair loss without any apparent preceding skin disease.

Diffuse hair loss

Hair is lost evenly from the whole scalp; this may, or may not, be accompanied by a thinning visible to others (Fig. 8.9). Some of the commonest causes are listed in Table 8.2, but often a simple explanation cannot be found.

Telogen effluvium

Cause

Each hair follicle goes through its growth cycles out of phase with its neighbours. However, if many pass into the resting phase (telogen) at the same time, then a correspondingly large number will be shed two to three months later. This process is known as telogen effluvium. It can be triggered by any severe illness, particularly if bouts of fever occur, and by childbirth.

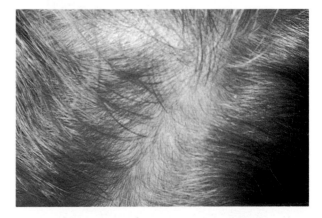

Fig. 8.9 Diffuse hair loss causing much anxiety but with minor thinning only.

Table 8.2 Some causes of diffuse hair loss

Telogen effluvium

Endocrine
   hypopituitarism, hypo- or hyperthyroidism
   hypoparathyroidism

Drug-induced
   antimitotic agents, anticoagulants, vitamin A
   excess, oral contraceptives

Androgenetic

Iron deficiency

Severe chronic illness

Malnutrition

Diffuse type of alopecia areata

Presentation and course

The diffuse hair fall, two to three months after the provoking illness, can be mild or severe. In the latter case Beau's lines (p. 82) may be seen on the nails. Regrowth, not always complete, usually occurs within a few months.

Differential diagnosis

This is from other types of diffuse hair loss (Table 8.2).

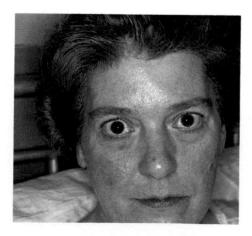

Fig. 8.10 Patient with hyperthyroidism, exophthalmos and diffuse hair loss most marked at the parting.

Treatment

This condition is unaffected by therapy.

Other causes of diffuse hair loss

The causes mentioned in Table 8.2 should be considered, and the exclamation-mark hairs seen in the diffuse type of alopecia areata should be looked for. If no cause is obvious it is worth checking the haemoglobin, ESR, ANF, serum iron and thyroxine (Fig. 8.10). It is true to say that often no cause for diffuse alopecia can be found.

> **LEARNING POINTS**
> *1 Be sympathetic even if the hair loss seems trivial to you.*
> *2 Reassure your patient that total baldness is not imminent.*

Hypotrichosis

The *ectodermal dysplasias* are a group of rare inherited disorders characterized by sparse hair, scanty sweat glands, and poor development of the nails and teeth. (Figs 8.11 & 8.12). One type is inherited as an X-linked recessive. Heat stroke may follow inadequate sweat production.

In other inherited disorders the hair may be beaded and brittle (*monilethrix*); flattened and twisted (*pili torti*); kinky (*Menke's syndrome* in association with abnormalities of copper metabolism); like bamboo (*Netherton's syndrome*); partly broken in many places (*trichorrhexis nodosa*); wooly or uncombable.

Hirsutism and hypertrichosis

Hirsutism is the growth of terminal hair in a female, but distributed in the pattern normally seen in a male. Hypertrichosis is an excessive growth of terminal hair but one which does not follow an androgen-induced pattern.

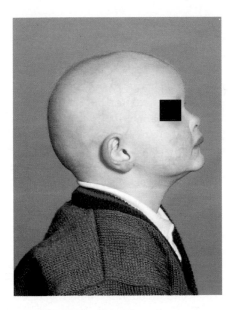

Fig. 8.11 Hypohidrotic ectodermal dysplasia: minimal scalp hair and characteristic facies.

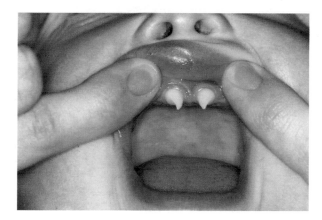

Fig. 8.12 The cone-shaped incisors of hypohidrotic ectodermal dysplasia.

Hirsutism

Cause

Some degree of hirsutism may be a racial or familial trait, and some increase of facial hair is common after the menopause. In addition, some patients, without a family background of hirsutism, become hirsute in the absence of any demonstrable hormonal cause (idiopathic hirsutism). Finally, a few patients with hirsutism will have one of the disorders listed in Table 8.3.

Presentation

An excessive growth of hair may be seen in the beard area, on the chest and shoulder-tips, around the nipples and in the male pattern of pubic hair. An androgenetic alopecia may complete the picture.

Course

Familial, racial, or idiopathic hirsutism tends to start at puberty and to worsen with age.

Complications

Infertility will follow virilization; psychological disturbances are common.

Investigations

Significant hormonal abnormalities are not usually found in patients with a normal menstrual cycle. Investigations are needed:
- If hirsutism occurs in childhood.
- If there are other features of virilization.
- If the hirsutism is of sudden or recent onset.
- If there is menstrual irregularity or cessation.

The tests used will include measurement of the serum testosterone, sex-hormone-binding globulin, dehydroepiandrosterone sulphate, androstenedione and prolactin. Ovarian ultrasound is a useful test when polycystic ovaries are suspected.

Treatment

Any underlying disorder must be treated on its

Table 8.3 Some causes of hirsutism

1 Ovarian	Polycystic ovaries
	Arrhenoblastoma
2 Adrenal	Cushing's syndrome
	Virilizing tumours
	Adrenogenital syndromes
3 Pituitary	Acromegaly
	Hyperprolactinaemia
4 Iatrogenic	Anabolic steroids
	Progesterones

merits. Otherwise the abnormally active follicles, if relatively few, may be destroyed by electrolysis. If the hairs are too numerous for this, the excess may be removed by waxing or shaving, or rendered less obvious by bleaching. Oral anti-androgens (e.g. cyproterone acetate, Formulary, p. 302) may sometimes be helpful, but will be needed long term. Spironolactone cannot now be recommended.

LEARNING POINTS
1 Full endocrinological assessment is needed for hirsutism plus virilization.
2 Significant hormonal abnormalities are rarely found in patients with a normal menstrual cycle.

Hypertrichosis

The localized type is most commonly seen over congenital melanocytic naevi. It can also affect the sacral area (a satyr's tuft) in some patients with spina bifida. Excessive amounts of hair may grow near chronically inflamed joints or under a plaster cast. Repeated shaving does not bring on hypertrichosis though occupational pressure may do so, for example from carrying weights on the shoulder.

Generalized hypertrichosis is much less common. Some causes are listed in Table 8.4.

Hair cosmetics

Hair may be made more attractive by dyeing, bleaching and waving, but there is often a price to be paid for beauty. Some hair dyes based on paraphenylenediamine are allergens. Bleaches may weaken the hair shafts, and hair damaged in this way is especially susceptible to further damage by permanent waving.

Table 8.4 Some causes of generalized hypertrichosis

Drug-induced (minoxidil, diazoxide, cyclosporin A)
Starvation, anorexia nervosa
Hepatic cutaneous porphyria
Fetal alcohol and fetal phenytoin syndromes
Hypertrichosis lanuginosa (congenital or acquired)
Some rare syndromes, e.g. Cornelia de Lange syndrome
   (hypertrichosis, microcephaly and mental deficiency)

Permanent waving solutions reduce disulphide bonds within hair keratin and so allow the hair to be deformed before being reset in a new position. The thioglycollates used to dissolve disulphide bonds are also popular as chemical hair removers. If used incorrectly, either too strong or for too long a time, or on hair already damaged by excessive bleaching or waving, thioglycollate waving lotions can cause hair to break off flush with the scalp. Accompanying this hair loss, which may be severe though temporary, may be an irritant dermatitis of the scalp.

The nails

The anatomy of the nails is described on p. 16. Nails vary with age, from the thin, sometimes spooned nails of early childhood to the duller, paler and more opaque nails of the very old. Longitudinal ridging and beading are particularly common in the elderly.

Congenital abnormalities

A few people are born with one or more nails missing. In addition there are many conditions, either inherited or associated with chromosomal abnormalities, and usually rare, in which nail changes form a minor part of the clinical picture. Most cannot be dealt with here.

In the rare *nail–patella syndrome*, the thumb nails, and to a lesser extent those of the fingers, are smaller than normal. Rudimentary patellae and iliac spines complete the syndrome which is inherited as an autosomal dominant trait linked with the locus controlling ABO blood groups.

Pachyonychia congenita is also rare and inherited as an autosomal dominant. The nails are grossly thickened, especially peripherally, and have a curious triangular profile (Fig. 8.13). Hyperkeratosis may occur on areas of friction on the legs and feet.

Permanent loss of the nails may be seen with the dystrophic types of *epidermolysis bullosa*.

In the *yellow nail syndrome* (Fig. 8.14) the nail changes begin in adult life, against a background of hypoplasia of the lymphatic system. Peripheral oedema is usually present and pleural effusions may occur. The nails grow very slowly and become thickened and greenish-yellow; their surface is smooth but they are over-curved from side to side.

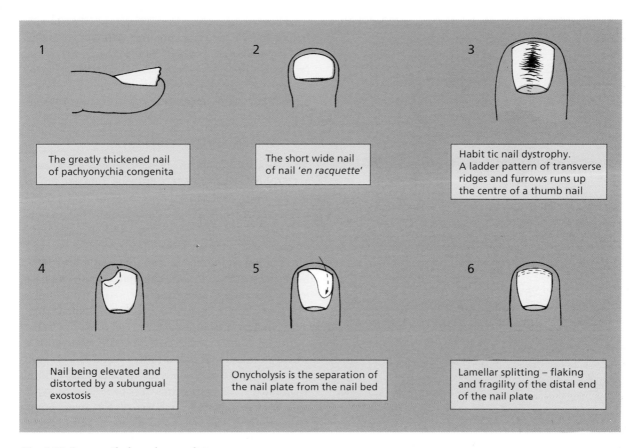

1

The greatly thickened nail
of pachyonychia congenita

2

The short wide nail
of nail 'en racquette'

3

Habit tic nail dystrophy.
A ladder pattern of transverse
ridges and furrows runs up
the centre of a thumb nail

4

Nail being elevated and
distorted by a subungual
exostosis

5

Onycholysis is the separation of
the nail plate from the nail bed

6

Lamellar splitting – flaking
and fragility of the distal end
of the nail plate

Fig. 8.13 Some nail plate abnormalities.

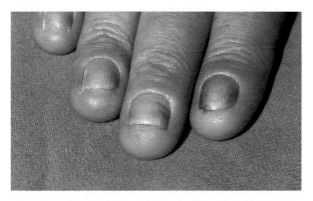

Fig. 8.14 The curved, slow growing greenish-yellow nails of the yellow nail syndrome.

The *nail 'en racquette'* is a short broad nail (Fig. 8.13), usually a thumb nail, which is seen in some 1–2% of the population and may be inherited as an autosomal dominant trait. The basic abnormality is shortness of the underlying terminal phalanx.

Effects of trauma

Damage to the nail matrix may be followed by permanent ridges or splits in the nail plate. *Splinter haemorrhages*, the linear nature of which is determined by longitudinal ridges and grooves in the nail bed, are commonly seen under the nails of manual workers and are due to minor trauma. They may also be a feature of psoriasis of the nail and of subacute bacterial endocarditis. Larger *subungual haematomas* (Fig. 8.15) are usually easy to identify but trauma to nails may have escaped notice and dark areas of altered blood may raise worries about the presence of a subungual melanoma.

Chronic trauma from sport and from ill-fitting shoes contributes to haemorrhage under the nails of the big toes, to the gross thickening of toe nails known as *onychogryphosis* (Fig. 8.16), and to *ingrowing nails. Onycholysis*, a separation of the nail plate from the nail bed (Fig. 8.13), may be due to

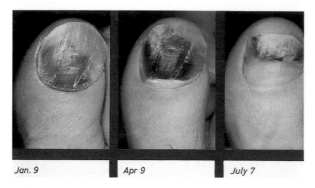

Fig. 8.15 A subungual haematoma of the big toe. Although there was no history of trauma we were happy to watch this grow out over six months as the appearance was sudden, the colour was right, and the nail folds showed no pigment.

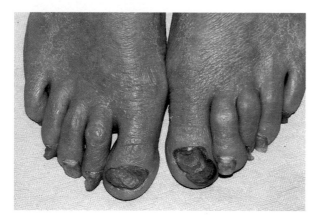

Fig. 8.16 Onychogryphosis.

minor trauma though it is also seen in nail psoriasis (see Fig. 6.11), and possibly in thyroid disease.

Some nervous habits can damage the nails. *Bitten nails* are short and irregular; some also bite their cuticles and the skin around the nails. Viral warts can be seeded rapidly in this way. In the common *habit tic nail dystrophy*, the cuticle of the thumb nail is the target for picking or rubbing. This repetitive trauma causes a ladder pattern of transverse ridges and grooves to run up the centre of the nail plate (Fig. 8.13).

Lamellar splitting of the distal part of the finger nails, so commonly seen in housewives, has been attributed to repeated wetting and drying (Fig. 8.13).

Attempts to beautify nails may lead to contact allergy. Common culprits are the acrylate adhesive used with artificial nails and formaldehyde in nail hardeners. In contrast, contact dermatitis due to allergens in nail polish itself seldom affects the fingers but presents as small itchy eczematous areas where the nail plates rest against the skin during sleep. The eyelids, face, and neck are favourite sites.

The nail in systemic disease

The nails provide useful clues for general physicians.

Clubbing (Fig. 8.17) is a bulbous enlargement of the terminal phalanx with an increase in the angle between the nail plate and the proximal fold to over 180° (Fig. 8.18). Its association with chronic lung disease and with cyanotic heart disease is well known. Rarely clubbing may be familial with no underlying cause. The mechanisms involved in its formation are still not known.

Koilonychia, a spooning and thinning of the nail plate, indicates iron deficiency (Fig. 8.19).

Colour changes: the 'half-and-half' nail, with a white proximal and red or brown distal half, is seen in a minority of patients with chronic renal failure. Whitening of the nail plates may be related to hypoalbuminaemia, as in cirrhosis of the liver. Some drugs, notably antimalarials, antibiotics and phenothiazines, may discolour the nails.

Beau's lines are transverse grooves which appear synchronously on all nails a few weeks after an acute illness, and which grow steadily out to the free margin (Fig. 8.19).

Connective tissue disorders (Fig. 8.20): nail fold telangiectasia or erythema is a useful physical sign

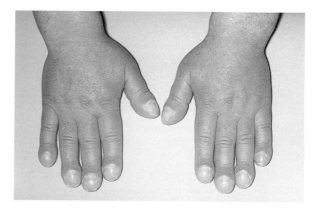

Fig. 8.17 In this case severe clubbing was accompanied by hypertrophic pulmonary osteoarthropathy.

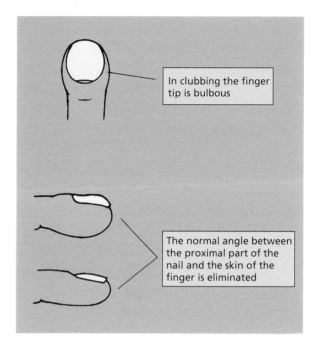

In clubbing the finger tip is bulbous

The normal angle between the proximal part of the nail and the skin of the finger is eliminated

Fig. 8.18 Clubbing.

in dermatomyositis, systemic sclerosis and systemic lupus erythematosus (Figs 8.19 & 12.7). In dermatomyositis the cuticles may become shaggy, and in systemic sclerosis loss of finger pulp may lead to over curvature of the nail plates. An impaired peripheral circulation, as in Raynaud's phenomenon, will lead to thinning and longitudinal ridging of the nail plate, sometimes with partial onycholysis.

Nail changes in the common dermatoses

Psoriasis

Most patients with psoriasis have nail changes at some stage: severe nail involvement correlates to some extent with the presence of arthritis. The best known nail change is pitting of the surface of the nail plate (see Fig. 6.10). Almost as common is psoriasis under the nail plate, showing up as red or brown areas, often with onycholysis bordered by obvious discoloration (see Fig. 6.11). There is no effective treatment for psoriasis of the nails.

Eczema

Patients with itchy chronic eczema may bring their nails to a high state of polish by scratching. In addition, eczema of the nail folds may lead to a coarse irregularity with transverse ridging of the adjacent nail plates.

Lichen planus

Some 10% of patients with lichen planus have nail changes, most often this is a reversible thinning of the nail plate with irregular longitudinal grooves and ridges. More severe involvement may lead to pterygium in which the cuticle grows forward over the base of the nail and attaches itself to the nail plate (Fig. 8.19). The threat of severe and permanent nail changes may rarely justify treatment with systemic steroids.

Alopecia areata

The more severe the hair loss, the more likely there is to be nail involvement. A roughness or fine pitting is seen on the surface of the nail plates and the lunulae may appear mottled.

> **LEARNING POINT**
> *Do not waste time and money treating nail psoriasis or onycholysis with antifungals.*

Infections

Acute paronychia

The portal of entry for the organisms concerned, usually staphylococci, is a break in the skin or cuticle due to minor trauma. The acute inflammation, often with the formation of pus in the nail fold or under the nail, requires systemic treatment with flucloxacillin or erythromycin (Formulary, p. 298) and appropriate surgical drainage.

Chronic paronychia

Cause

A combination of circumstances allows a mixture of opportunistic pathogens (yeasts, Gram-positive cocci and Gram-negative rods) to colonize the space

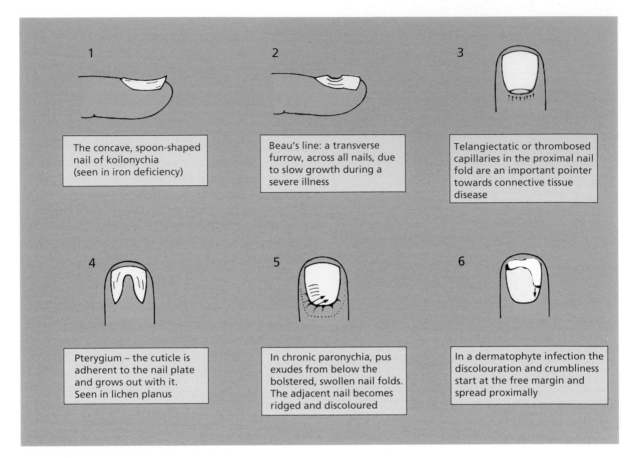

Fig. 8.19 Some other nail changes.

---

between the nail fold and nail plate. Predisposing factors include a poor peripheral circulation, wet work, working with flour, diabetes, vaginal candidosis, and overvigorous cutting back of the cuticles.

Presentation and course

The nail folds are tender and swollen (Fig. 8.19) and small amounts of pus are discharged at intervals. The cuticular seal is damaged and the adjacent nail plate becomes ridged and discoloured. The condition may last for many years.

Differential diagnosis

In atypical cases consider the outside chance of an amelanotic melanoma. Paronychia should not be confused with a dermatophyte infection in which the nail folds are not primarily affected.

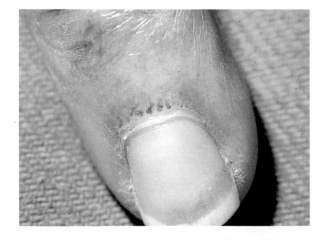

Fig. 8.20 Large tortuous capillary loops of the proximal nail fold signal the presence of a connective tissue disorder.

Investigations

Test the urine for sugar, check for vaginal candidosis. Pus should be cultured.

Treatment

Manicuring of the cuticle should cease. The hands should be kept as warm and as dry as possible, and the damaged nail folds may be packed several times a day with an imidazole cream (Formulary, p. 292). If there is no response, and swabs confirm that candida is present, a two week course of itraconazole should be considered (Formulary, p. 300).

Dermatophyte infections

Cause

The common dermatophytes which cause tinea pedis can also invade the nails (p. 184).

Presentation

Toe nail infection is common and associated with tinea pedis. The early changes occur at the free edge of the nail and spread proximally. The nail plate becomes yellow, crumbly and thickened. Usually only a few nails are infected but occasionally all are. The finger nails are involved less often, and the changes, in contrast to those of psoriasis, are usually confined to one hand.

Clinical course

The condition seldom clears spontaneously.

Differential diagnosis

Psoriasis has been mentioned. Yeast infections of the nail plate, much more rare than dermatophyte infections, can look similar.

Investigations

Microscopic examination of a nail clipping is a simple procedure (p. 39). Cultures should be carried out in a mycology laboratory.

Treatment

This is given on p. 188. Remember that symptom-free fungal infections of the toe nails may need no treatment at all.

Tumours

Peri-ungual warts are common and differ in no way from warts elsewhere. Cryotherapy must be used carefully to avoid damage to the nail matrix; it is painful but effective.

Peri-ungual fibromas (see Fig. 22.4) arise from the nail folds, usually in late childhood, in patients with tuberous sclerosis.

Glomus tumours may occur beneath the nail plate. The small red or bluish lesions are exquisitely tender and also hurt with changes in temperature. Treatment is surgical.

Subungual exostoses (Fig. 8.13) protrude painfully under the nail plate. Usually secondary to trauma to the terminal phalanx, the bony abnormality can be seen on X-ray and treatment is surgical.
Myxoid cysts occur on the proximal nail folds, usually of the fingers. The smooth domed swelling contains a clear jelly-like material which transilluminates well. A groove may form on the adjacent nail plate. Cryotherapy, injections of triamcinolone, and surgical excision all have their advocates.

Malignant melanoma should be suspected in any subungual pigmented lesion, particularly if the pigment spreads to the surrounding skin. Subungual haematomas may cause confusion but 'grow out' with the nail (see Fig. 8.15). The risk of misdiagnosis is highest with an amelanotic melanoma which may mimic chronic paronychia or a pyogenic granuloma.

LEARNING POINT
Do not let the nail stop you from biopsying suspicious lesions under it promptly.

CHAPTER 9

Eczema and dermatitis

The conditions grouped under this heading are the most common to be referred to our clinics, making up some 20% of all new patients.

Terminology

Too much time has been devoted in the past to trying to distinguish between eczema and dermatitis. This exercise in hair-splitting semantics can be avoided by accepting that the two terms mean the same thing. Such an approach has now been adopted by most dermatologists, and will be used in this book. Contact eczema, therefore, is here the same as contact dermatitis; seborrhoeic eczema the same as seborrhoeic dermatitis, etc.

It may, however, be wise to stick to the term eczema when talking to patients as, to them, 'dermatitis' may carry industrial and compensation overtones which sometimes stir up unnecessary legal battles.

> **LEARNING POINT**
> *'When I use a word it means just what I choose it to mean' said Humpty Dumpty. Choose to make the words eczema and dermatitis mean the same to you.*

Classification of eczema

This remains difficult and unsatisfactory. Eczema is a reaction pattern which has many causes (Fig. 9.1). Some terms are based on the appearance of lesions, e.g. discoid eczema and hyperkeratotic eczema, while others reflect outmoded or unproven theories

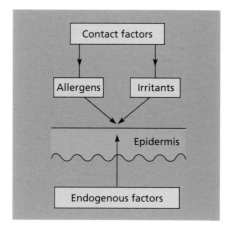

Fig. 9.1 The causes of eczema.

of causation, e.g. infective eczema and seborrhoeic eczema. Classification by site, e.g. flexural eczema and hand eczema, is equally unhelpful. Perhaps the most acceptable subdivision is into:
1 Exogeneous (or contact) eczema.
2 Endogeneous (or constitutional) eczema.

Any rational approach to therapy depends upon making this distinction, but even experienced dermatologists admit that they can only classify some two-thirds of the cases they see. Further confusion can occur when the groups overlap, e.g. when a contact eczema is superimposed on a gravitational eczema. A convenient working classification is shown in Table 9.1.

Pathogenesis

The pathways leading to an eczematous reaction are likely to be common to all subtypes and to involve similar inflammatory mediators (prostaglandins,

Table 9.1 Eczema — a working classification

Exogenous (contact)	Irritant
	Allergic
	Photodermatitis (Chapter 17)
Endogenous (constitutional)	Atopic
	Seborrhoeic
	Discoid (nummular)
	Pompholyx
	Gravitational (stasis)
Unclassified	Asteatotic
	Neurodermatitis
	Juvenile plantar dermatosis

leukotrienes and cytokines; p. 30). Helper T cells predominate in the inflammatory infiltrate. One current view is that these are mainly of the TH-2 subset in atopic dermatitis, stimulating an excessive production of IgE (p. 25; Fig. 3.6).

Histology (Fig. 9.2)

The clinical appearance of the different stages of eczema mirrors their histology. In the acute stage, oedema in the epidermis (spongiosis) progresses to the formation of intra-epidermal vesicles, which may coalesce into larger blisters or rupture. The chronic stages of eczema show less spongiosis and vesication but more thickening of the prickle cell (acanthosis) and horny layers (hyperkeratosis and parakerotisis). These changes are accompanied by a variable degree of vasodilatation and infiltration with lymphocytes.

Clinical features common to most patterns of eczema

The different types of eczema have their own distinguishing marks, and these will be dealt with later; but most share certain general features which it is convenient to consider here.

Acute eczema

Acute eczema (Figs 9.3 & 9.4) is recognized by its:

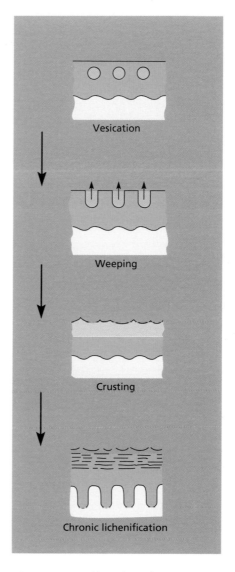

Fig. 9.2 The sequence of histological events in eczema.

● Redness and swelling, usually with an ill-defined border.
● Papules, vesicles and, in fierce cases, large blisters (Fig. 9.5).
● Exudation and crusting.
● Scaling.

Chronic eczema

Chronic eczema may show all of the above changes but in general is:

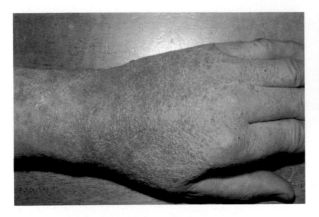

Fig. 9.3 Acute vesicular contact eczema of the hand.

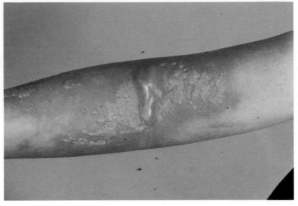

Fig. 9.5 Acute bullous photodermatitis of plant origin.

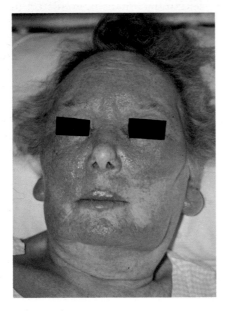

Fig. 9.4 Vesicular and crusted contact eczema of the face (cosmetic allergy).

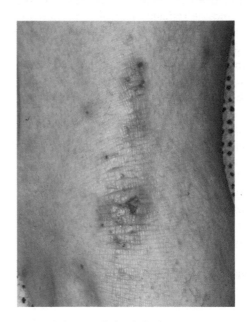

Fig. 9.6 Lichenification behind the knee in chronic atopic eczema.

- Less vesicular and exudative.
- More scaly, pigmented and thickened.
- More likely to be lichenified (Fig. 9.6) (a dry leathery thickened state, with increased skin markings, secondary to repeated scratching or rubbing).
- More likely to develop painful fissures.

Complications

1 Heavy bacterial colonization is common in all types of eczema but overt infection is most troublesome in the seborrhoeic and atopic types.

2 Reactions to medicaments may provoke dissemination, especially in gravitational eczema.

3 Anxiety states may develop with all severe forms of eczema.

Differential diagnosis

This falls into two halves. Eczema has first to be

separated from other skin conditions which look like it:

• *Psoriasis* (Chapter 6). This presents problems on the scalp (neurodermatitis and seborrhoeic eczema), in the flexures (seborrhoeic eczema), on the hands (all chronic eczemas) and on the limbs (discoid eczema). Psoriasis tends to be less itchy and more marginated. One should look for signs of psoriasis elsewhere, particularly on the nails, elbows and knees.

• *Fungal infections* (Chapter 15). These must be considered in any apparent eczema of the groin, feet and hands, particularly if asymmetrical and not doing well with topical steroids. In addition tinea pedis can provoke a secondary pompholyx-like eruption of the hands. Pityriasis versicolor (p. 191) may look like seborrhoeic eczema of the trunk but is browner and depigments in the sun. In all of these instances examination of scales made transparent with potassium hydroxide solution should settle the issue (p. 39).

• *Scabies* (Chapter 16). Beware of the patient with no past history of skin trouble who suddenly develops itchy lesions mimicking infected eczema, especially if there are also itchy contacts.

• Also consider the following:

Head lice in infected eczema of the scalp.

Angio-oedema and erysipelas in facial contact eczema.

Lichen planus in palmar eczema.

Pityriasis rosea and secondary syphilis in seborrhoeic eczema of the trunk.

Drug reactions in photodermatitis.

It is also important to try to distinguish between exogenous and endogenous eczema on clinical grounds, as this will determine both the need for investigation and the best line of treatment. Sometimes an eruption will follow one of the well-known patterns of eczema, and the distinction can then be made readily enough; often, however, this is not the case, and the history then becomes especially important. A contact element is more likely if:

• There is obvious contact with known irritants or allergens.

• The eruption clears when the patient goes on holiday, or at the weekends.

• The eczema is asymmetrical, or with a linear or rectilinear configuration.

• The rash picks out the eyelids, external ear canals,

hands and feet, the skin around stasis ulcers, and peri-anal skin.

Investigations

Each eczema pattern needs a different line of enquiry.

Exogenous eczema

Here the main decision is whether or not to undertake patch testing (p. 40). This is of no value in irritant eczema but may be helpful in allergic contact eczema. The technique is not easy: its problems include separating irritant from allergic patch test reactions, and picking the right allergens to test. If legal issues depend on the results, the testing should be done by a dermatologist who will have the standard equipment and suitably selected allergens (Fig. 4.5). Patch testing can be used to confirm a suspected allergy, or, by the use of a battery of common sensitizers, to uncover allergies which then have to be assessed in the light of the history and the clinical picture. Photopatch-testing is more specialized and facilities are only available in a few centres. A visit to the home or workplace may be invaluable in investigating contact eczema.

Endogenous eczema

The only indication for patch testing here is when an added contact allergic element is suspected. This is most common in stasis eczema where neomycin, soframycin, lanolin or preservative allergy may perpetuate the condition or trigger dissemination. Ironically rubber gloves, so often used to protect eczematous hands, can themselves sensitize.

The role of prick testing in atopic eczema is discussed on p. 40.

Some find the measurement of serum total IgE and IgE antibodies specific to certain antigens not only useful in diagnosing the atopic state, but also helpful when investigating and advising on the role of dietary and environmental allergens in causing or perpetuating atopic dermatitis. Specific IgE antibodies are measured by a radioallergosorbent test (RAST). Prick and RAST testing should give similar results but many now prefer the more expensive

RAST test as it is easier to perform and less time consuming in the clinic, especially when dealing with children.

Specimens should be cultured for bacterial pathogens or *Candida* if superinfection is suspected or if eczema is worsening despite treatment. Scrapings for fungal culture can be used to rule out tinea if there is clinical doubt — as in some cases of discoid eczema.

Finally, malabsorption should be considered and looked for in otherwise unexplained, widespread pigmented atypical patterns of endogenous eczema.

Treatment

Acute weeping eczema

This does best with liquid applications. Non-steroidal preparations are helpful at this stage and the technique used will vary with the facilities available and the site of the lesions. In general practice a simple and convenient way of dealing with weeping eczema of the hands or feet is to use thrice daily 10 minute soaks in a cool 0.01% solution of potassium permanganate or 0.65% aluminium acetate solution (Formulary, p. 288), each soaking being followed by a smear of a corticosteroid cream or lotion and the application of a non-stick dressing or cotton gloves. One disadvantage is that permanganate stains the skin and nails brown — patients should be told about this.

Wider areas on the trunk respond well to corticosteroid creams and lotions. However, traditional remedies such as exposure and frequent applications of calamine lotion, and the use of half-strength magenta paint for the flexures, are also very effective.

An experienced doctor or nurse can supervise or teach the patient how to use wet dressings. The dilute potassium permanganate solution, aluminium acetate solution, saline, 0.5% silver nitrate, or even tap water, can be applied on cotton gauze, under a polythene covering, and changed twice daily. Rest at home will help too.

Subacute eczema

Steroid lotions or creams form the mainstay of treatment; their strength is determined by the severity of the attack. Neomycin or vioform can be incorporated into the application if an infective element is present, but preferably should not be used on stasis eczema as sensitization is so often induced.

Chronic eczema

This responds best to steroids in an ointment base, but is also often helped by non-steroid applications such as ichthammol and zinc cream.

The strength of the steroid is important (Fig. 9.7). Nothing stronger than 0.5 or 1% hydrocortisone ointment should be used on the face or in infancy. Even in adults one should be reluctant to prescribe more than 200 g of a mildly potent steroid, 50 g of a moderately potent or 30 g of a potent one, per week for long periods. Very potent topical steroids should not be used long term.

Bacterial superinfection may need systemic antibiotics but can often be controlled by the incorporation of antibiotics, e.g. neomycin or chlortetracycline, or antiseptics, e.g. vioform, into the steroid formulation. Many proprietary mixtures of this type are available in the UK. Chronic localized hyperkeratotic eczema of the palms or soles can be helped by salicylic acid (1–6% in emulsifying ointment) or stabilized urea preparations (Formulary, p. 287).

Systemic treatment

Short courses of systemic steroids may occasionally be justified in extremely acute and severe eczema

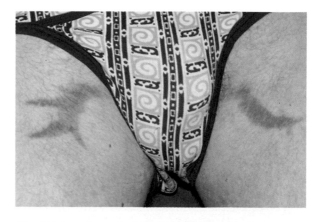

Fig. 9.7 Stretch marks following the use of too potent topical steroids to the groin.

but prolonged systemic steroid treatment should be avoided in chronic cases, particularly in atopic eczema. Hydroxyzine, trimeprazine and other anti-histamines (Formulary, p. 301) may be helpful at night. Systemic antibiotics may be needed in wide-spread bacterial superinfection.

Common patterns of eczema

Irritant contact eczema

This accounts for the majority of industrial cases.

Cause

Strong irritants elicit an acute reaction after brief contact and the diagnosis is then usually obvious. Prolonged exposure, sometimes over a period of years, is needed for weak irritants to cause eczema, usually of the hands and forearms (Fig. 9.8). Deter-gents, alkalis, solvents, cutting oils and abrasive dusts are common culprits. There is a wide range of susceptibility, those with dry skins or atopy being especially vulnerable.

Course

The need to continue at work, or with housework, seldom allows the skin to regain its normal barrier function. This may take several months. All too often, therefore, this condition, potentially reversible in the early stages, becomes chronic.

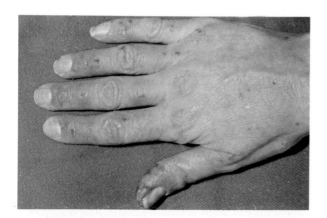

Fig. 9.8 Chronic irritant housewife's hand eczema.

Complications

The condition may lead to loss of work.

Differential diagnosis

It is often hard to differentiate from allergic contact dermatitis and from atopic eczema of the hands. Atopic patients are especially prone to develop irritant eczema.

Investigations

Patch testing with irritants is not helpful and indeed may be misleading: patch testing to a battery of common allergens (p. 93) may be worthwhile if an allergic element is suspected.

Treatment

Management is based upon avoidance of the irritants responsible but often this is not possible and the best that can be achieved is reduced exposure and the use of protective gloves and clothing. The factory doctor or nurse can often advise here. Barrier creams seldom help established cases. Moderately potent topical corticosteroids are valuable but are secondary to the avoidance of irritants and protective measures. A wiser choice of career might have prevented the trouble arising in the first place in those with vulner-able skins. Some jobs to beware of are listed in Table 9.2.

Allergic contact dermatitis

Cause

The mechanism is that of delayed (type IV)

Table 9.2 Jobs carrying a high risk of chronic irritant contact dermatitis

Building site workers	Hairdressing
Car mechanics	Horticulture
Catering	Housework
Cleaning	Labouring
Engineering	Metal work
Farming	Mining

hypersensitivity. This is dealt with in detail on p. 33. It has the following features:

- Previous contact is needed to induce allergy.
- Specificity to one chemical or its close relatives.
- All areas of skin react to the allergen.
- Sensitization persists indefinitely.
- Desensitization is seldom possible.

Allergens

It is not easy to guess whether a substance is likely to sensitize or not just by looking at its formula. A whole new industry has arisen around the need for predictive patch testing before new substances or cosmetics are let out into the community. Most allergens are relatively simple chemicals (Chapter 3; see p. 28) which must bind to protein before becoming a 'complete antigen'. The ability to sensitize varies from substances which often do so after a single exposure (e.g. poison ivy) to those which need prolonged exposure (e.g. brick layers take an average of 10 years to become allergic to chrome).

Presentation and clinical course

The original site of the eruption gives a clue to the likely allergen which secondary spread may later obscure. The lax skin of the eyelids and genitalia is especially likely to become oedematous.

Easily recognizable patterns exist. Nickel allergy, for example, gives rise to eczema under jewellery, bra clips and jean studs (Fig. 9.9). Possible allergens are numerous and to spot the less common ones

in the environment needs specialist knowledge. Table 9.3 lists some common allergens and their distribution.

Investigations

Questioning should cover both occupational and domestic exposure to allergens. The indications for patch testing have already been discussed on p. 89. The techniques are constantly improving: dermatologists will have access to a battery of common allergens, commercially available, suitably diluted in a bland vehicle. They are applied in aluminium cups held in position on the skin for two or three days (Fig. 4.5) by tape. Patch testing will often start with a standard series (battery) of allergens whose selection is based on local experience. Extra allergens will be used as appropriate, and especially for those in jobs, like dentistry or hairdressing, which carry unusual risks. Table 9.3 shows the battery we use and how it helps us with the commonest types of contact allergy.

Treatment

Simply to reduce exposure to the offending allergen is usually not enough and active steps have to be taken to avoid it completely. Job changes are sometimes necessary to achieve this. Some believe that reactions to nickel may be kept going by nickel in the diet, released from cans or steel saucepans — changes in diet and cooking utensils may occasionally be helpful.

Atopic eczema

The word 'atopy' comes from the Greek (a-topos: without a place). It was introduced by Coca and Cooke in 1923 and refers to the lack of a niche for the grouping of asthma, hayfever and eczema in the medical classifications then in use. Atopy is a state in which an exuberant production of IgE occurs as a response to common environmental allergens. Atopic subjects may, or may not, develop one or more of the atopic diseases such as asthma, hayfever, eczema and food allergies. Some 15% of the population have at least one atopic manifestation and the prevalence of atopy is steadily rising. The reasons for this are not clear.

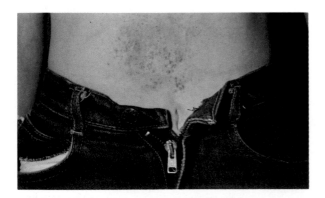

Fig. 9.9 Contact eczema due to allergy to nickel in a jean stud.

Table 9.3 The allergens in our battery and what they mean

Allergen	Common sources	Comments

Metals
The classic metal allergy for men is still to chrome, present in cement. In the past, more women than men have been nickel allergic but the current fashion for men to have their ears pierced will change this.

Allergen	Common sources	Comments
Chrome	Cement; chromium plating processes; anti-rust paints; tattoos (green) and some leathers. Sensitization follows contact with chrome salts rather than chromium metal.	A common problem for building site workers. In Scandinavia putting iron sulphate into cement has been shown to reduce its allergenicity by making the chrome salts insoluble.
Nickel	Nickel plated objects especially cheap jewellery. Remember jean studs.	The best way of becoming sensitive is to pierce your ears. Nickel is being taken out of some good costume jewellery.

Cosmetics
Despite attempts to design 'hypoallergenic' cosmetics, allergic reactions are still seen. The commonest culprits are fragrances, followed by preservatives, dyes and lanolin.

Allergen	Common sources	Comments
Fragrance mix	An infinite variety of cosmetics, sprays and toiletries.	Any perfume will contain many ingredients. This convenient mix picks up only some 80% of perfume allergies. Some sensitive subjects also react to Balsam of Peru, tars or colophony.
Balsam of Peru	Used in some scented cosmetics. Also in some spices and suppositories e.g. Anusol.	May indicate allergy to perfumes also. Can cross-react with colophony, orange peel, cinnamon and benzyl benzoate.
Formaldehyde	Used as a preservative in some shampoos and cosmetics. Also in pathology laboratories and white shoes.	Too many pathologists are allergic to it. Quaternium 15 (see below) releases formaldehyde as do some formaldehyde resins.
Parabens-mix	Preservatives in a wide variety of creams and lotions, both medical and cosmetic.	Common cause of allergy in those who react to a number of seemingly unrelated creams.
Kathon	Preservative in many cosmetics, shampoos, soaps and sunscreens.	Also found in some odd places such as moist toilet papers, and washing-up liquids.
Quaternium 15	Preservative in many topical medicaments and cosmetics.	Releases formaldehyde and may cross-react with it.
Paraphenylene diamine (PPD)	Dark dyes for hair and clothing.	Few heed the manufacturer's warning to patch test themselves before dyeing their hair. May cross-react with other chemicals containing the 'para' group e.g. some local anaesthetics, sulphonamides, para-aminobenzoic acid (in some sunscreens).
Wool alcohols	Anything with lanolin in it.	Common cause of reaction to cosmetics and topical medicaments.

Medicaments
These may share allergens, such as preservatives and lanolin, with cosmetics (see above). In addition the active ingredients can sensitize, especially when applied long term to venous ulcers, pruritus ani or eczema, otitis externa.

Allergen	Common sources	Comments
Neomycin	Popular topical antibiotic. Safe in short bursts e.g. for impetigo.	Common sensitizer in those with venous ulcers. Simply swapping to another antibiotic may not always help as it cross-reacts with framycetin and gentamycin.

(continued)

Table 9.3 Continued

Allergen	Common sources	Comments
Quinoline mix	Used as an antiseptic in creams, often in combination with a corticosteroid.	Its aliases include vioform and chinoform.
Ethylenediamine dihydrochloride	Stabilizer in some topical steroid mixtures (e.g. mycolog and the alleged active ingredient in fat removal creams). A component in aminophylline. A hardener for epoxy resin.	Cross-reacts with some antihistamines e.g. hydroxyzine.
Benzocaine	A local anaesthetic which lurks in some topical applications e.g. for piles.	Dermatologists seldom recommend using these preparations — they have seen too many reactions.

Rubber
Rubber itself is often not the problem: but it has to be converted from soft latex to usable rubber by adding vulcanizers to make it harder, accelerators to speed up vulcanization, and antioxidants to stop it perishing in the air. These additives are allergens.

Mercapto-mix	Chemicals used to harden rubber.	Diagnosis is often obvious; sometimes less so. Remember shoe soles, rubber bands, golf club grips.
Thiuram-mix	Another set of rubber accelerators.	Common culprit in rubber glove allergy.
Black rubber mix	All black heavy duty rubber e.g. tyres, rubber boots, squash balls.	These are paraphenylene diamine derivatives, cross-reacting with PPD dyes (see above).

Plants
In the USA, the Rhus family (poison ivy and poison oak) are important allergens: in Europe, *Primula obconica* holds pride of place. Both cause severe reactions with streaky erythema and blistering. The Rhus antigen is such a potent sensitizer that patch testing with it is unwise. Other reaction patterns include a lichenified dermatitis of exposed areas from chrysanthemums, and a finger tip dermatitis from tulip bulbs.

Primin	Allergen in *Primula obconica*.	Can patch test to primula leaf, but primin is more reliable.

Resins
Common sensitizers such as epoxy resins can cause trouble both at home, as adhesives, and in industry.

Epoxy resin	Common in 'two-component' adhesive mixtures (e.g. Araldite). Also used in electrical and plastics industries.	'Cured' resin does not sensitize. A few become allergic to the added hardener rather than to the resin itself.
Paratertiary butylphenol formaldehyde resin	Used as an adhesive e.g. in shoes, wrist watch straps, prostheses, hobbies.	Cross-reacts with formaldehyde. Depigmentation has been recorded.
Colophony	Naturally occurring and found in pine sawdust. Used as an adhesive in sticking plasters (bandages). Also found in various varnishes, paper and rosin.	The usual cause of sticking plaster allergy; also of dermatitis of the hands of violinists who handle rosin.

Inheritance

A strong genetic component is obvious. The concordance rates from atopic eczema in monozygotic and dizygotic twins are 0.86 and 0.21 respectively. Atopic diseases tend to run true to type within each family: in some, most of the affected members will have eczema, in others respiratory allergy will predominate.

Another odd feature is that atopic diseases are inherited more often from the mother than the father. This fits with the suggestion that a gene important in atopy lies on chromosome 11q13, and is responsible for about 60% of atopy but is inherited in an unusual way as an autosomal dominant passing only through the female line. It has to be said, however, that several groups have failed to confirm this linkage either in the families of those with atopic eczema or respiratory allergy.

Nevertheless, the candidate for the gene on chromosome 11q13 is a plausible one. The high affinity receptor for IgE is composed of alpha, beta, and gamma subunits. The beta subunit gene lies on chromosome 11q13 and is closely linked to the suspected gene for atopy. The high affinity IgE receptor is found both on mast cells (Fig. 3.8, p. 31), important in immediate hypersensitivity, and on Langerhans cells (Fig. 3.1, p. 22), important as antigen presenting cells within the skin. It seems to provide a bridge between the immediate and delayed hypersensitivity components of atopy.

Presentation and course

Atopic eczema often begins before the age of six months. It affects at least 3% of infants, but the onset may be delayed until childhood or adult life. The distribution and character of the lesions vary with age (Fig. 9.10); but a general dryness of the skin may persist throughout life.
• In infancy, atopic eczema tends to be vesicular and weeping. It often starts on the face (Fig. 9.11) with a non-specific distribution elsewhere, commonly sparing the napkin (diaper) area.
• In childhood, the eczema becomes leathery, dry and excoriated, affecting mainly the elbow and knee flexures (Fig. 9.12), wrists and ankles. A stubborn 'reverse' pattern affecting the extensor aspects of the limbs is also recognized.
• In adults, the distribution is as in childhood with a marked tendency towards lichenification and a more widespread but low-grade involvement of the trunk (Fig. 9.13), face and hands.

The cardinal feature of atopic eczema is itching; and scratching may account for most of the clinical picture. Affected children may sleep poorly, and be hyperactive, and sometimes manipulative, using the state of their eczema to get what they want from their parents. Luckily the condition remits spontaneously before the age of 10 in at least two-thirds of affected children, though it may come back at

times of stress. Eczema and asthma may see-saw so that while one improves the other may get worse.

Complications

Overt bacterial infection is troublesome in many patients with atopic eczema (Fig. 9.14). They are also especially prone to viral infections, most dangerously with widespread herpes simplex (eczema herpeticum), but also with molluscum contagiosum and warts. Growth hormone levels rise during deep sleep (stages 3 and 4), but these stages may not be reached during the disturbed sleep of children with severe atopic eczema. As a consequence they may grow poorly. The absorption of topical steroids can contribute to this too.

Investigation

Prick testing demonstrates immediate-type hypersensitivity and is helpful in the investigation of asthma and hay fever. The value of prick testing in atopic eczema, however, remains controversial; often the finding of multiple positive reactions, and a high IgE level, does little more than support a doubtful clinical diagnosis without leading to fruitful lines of treatment.

Treatment

Management here is complex and should include:
• Explanation, reassurance and encouragement.
• The avoidance of irritants, e.g. woollen clothing, and later of careers, such as hairdressing and engineering, which would inevitably lead to much exposure to irritants.
• The judicious use of topical steroids and other applications as for other types of chronic eczema (p. 90).
• The regular use of bland emollients, either directly to the skin or in the form of oils to be used in the bath. Some of these can also be used as soap substitutes. A list of suitable preparations is given in the Formulary (p. 287).
• Those with an associated ichthyosis generally should use ointments rather than creams.
• The scratch/itch cycle can often be interrupted by occlusive bandaging, e.g. with 1% ichthammol paste.
• Sedative antihistamines, e.g. trimeprazine or

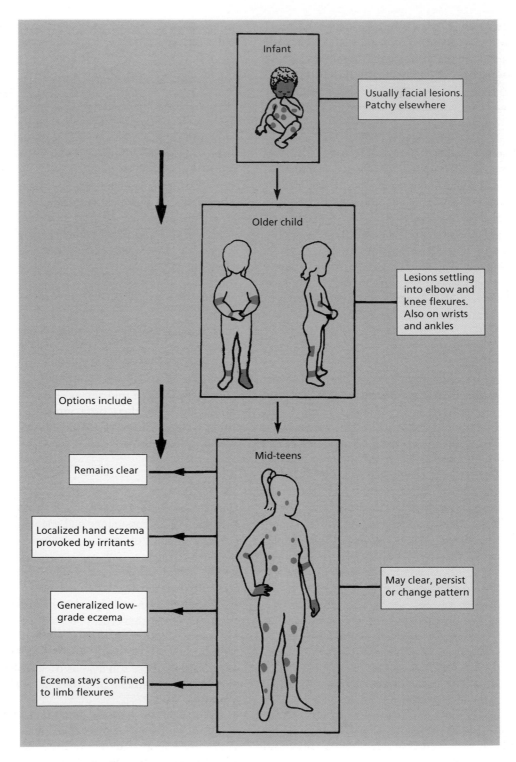

Fig. 9.10 The pattern of atopic eczema varies with age. It may clear at any stage.

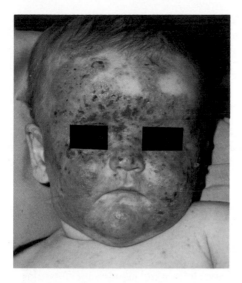

Fig. 9.11 Acute crusted infantile atopic eczema.

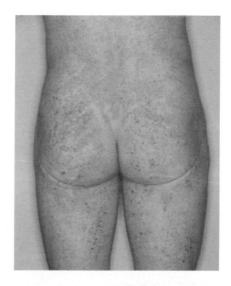

Fig. 9.13 Widespread excoriated adult atopic eczema.

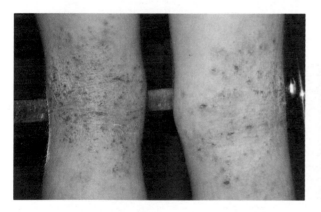

Fig. 9.12 Chronic excoriated atopic eczema behind the knees.

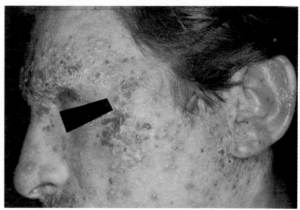

Fig. 9.14 Bacterial superinfection of facial atopic eczema.

hydroxyzine (Formulary, p. 301) are of value if sleep is interrupted. The newer non-sedative anti-histamines do not help so much with pruritus.
• Those with active herpes simplex infections should be avoided to cut the risk of developing eczema herpeticum.
• The role of diet is still debated. It is not certain that the avoidance of dietary allergens (e.g. cow's milk and eggs) by a pregnant or lactating woman lessens the risk of her baby developing eczema. It may still be wise to breast feed children at special risk, for six months.
• House dust mite avoidance: prick tests confirm that nearly all sufferers from atopic eczema have immediate hypersensitivity responses to allergens in the faeces of house dust mites. Sometimes, but not always, measures to reduce contact with these allergens seem to help eczema. These measures may include barrier materials on mattresses, thorough and regular vacuuming in the bedroom, where carpets should preferably be avoided, and the use of anti-mite sprays.
• Even without frank sepsis, a proliferation of bacterial pathogens may exacerbate atopic eczema. A month's course of a systemic antibiotic, e.g. erythromycin, may then be helpful.
• Routine inoculations are permissible during quiet phases of the eczema. However, children who are

allergic to eggs should not be inoculated against measles, influenza and yellow fever.

• In stubborn cases UVB or even PUVA therapy may be useful.

• A course of oral evening primrose oil lasting at least three months helps some patients.

• Cyclosporin: severe and unresponsive cases may be helped by short courses under specialist supervision (p. 303).

• Chinese herbal remedies: properly conducted trials have given promising results but difficulties remain. The active ingredients within these complex mixtures of herbs have still not been identified. We have some hope for the future but currently do not prescribe these treatments for our patients.

Seborrhoeic eczema

Cause

This condition is unrelated to seborrhoea. It may run in some families and often affects those with a tendency to dandruff. Some believe that the over-growth of pityrosporum yeasts plays an important part in the development of seborrhoeic eczema.

Presentation and course

The term covers at least three common patterns of endogenous eczema which may merge together (Fig. 9.15):

1 A red, scaly or exudative eruption of the scalp, ears (Fig. 9.16), face (Fig. 9.17) and eyebrows. May be associated with chronic blepharitis and otitis externa.

2 Dry, scaly, 'petaloid' lesions of the presternal (Fig. 9.18) and interscapular areas. There may also be extensive follicular papules or pustules on the trunk (seborrhoeic folliculitis or pityrosporum folliculitis).

3 Intertriginous lesions of the armpits, umbilicus or groins, or under spectacles or hearing aids.

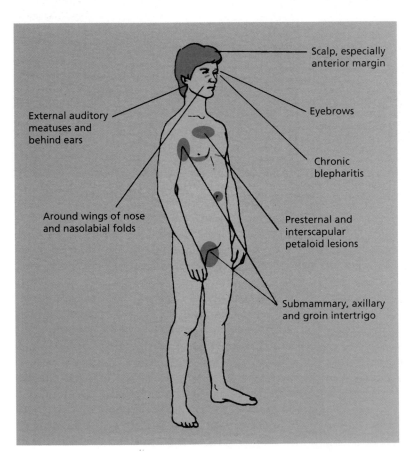

External auditory meatuses and behind ears

Around wings of nose and nasolabial folds

Scalp, especially anterior margin

Eyebrows

Chronic blepharitis

Presternal and interscapular petaloid lesions

Submammary, axillary and groin intertrigo

Fig. 9.15 Areas most often affected by seborrhoeic eczema.

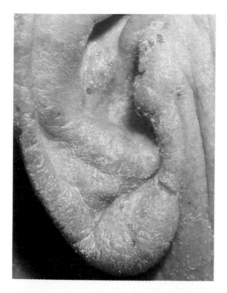

Fig. 9.16 Dry scaly seborrhoeic eczema of the ear.

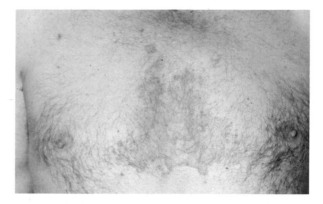

Fig. 9.18 Typical presternal patch of seborrhoeic eczema.

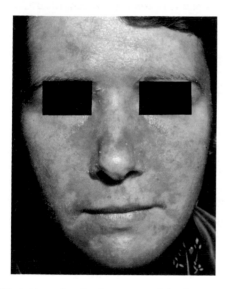

Fig. 9.17 Active seborrhoeic eczema of the face.

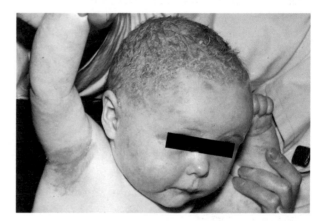

Fig. 9.19 Infantile seborrhoeic eczema.

Seborrhoeic eczema may affect infants (Fig. 9.19) but is most common in adult males. In infants it clears quickly but in adults its course is unpredictable and may be chronic or recurrent. Some particularly severe cases have occurred in patients with AIDS (p. 182; Fig. 15.30).

Complications

May be associated with furunculosis. In the intertriginous type superadded *Candida* infection is common.

Investigations

None are usually needed. Bear possible HIV infection in mind.

Treatment

Therapy is suppressive rather than curative and patients should be told this. Topical imidazoles (Formulary, p. 292) are perhaps the first line of treatment. Two per cent sulphur and 2% salicylic acid in aqueous cream is often helpful and avoids the problem of topical steroids. It may be used to the scalp overnight and removed by a medicated shampoo which may contain ketoconazole, tar, salicylic acid, sulphur, zinc or selenium sulphide (Formulary, p. 287). A topical lithium preparation (Formulary, p. 296) may help the facial rash. For intertriginous lesions a weak steroid–antiseptic or steroid–antifungal combination (Formulary, p. 291) is often effective. For very severe and unresponsive cases a short course of oral itraconazole may be helpful.

Discoid (nummular) eczema

Cause

No cause has been established but chronic stress is often present. A reaction to bacterial antigens has been suspected as the lesions often yield staphylococci on culture, and as steroid–antiseptic or antibiotic mixtures do better than either separately.

Presentation and course

This common pattern of endogenous eczema classically affects the limbs of middle-aged males. The lesions are multiple, coin-shaped, vesicular or crusted, highly itchy plaques (Fig. 9.20), usually less than 5 cm across. The condition tends to persist for many months.

Investigations

None are usually needed.

Treatment

With topical steroid antiseptic or antibiotic combinations (see above).

Pompholyx

Cause

Usually unknown but sometimes provoked by heat or emotional upsets. In allergic subjects the ingestion of small amounts of nickel in food may trigger pompholyx. The vesicles are not plugged sweat ducts.

Presentation and course

In this tiresome and sometimes very unpleasant form of eczema, recurrent bouts of vesicles or larger blisters appear on the palms (Fig. 9.21), fingers (Fig. 9.22) and/or the soles of adults. Bouts lasting a few weeks recur at irregular intervals. Secondary infection and lymphangitis are a recurrent problem for some patients.

Investigations

None are usually needed: sometimes a pompholyx-like eruption of the hands can follow acute tinea pedis. If this is suspected, scrapings or blister roofs from the feet should be sent for mycological examination. Swabs from infected vesicles should be cultured for bacterial pathogens.

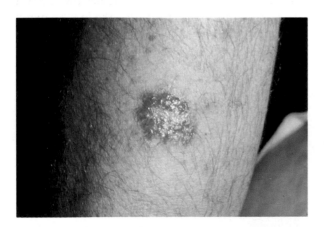

Fig. 9.20 Vesicular and weeping patch of discoid eczema.

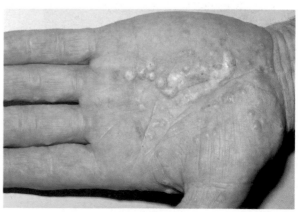

Fig. 9.21 Pompholyx of the palm with early secondary infection.

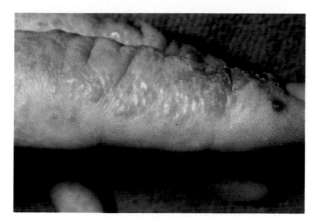

Fig. 9.22 Pompholyx vesicles along the side of a finger.

Treatment

As for acute eczema of the hands and feet (p. 90). Appropriate antibiotics should be given for bacterial infection. Potassium permanganate soaks followed by a very potent corticosteroid cream are often helpful.

Gravitational (stasis) eczema

Cause

Often, but not always, accompanied by obvious venous insufficiency.

Presentation and course

A chronic patchy eczematous condition of the lower legs, sometimes accompanied by varicose veins, oedema, and haemosiderin deposition (Fig. 9.23). When severe it may spread to the other leg or even become generalized.

Complications

Patients often become sensitized to local antibiotic applications or to the preservatives in medicated bandages. Excoriations may lead to ulcer formation.

Treatment

This should include the elimination of oedema by elevation, pressure bandages or diuretics. A

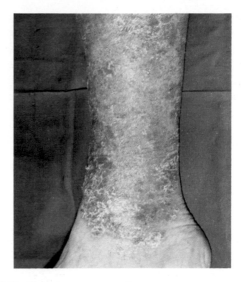

Fig. 9.23 Chronic gravitational eczema.

moderately potent topical steroid may be helpful but stronger ones are best avoided. Bland applications, e.g. Lassar's paste or zinc cream BNF, or medicated bandages (Formulary, p. 296), are useful but stasis eczema is liable to persist, despite surgery to the underlying veins.

Asteatotic eczema

Cause

Many who develop asteatotic eczema in old age will always have had a dry skin and a tendency to chap. Other contributory factors may include the removal of surface lipids by overwashing, the low humidity of winter and central heating, the use of diuretics, and hypothyroidism.

Presentation and course

Often unrecognized, this common and itchy pattern of eczema occurs on the legs of elderly patients. Against a background of dry skin, a network of fine red superficial fissures causes a 'crazy paving' appearance (Fig. 9.24).

Investigations

None are usually needed. Very extensive cases may

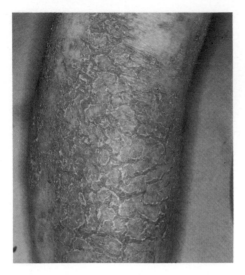

Fig. 9.24 Asteatotic eczema with network of fine fissures in the stratum corneum.

be part of malabsorption syndromes or internal malignancy.

Treatment

Can be cleared by the use of a mild or moderately potent topical steroid in a greasy base, and aqueous cream as a soap substitute for the area. Once clear, daily use of unmedicated emollients (Formulary, p. 287) usually prevents recurrence.

Localized neurodermatitis (lichen simplex)

Cause

The skin is damaged as a result of repeated rubbing or scratching, as a habit or in response to stress, but there is no underlying skin disorder.

Presentation and course

Usually occurs as a single, fixed, lichenified plaque. Favourite areas are the nape of the neck in women, the legs in men, and the anogenital area in both sexes. Lesions may resolve with treatment but tend to recur either in the same place or elsewhere.

Investigations

None are usually needed.

Treatment

Potent topical steroids or occlusive bandaging, where feasible, help to break the scratch/itch cycle. Tranquillizers are often disappointing.

Pruritus ani and vulvae

These terms are simply descriptive. Their many causes include lichen simplex, allergic contact dermatitis, psoriasis, candidiasis, threadworms and poor hygiene with maceration from sweating and faecal seepage. Psychosexual factors may be important.

Juvenile plantar dermatosis

Cause

This condition is thought to be related to the impermeability of modern socks and shoe linings with subsequent sweat gland blockage and so has been called the 'toxic sock syndrome'! Some feel the condition is a manifestation of atopy.

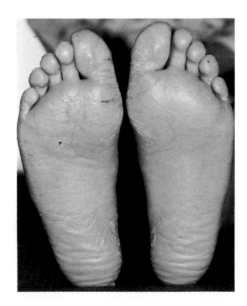

Fig. 9.25 The shiny skin and fissures of juvenile plantar dermatosis.

Presentation and course

The skin of the weight-bearing areas of the feet, particularly the forefeet and undersides of the toes, becomes dry and shiny with deep painful fissures which make walking difficult (Fig. 9.25). The toe webs are spared. Onset can be at any time after shoes are first worn, and even if untreated the condition clears in the early teens.

Investigations

Much time has been wasted in patch testing and scraping for fungus.

Treatment

The child should use a commercially available cork insole in all shoes, and stick to cotton or wool socks. An emollient such as emulsifying ointment or 1% ichthammol paste, or an emollient containing lactic acid, is as good as a topical steroid.

Napkin (diaper) dermatitis

Cause

The commonest type of napkin eruption is irritant in origin, and is aggravated by the use of waterproof plastic pants. The mixture of faeces and ammonia produced by urea-splitting bacteria, if allowed to remain in prolonged contact with the skin, leads to a severe reaction.

Presentation

The moist, often glazed and sore erythema affects the napkin area generally, with the exception of the skin folds which tend to be spared (Fig. 9.26).

Complications

Superinfection with *Candida albicans* is common, and this may lead to small erythematous papules or vesicopustules appearing around the periphery of the main eruption.

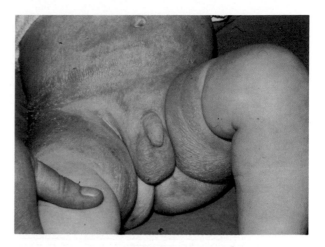

Fig. 9.26 Irritant napkin erythema with some sparing of skin folds.

Differential diagnosis

The sparing of the folds helps to separate this condition from infantile seborrhoeic eczema and candidiasis.

Treatment

It is never easy to keep the area clean and dry, but to do so remains the basis of all treatment. Theoretically, the child should be allowed to be free of napkins as much as possible but this may become a messy nightmare. On both sides of the Atlantic disposable nappies (diapers) have largely replaced washable ones. The super absorbent type is best and should be changed regularly, especially in the middle of the night. When towelling napkins are used they should be washed thoroughly and changed frequently. The area should be cleaned at each nappy change with aqueous cream and water. Protective ointments, e.g. zinc and castor oil ointment, or silicone protective ointments, are often useful (Formulary, p. 288). Potent steroids should be avoided but combinations of hydrocortisone with antifungals or antiseptics (Formulary, p. 291) are often useful.

LEARNING POINTS

1 Do not accept 'eczema' as an adequate diagnosis: treatment hinges on establishing its cause and type.

2 Keep fluorinated steroids off the face of adults and off the skin of infants.

3 Monitor repeat prescriptions of topical steroids, keeping an eye on the amount used and their potency.

4 Do not promise that atopic eczema will be clear by any particular age: guesses are always wrong and the patients lose faith.

CHAPTER 10

Reactive erythemas and vasculitis

Blood vessels can be affected by a variety of insults, both exogenous and endogenous. When this occurs the epidermis is usually normal, but the skin becomes red or pink and often oedematous. This is a reactive erythema. If the blood vessels are damaged more severely, as in vasculitis, purpura or haemorrhage masks the erythematous colour.

Urticaria (hives)

Cause

The characteristic wheals of this common condition are due to vasodilatation and leakage of fluid into the surrounding tissues. Urticaria is sometimes caused by an allergy, but is often mediated by non-allergic mechanisms. The various types of urticaria are listed in Table 10.1.

Physical urticarias

Cold urticaria

Patients develop wheals in areas exposed to cold, for example when cycling in the face of a cold wind.

A useful test in the clinic is to reproduce the reaction by immersing an extremity in cold water or holding an ice cube against forearm skin. A few cases are associated with the presence of cryoglobulins, cold agglutinins, or cryofibrinogens.

Solar urticaria

Wheals occur within minutes of sun exposure. Some patients with solar urticaria have erythropoietic protoporphyria (p. 251); most have an IgE-mediated urticarial reaction to sunlight.

Table 10.1 The main types of urticaria

Physical
cold
solar
heat
cholinergic
dermographism
delayed pressure
Inherited
hereditary angioedema
Hypersensitivity
Pharmacological
Contact

Heat urticaria

In this condition wheals arise in areas in contact with hot objects or solutions.

Cholinergic urticaria

Anxiety or strenuous exercise elicits this characteristic response. Transient, 2–5 mm follicular macules or papules resemble a blush or viral exanthem. The condition is mediated by acetyl choline released from sympathetic nerves in the skin. In patients with cholinergic urticaria, vessels overdilate in response to this neuromediator, and the overlying skin becomes pink.

Dermographism

This is a physical urticaria in which skin mast cells release extra histamine after rubbing or scratching. The linear wheals are therefore an exaggerated triple response of Lewis (Fig. 10.1).

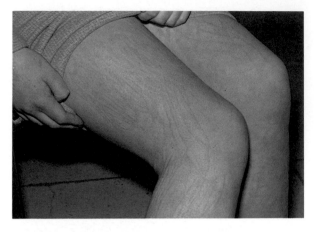

Fig. 10.1 Dermographism: linear wheals on the legs after scratching.

Delayed pressure urticaria

Sustained pressure causes oedema of the underlying skin and subcutaneous tissue 3–6 hours later. The swelling may last up to 48 hours and it is probably mediated by kinins or prostaglandins rather than histamine. It occurs particularly on the feet after walking, on the hands after clapping and on the buttocks after sitting.

Other types of urticaria

Hereditary angioedema

This autosomal dominant condition is characterized by recurrent attacks of abdominal pain and vomiting, or massive oedema of soft tissues which may involve the larynx. Tooth extraction, cheek biting, and other forms of trauma may precipitate an attack. A deficiency of an inhibitor to C1 esterase allows complement consumption to go unchecked so that vasoactive mediators are generated. To confirm the diagnosis, a serum C1 esterase inhibitor level and a C4 level should both be checked as the level of C1 esterase inhibitor is not always depressed (there is a type where the inhibitor is present but does not work).

Hypersensitivity urticaria

This most common form of urticaria is due to hypersensitivity, often an IgE-mediated (type I) allergic

Table 10.2 The eight Is of antigen encounter in hypersensitive urticaria

Ingestion
Inhalation
Instillation
Injection
Insertion
Insect bites
Infestations
Infections

reaction (Chapter 3). Allergens may be encountered in eight different ways (the eight I's listed in Table 10.2).

Pharmacological urticaria

This occurs when drugs cause mast cells to release histamine in a non-allergic manner (e.g. aspirin and morphine).

Contact urticaria

This type of urticaria may be IgE mediated or a pharmacological effect. Wheals occur most often around the mouth. Foods and food additives are the most common culprits but the reaction may be caused by drugs, animal saliva, caterpillars, and plants.

Presentation

Most types of urticaria share the sudden appearance of pink, itchy wheals, which may come up anywhere on the skin surface (Fig. 10.2). Each lasts less than a day, and most disappear within a few hours. Lesions may enlarge rapidly and some resolve centrally to take up an annular shape (Fig. 10.3). In an acute anaphylactic reaction, wheals may cover most of the skin surface. In contrast, in chronic urticaria, only a few wheals may develop each day.

Angioedema describes a variant of urticaria which primarily affects the subcutaneous tissues so that the swelling is less demarcated and less red than an urticarial wheal. Angioedema most commonly occurs at junctions between skin and mucous membranes (e.g. peri-orbital, peri-oral and genital) (Fig. 10.4). It may be associated with swelling of

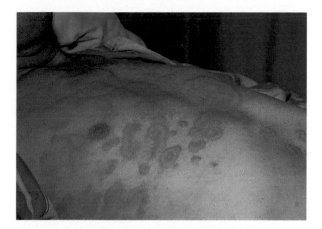

Fig. 10.2 Severe and acute urticaria due to penicillin allergy.

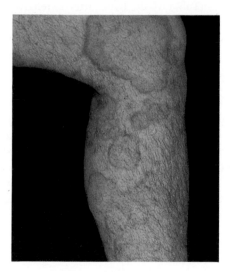

Fig. 10.3 Giant annular wheals in chronic urticaria.

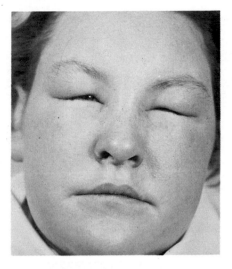

Fig. 10.4 Angiodema of the face: note lack of erythema and marked swelling of the eyelids.

end of the scale, some patients have chronic urticaria for years without any discernible cause.

Complications

Urticaria is normally uncomplicated, although its itch may be enough to interfere with sleep or daily activities. In acute anaphylactic reactions, oedema of the larynx may lead to asphyxiation and oedema of the tracheobronchial tree to asthma.

Differential diagnosis

There are two aspects to the differential diagnosis of urticaria. The first is to tell urticaria from other eruptions which are not urticaria at all. The second is to define the type of urticaria, according to Table 10.1. Insect bites and infestations commonly elicit urticarial papules, but these may have a central punctum. Erythema multiforme can also look like an annular urticaria (Fig. 10.5). A form of vasculitis (urticarial vasculitis) may resemble urticaria, but individual lesions last for longer than 24 hours and may leave bruising in their wake. Some bullous diseases, such as dermatitis herpetiformis, pemphigoid and herpes gestationis begin as urticarial areas, but later bullae make the diagnosis obvious. On the face, erysipelas can be distinguished from angioedema by its sharp margin and accompanying pyrexia (Fig. 10.6).

the tongue and laryngeal mucosa. It frequently accompanies chronic urticaria and its causes may be the same. Some patients have an underlying lymphoma or hypereosinophilic syndrome.

Course

The course of an urticarial reaction depends on its cause. If the urticaria is allergic, it will continue until the allergen is removed, tolerated or metabolized. Most such patients clear up within a day or two, even if the allergen is not identified. Urticaria may recur if the allergen is met again. At the other

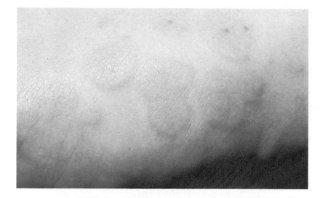

Fig. 10.5 Urticarial lesions simulating the target lesions of erythema multiforme.

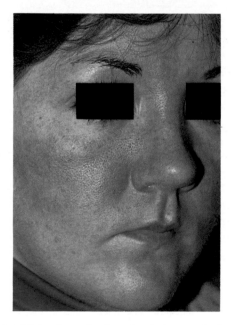

Fig. 10.6 Urticaria on the face simulating erysipelas: note the ill-defined margin and lack of surface change.

Investigations

The investigations will depend upon the presentation and type of urticaria. As noted above, many of the physical urticarias can be reproduced by appropriate tests.

Almost invariably, more is learned from the history than from the laboratory. It should include details of the events surrounding the onset of the eruption. A review of systems may uncover evidence of an underlying disease. Careful attention should be paid to drugs, remembering that self-prescribed ones can also cause urticaria. Over-the-counter medications (such as aspirin) and medications given by other routes (Table 10.2) can produce wheals. If a patient has acute urticaria, and its cause is not obvious, investigations are often deferred until it has persisted for a few weeks; then a physical examination (if it has not already been done) and screening tests such as a complete blood count, erythrocyte sedimentation rate, routine biochemical screen, chest X-ray, and urine analysis are worthwhile. If the urticaria continues for two to three months, the patient should probably be referred to a dermatologist for further evaluation. In general the focus of such investigations will be on internal disorders associated with urticaria (Table 10.3) and on external allergens (Table 10.4). Even after extensive evaluation and environmental change, the cause cannot always be found.

Treatment

The ideal is to find a cause and then to eliminate it. Aspirin, in any form, should be banned. The treatment for each type of urticaria is outlined in Table 10.5. In general, antihistamines are the mainstay of symptomatic treatment. Terfenidine 60 mg

Table 10.3 Some endogenous causes of urticaria

Infection
Connective tissue disorders
Hyperthyroidism
Diabetes
Pregnancy
Intestinal parasites
Cancer
Lymphomas

Table 10.4 Some exogenous causes of urticaria

Drugs, both topical and systemic
Foods and food additives
Bites
Inhalants
Pollens
Insect venoms
Animal dander

Table 10.5 Some types of urticaria and their management

Type	Treatment
Cold urticaria	Avoid cold Protective clothing Antihistamines
Solar urticaria	Avoid sun exposure Protective clothing Sunscreens and sunblocks Beta-carotene Antihistamines
Cholinergic urticaria	Avoid heat Minimize anxiety Avoid excessive exercise Anticholinergics Antihistamines Tranquillizers
Dermographism	Avoid trauma Antihistamines
Hereditary angioedema	Avoid trauma Attenuated androgenic steroids as prophylaxis Tracheostomy may be necessary
Hypersensitivity urticarias	Remove cause Antihistamines (H1 + H2) Sympathomimetics Systemic steroids (rarely justified) Avoid drugs containing aspirin

twice daily, cetirizine 10 mg daily, loratadine 10 mg daily or hydroxyzine, 10–25 mg up to every six hours, are useful treatments. Sometimes they can be combined with a longer acting antihistamine (such as chlorpheniramine maleate 12 mg sustained release tablets every 12 hours) so that peaks and troughs are blunted, and histamine activity is blocked throughout the night. If the eruption is not controlled, the dose of a short acting antihistamine like hydroxyzine can often be increased and still tolerated. H2-blocking antihistamines (e.g. cimetidine) may add a slight benefit if used in conjunction with an H1 histamine antagonist. Sympathomimetic agents can help urticaria, although the effects of adrenaline (epinephrine) are short lived. Pseudoephedrine, 30 or 60 mg every four hours, or terbutaline, 2.5 mg every eight hours, can sometimes be useful adjuncts. A tapering course of systemic corticosteroids may be used, but only when the cause is known and there are no contra-indications, and certainly not as a panacea to control chronic urticaria or urticaria of unknown cause. For treatment of anaphylaxis see p. 274.

> **LEARNING POINTS**
> *1 Avoid aspirins and systemic steroids in chronic urticaria.*
> *2 Do not promise patients that all will be solved by allergy tests.*
> *3 Alert those with cold urticaria to the dangers of swimming and ice cream.*
> *4 Take respiratory tract blockage seriously.*

Erythema multiforme

Cause

In erythema multiforme, the victim has usually reacted to an infection, often herpes simplex, or to a drug, but other factors have occasionally been implicated (Table 10.6).

Presentation

The symptoms of an upper respiratory tract infection may precede the eruption. Typically, annular non-scaling plaques appear on the palms, soles, forearms,

Table 10.6 Some causes of erythema multiforme

Viral infections, especially:
  herpes simplex
  hepatitis A and B
  mycoplasma
  orf

Bacterial infections

Fungal infections
  coccidioidomycosis

Parasitic infestations

Drugs

Pregnancy

Malignancy, or its treatment with
  radiotherapy

Idiopathic

and legs. They may be slightly more purple than the wheals of ordinary urticaria. Individual lesions enlarge but clear centrally. A new lesion may begin at the same site as the original one, so that the two concentric plaques look like a target (Figs 10.7 & 10.8). Occasionally lesions may blister. The Stevens—Johnson syndrome is a severe variant of erythema multiforme associated with fever and mucous membrane lesions. The oral mucosa, lips and bulbar conjunctivae are most commonly affected, but the nares, penis, vagina, pharynx, larynx, and tracheobronchial tree may also be involved (Fig. 10.9).

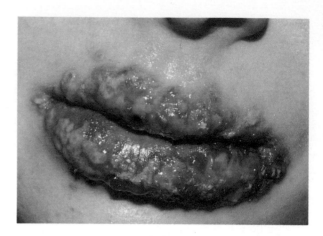

Fig. 10.9 Stevens—Johnson type of erythema multiforme. The eyelids were also severely involved.

Course

Crops of new lesions appear for one or two weeks, or until the responsible drug or other factor has been eliminated. Individual lesions last several days, and this differentiates them from the more fleeting lesions of an annular urticaria. The site of resolved lesions is marked transiently by hyperpigmentation, particularly in pigmented individuals.

Complications

There are usually no complications. However, severe lesions in the tracheobronchial tree of patients with Stevens—Johnson syndrome may lead to asphyxia, and ulcers of the bulbar conjunctiva to blindness. Corneal ulcers, anterior uveitis, and panophthalmitis may also occur. Genital ulcers may cause urinary retention and phimosis or vaginal sticture after they heal.

Differential diagnosis

Erythema multiforme can mimic the annular variant of urticaria as described above. However, target lesions are pathognomonic of erythema multiforme. Its acral distribution, the way individual lesions last for more than 24 hours, their purple colour, and the involvement of mucous membranes, all help to identify erythema multiforme. Other bullous disorders may enter the differential diagnosis (Chapter 11).

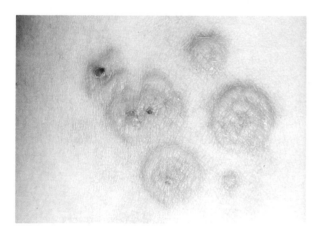

Fig. 10.7 Erythema multiforme: close-up of typical target lesions, tending to become bullous around their edges.

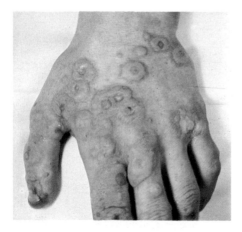

Fig. 10.8 Bullous target lesions occurring in a favourite site. In this patient recurrent attacks or erythema multiforme followed episodes of herpes simplex.

Investigations

The histology of erythema multiforme is distinctive. Epidermal necrosis and dermal changes, consisting of endothelial swelling, a mixed lymphohistiocytic perivascular infiltrate and papillary dermal oedema are seen. The abnormalities may be predominantly epidermal or dermal or a combination of both; they probably depend on the age of the lesion biopsied.

Most investigations are directed towards identifying a cause. A careful history helps rule out a drug reaction. Tzanck smears (p. 40) or culture of suspicious prodromal vesicles may identify a precipitating herpes simplex infection. A chest X-ray and serological tests should identify mycoplasmal pneumonia. A search for other infectious agents, neoplasia, endocrine causes, or collagen disease is sometimes necessary, especially when the course is prolonged or recurrent. About 50% of cases have no demonstrable provoking factor.

Treatment

The best treatment for erythema multiforme is to identify and remove its cause. In mild cases, only symptomatic treatment is needed and this includes the use of antihistamines.

The Stevens–Johnson syndrome, on the other hand, may demand immediate consultation between dermatologists and specialists in other fields such as ophthalmology, urology, and infectious diseases, depending on the particular case. The use of systemic steroids to abort Stevens–Johnson syndrome is debatable, but many believe that a short course (e.g. prednisolone 80 mg/day in divided doses in an adult) helps. However, the dose should be tapered rapidly or stopped because prolonged treatment in the Stevens–Johnson syndrome has been linked, controversially, with a high complication rate. Good nursing care with attention to the mouth and eyes is essential. The prevention of secondary infection, maintenance of a patent airway, good nutrition, and proper fluid and electrolyte balance, are important.

Herpes simplex infections should be suspected in recurrent erythema multiforme of otherwise unknown cause. Treatment with oral acyclovir 200 mg three to five times daily may prevent attacks, both of herpes simplex and of the recurrent erythema multiforme which follows it.

LEARNING POINTS
1 Look for target lesions and involvement of the palms.
2 Herpes simplex infection is the commonest provoking factor, but do not forget drugs.

Erythema nodosum

Erythema nodosum is an inflammation of the subcutaneous fat (a panniculitis). It is an immunological reaction, elicited by various bacterial, viral, and fungal infections, malignant disorders, drugs, and by a variety of other causes (Table 10.7).

Presentation

The characteristic lesion is a tender, red nodule developing alone or in groups on the legs and forearms or, rarely, on other areas such as the thighs, face, breasts, or other areas where there is fat (Fig. 10.10). Some patients also have painful joints and fever.

Course

Lesions usually resolve in six to eight weeks. In the interim, lesions may enlarge and new ones may occur at other sites. Like other reactive erythemas, erythema nodosum may persist if its cause is not removed.

Table 10.7 Some causes of erythema nodosum

Infections
    bacteria (e.g. streptococci, tuberculosis, brucellosis, leprosy)
    viruses
    Mycoplasma
    Rickettsia
    Chlamydia
    fungi (especially coccidioidomycosis)

Drugs (e.g. sulphonamides, oral contraceptive agents)

Systemic disease (e.g. sarcoidosis, ulcerative colitis, Crohn's disease, Behçet's disease)

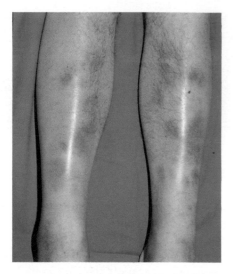

Fig. 10.10 Erythema nodosum: large painful dusky plaques on the shins. Always investigate this important reaction pattern (see text).

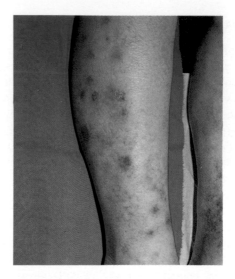

Fig. 10.11 The smaller lesions of nodular vasculitis, the causes of which overlap with erythema nodosum.

Complications

The nodules may be so tender that walking is difficult. Erythema nodosum leprosum occurs when lepromatous leprosy patients establish cell-mediated immunity to *Mycobacterium leprae*. These patients have severe malaise, arthralgia, and fever.

Differential diagnosis

The differential diagnosis of a single, tender, red nodule is extensive and includes trauma, infection (early cellulitis or abscess), and phlebitis.

When lesions are multiple, infection becomes less likely unless the lesions are developing in a sporotrichoid manner (p. 193). Other causes of a nodular panniculitis which may appear like erythema nodosum include panniculitis from pancreatitis, cold, trauma, injection of drugs or other foreign substances, withdrawal from systemic steroids, lupus erythematosus, superficial migratory thrombophlebitis, polyarteritis nodosa and a deficiency of alpha-1-antitrypsin. Some people use the term nodular vasculitis to describe a condition like erythema nodosum which lasts for more than six months (Fig. 10.11).

Investigations

Erythema nodosum demands a careful history, physical examination, a chest X-ray, throat culture for streptococcus, a Mantoux test, and an antistreptolysin-O (ASO) titre. If the results are normal, and there are no symptoms or physical findings to suggest other causes, extensive investigations can be deferred because the disease will resolve in most such patients.

Treatment

The ideal treatment for erythema nodosum is to identify and eliminate its cause if possible. For example, if a streptococcal infection is confirmed by culture or an ASO test, a suitable antibiotic will be recommended. Bed rest is also an important part of treatment. Non-steroidal anti-inflammatory agents such as aspirin, indomethacin, or ibuprofen may be helpful. Systemic steroids are usually not needed. For reasons which are not clear, potassium iodide in a dose of 400–900 mg/day can help, but should not be used for longer than six months.

Vasculitis

Whereas the reactive erythemas are associated with some inflammation around superficial or deep blood vessels, the term vasculitis is reserved for those showing inflammation within the vessel wall, with endothelial cell swelling, necrosis or fibrinoid change. The clinical manifestations depend upon the size of the blood vessel affected.

Leucocytoclastic (small vessel) vasculitis (Syn: allergic or hypersensitivity vasculitis, anaphylactoid purpura)

Cause

Immune complexes may lodge in the walls of blood vessels, activate complement, and attract polymorphonuclear leucocytes (Fig. 10.12). Enzymes released from these can degrade the vessel wall. Antigens in these immune complexes include drugs, auto-antigens, and infectious agents such as bacteria.

Presentation

The most common presentation of vasculitis is painful, palpable, purpura (Fig. 10.13). Crops of lesions arise in dependent areas (the forearms and legs in ambulatory patients, or on the buttocks and flanks in bedridden ones) (Fig. 10.14). Some have a small, livid or black centre, due to necrosis of the tissue

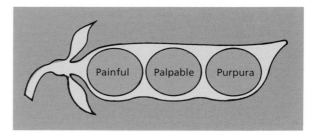

Fig. 10.13 The three Ps of small vessel vasculitis.

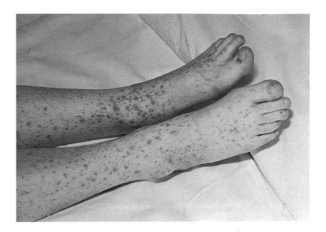

Fig. 10.14 Palpable purpuric lesions on both legs indicate small vessel vasculitis.

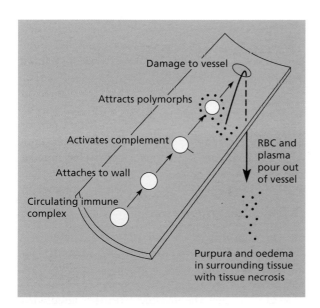

Fig. 10.12 Pathogenesis of vasculitis.

overlying the affected blood vessel. The purpura is palpable because the damaged vessel has leaked fluid.

Henoch–Schönlein purpura is a small vessel vasculitis associated with palpable purpura, arthritis, and abdominal pain, often preceded by an upper respiratory tract infection.

Course

The course of the vasculitis varies with its cause, its extent, the size of blood vessel affected, and the involvement of other organs.

Complications

Vasculitis may simply be cutaneous; alternatively it may be systemic, and then other organs will be damaged, including the kidney, central nervous system, gastrointestinal tract, and lungs.

Differential diagnosis

Small vessel vasculitis has to be separated from other causes of purpura (p. 148) such as abnormalities of the clotting system and sepsis (with or without vasculitis). Occasionally the vasculitis may look like urticaria if its purpuric element is not marked.

Investigations

Investigations should be directed toward identifying the cause and detecting internal involvement. A physical examination, chest X-ray, erythrocyte sedimentation rate, and biochemical tests monitoring the function of various organs are indicated. The most important test, however, is urine analysis, checking for proteinuria and haematuria, because vasculitis can affect the kidney subtly and so lead to renal insufficiency.

Skin biopsy will confirm the diagnosis of small vessel vasculitis. The finding of circulating immune complexes, or a lowered level of total complement (CH50) or C4, will implicate immune complexes as its cause. Tests for hepatitis virus, cryoglobulins, rheumatoid factor, and antinuclear antibodies may also be needed.

Direct immunofluorescence can be used to identify immune complexes in blood vessel walls, but is seldom performed because of false positive and false negative results as inflammation may destroy the complexes in a true vasculitis, and induce non-specific deposition in other diseases. Henoch–Schönlein vasculitis is confirmed if IgA deposits are found in the blood vessels of a patient with the clinical triad of palpable purpura, arthritis, and abdominal pain.

Treatment

The treatment of choice is to identify the cause and eliminate it. In addition, antihistamines and bed rest are sometimes helpful. Colchicine 0.6 mg twice daily or dapsone 100 mg daily may be worth a trial, but require monitoring for side effects (Formulary, p. 307). Patients whose vasculitis is damaging the kidneys or other internal organs may require systemic corticosteroids or immunosuppressive agents such as cyclophosphamide.

> **LEARNING POINT**
> *Leucocytoclastic vasculitis of the skin may indicate that the kidneys are being damaged. Be sure to analyse the urine.*

Polyarteritis nodosa

Cause

This necrotizing vasculitis of large arteries causes skin nodules, infarctive ulcers, and peripheral gangrene. Immune complexes may initiate this vasculitis, and sometimes contain hepatitis B antigen. Other known causes are adulterated drugs, B cell lymphomas, and immunotherapy.

Presentation

Tender subcutaneous nodules appear along the line of arteries. The skin over them may ulcerate or develop stellate patches of purpura and necrosis. Splinter haemorrhages and a peculiar, net-like vascular pattern (livedo reticularis) aid the clinical diagnosis. The disorder may be of the skin only (cutaneous polyarteritis nodosa), or also affect the kidneys, heart muscle, nerves, and joints (Fig. 10.15). Patients may be febrile, lose weight, and feel pain the muscles, joints, or abdomen. Some develop peripheral neuropathy, hypertension, and ischaemic heart disease. Renal involvement, with or without hypertension, is common.

Course

Untreated, systemic polyarteritis nodosa becomes chronic. Death, often from renal disease, is common, even in treated patients.

Differential diagnosis

Embolism, panniculitis, and infarctions can cause a similar clinical picture. Wegener's granulomatosis, allergic granulomatosis, temporal arteritis, and vasculitis which accompanies systemic lupus erythematosus and rheumatoid arthritis should be considered.

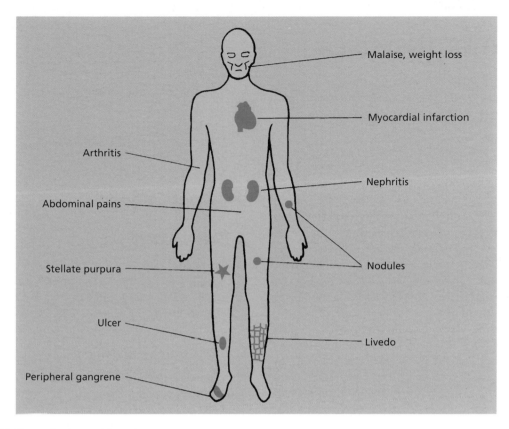

Fig. 10.15 Signs of polyarteritis nodosa.

Investigations

The laboratory findings are non-specific. An elevated ESR, neutrophil count, and gamma-globulin level are common. Investigations for cryoglobulins, rheumatoid factor, antinuclear antibody, and hepatitis B surface antigen are worthwhile, as are checks for disease in the kidney, heart, liver, and gut. Low levels of complement suggest active disease. The use of biopsy to confirm the diagnosis of large vessel vasculitis is not always easy as the arterial involvement may be segmental, and surgery itself difficult. Histological confirmation is most likely when biopsies are from a fresh lesion. Affected vessels show aneurysmal dilatation or necrosis, and fibrinoid changes in their walls, and an intense neutrophilic infiltrate around and even in the vessel wall.

Treatment

Systemic steroids and cyclophosphamide improve chances of survival. Low-dose systemic steroids alone are usually sufficient for the purely cutaneous form.

Wegener's granulomatosis

In this granulomatous vasculitis of unknown cause, fever, weight loss, and fatigue accompany naso-respiratory symptoms such as rhinitis, hearing loss, or sinusitis. Only half of the patients have skin lesions, usually symmetrical ulcers or papules on the extremities. Other organs can be affected, including the eye, joints, heart, nerves, lung, and kidney. Antineutrophil antibodies are present in most cases and are a useful but non-specific diagnostic marker. Cyclophosphamide is the treatment of choice, used alone or with systemic steroids.

CHAPTER 11

Bullous diseases

If fluid collects within the epidermis or immediately under it, blisters may form. These have many causes. Sometimes the morphology or distribution makes the diagnosis obvious, as in herpes simplex or zoster. Sometimes the history aids the diagnosis, as in cold or thermal injury, or in acute contact dermatitis. When the cause is not obvious, a biopsy can help by showing the level in the skin at which the blister has arisen (Fig. 11.1).

Subepidermal blisters occur between the dermis and the epidermis. Clinically these are thick-walled and may contain blood. Intra-epidermal bullae occur within the prickle cell layer of the epidermis: subcorneal blisters form just beneath the stratum corneum, at the outermost edge of the viable epidermis, and therefore have a particularly thin roof.

A list of differential diagnoses, based on histology, is given in Fig. 11.1 and some clinical and pathological distinguishing features are listed in Table 11.1. Only the most common conditions will be discussed here.

Subcorneal blisters

Bullous impetigo (p. 161)

This is a common cause of blistering in children. The bullae are flaccid, often contain pus, and are frequently grouped or located in body folds. Bullous impetigo is caused by *Staphylococcus aureus*.

Scalded skin syndrome (p. 163)

A toxin elaborated by some strains of *S. aureus* makes the skin painful and red; later it peels like a scald. The staphylococcus is usually hidden (e.g. conjunctiva, throat, wound, furuncle).

Miliaria crystallina (p. 160)

Here sweat accumulates under the stratum corneum leading to the development of thousands of uni-

Table 11.1 Distinguishing features of some bullous diseases

	Age	Site of blisters	General health	Blisters in mouth	Nature of blisters	Circulating antibodies	Fixed antibodies	Treatment
Pemphigus	Middle age	Trunk, flexures and scalp	Poor	Common	Superficial and flaccid	IgG to intercellular substance	IgG in intercellular substance	Steroids Immuno-suppressives
Pemphigoid	Old	Often flexural	Good	Rare	Tense and blood-filled	IgG to basement membrane region	IgG at basement membrane	Steroids Immuno-suppressives
Dermatitis herpetiformis	Primarily adults	Elbows, knees, upper back, buttocks	Itchy	Rare	Small, excoriated and grouped	IgG to the endomysium of muscle	IgA granular deposits in papillary dermis	Gluten-free diet Dapsone Sulpha-pyridine

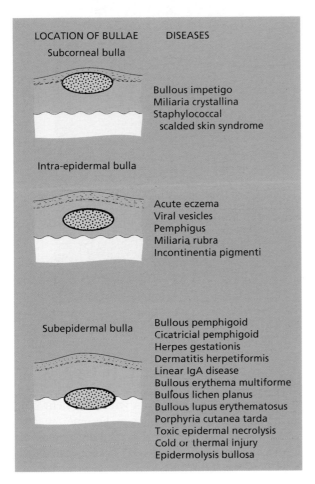

LOCATION OF BULLAE   DISEASES

Subcorneal bulla

Bullous impetigo
Miliaria crystallina
Staphylococcal
  scalded skin syndrome

Intra-epidermal bulla

Acute eczema
Viral vesicles
Pemphigus
Miliaria rubra
Incontinentia pigmenti

Subepidermal bulla   Bullous pemphigoid
Cicatricial pemphigoid
Herpes gestationis
Dermatitis herpetiformis
Linear IgA disease
Bullous erythema multiforme
Bullous lichen planus
Bullous lupus erythematosus
Porphyria cutanea tarda
Toxic epidermal necrolysis
Cold or thermal injury
Epidermolysis bullosa

Fig. 11.1 The differential diagnosis of bullous diseases based on the histological location of the blister.

formly spaced vesicles without underlying redness. Often this occurs after a fever or heavy exertion. The vesicles look like water droplets on the surface, but the skin is dry to the touch. The disorder is self-limiting and needs no treatment.

Subcorneal pustular dermatosis

As its name implies, the lesions are small groups of pustules rather than vesicles. However, the pustules pout out of the skin in a way that suggests they were once vesicles (like the vesico-pustules of chicken-pox). The cause of this rare disease is unknown, but oral dapsone (Formulary, p. 307) usually suppresses it.

Intra-epidermal vesicles or bullae

Acute dermatitis (Chapter 9)

Severe, acute eczema, especially the contact allergic type, can produce bullae (the name eczema suggests the bubbling of boiling water). Plants such as poison ivy, poison oak, or primula are common causes. The varying size of the vesicles, their close grouping, their asymmetry, their odd configurations (e.g. linear, square, rectilinear) and a history of contact with plants are helpful guides to the diagnosis.

Pompholyx (p. 100)

In pompholyx, highly itchy, small, eczematous vesicles occur along the sides of the fingers. Some physicians call this disorder 'dyshidrotic eczema', but the vesicles are not related to sweating or sweat ducts. The disorder is very common, but its cause is not known.

Viral infections (Chapter 15)

Some viruses create blisters in the skin by destroying epithelial cells. The vesicles of herpes simplex and zoster are the most common examples.

Pemphigus

Pemphigus is a severe, and often life-threatening blistering condition.

Cause

It is an autoimmune disease. IgG antibodies bind to complexes of polypeptides at the intercellular areas of the epidermis. The complexes vary with the type of pemphigus, for example, plakoglobin is important in both *P. foliaceus* and *P. vulgaris* and desmoglobin in *P. foliaceus* only. This antigen—antibody reaction induces the keratinocytes to release a proteolytic enzyme which dissolves the intercellular cement so that the keratinocytes fall apart. Rarely pemphigus may be associated with a thymoma or signify an underlying carcinoma (paraneoplastic pemphigus).

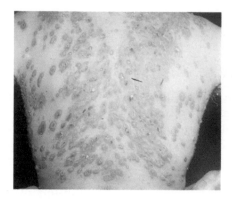

Fig. 11.2 Pemphigus vulgaris: widespread superficial blisters and erosions.

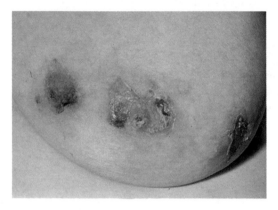

Fig. 11.3 Pemphigus vulgaris: thin-roofed blisters rupture easily leaving unhealing painful erosions.

Presentation

The disease is characterized by flaccid blisters of the skin (Figs 11.2 & 11.3), and mouth (Fig. 11.4) and, after the blisters rupture, by widespread erosions. Most patients develop lesions in the mouth first. The skin lesions are flaccid blisters from the outset. Shearing stresses on normal skin may cause a new erosion to form (positive Nikolsky sign).

There are several forms of pemphigus. The common type, pemphigus vulgaris, is a blistering and erosive disease. Pemphigus vegetans leads to the formation of heaped up, cauliflower-like, weeping areas, particularly in the groin and body folds. The blisters in pemphigus foliaceus are so superficial, and rupture so easily, that there are more weeping and crusting erosions than blisters.

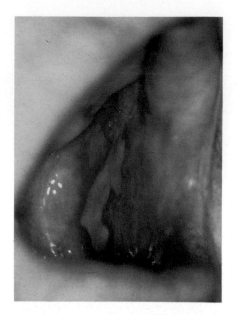

Fig. 11.4 Painful sloughy mouth ulcers in pemphigus vulgaris.

Course

The course is prolonged, even with treatment. The huge areas of denudation may become infected and smelly. However, with modern treatment, most patients can live relatively normal lives, with occasional exacerbations.

Complications

Infections are common. Complications are inevitable with the high doses of steroids and immunosuppressive drugs which are needed. Indeed, side effects of treatment are now the leading cause of death. Severe oral ulcers make eating painful.

Differential diagnosis

Widespread erosions may suggest a pyoderma, impetigo, epidermolysis bullosa, or ecthyma. Mouth ulcers may be mistaken for aphthae, Behçet's disease, or herpes simplex infection.

Investigations

Biopsy shows that the vesicles are intra-epidermal, with rounded keratinocytes floating free within

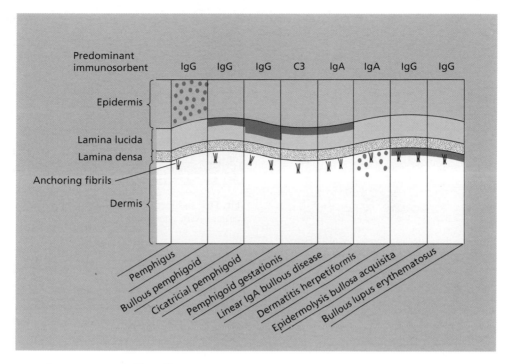

Fig. 11.5 Immunofluorescence in bullous diseases.

the blister cavity (acantholysis). Direct immuno-fluorescence (p. 42) of adjacent normal skin shows intercellular epidermal deposits of IgG and C3 (Fig. 11.5). The serum from a patient with pemphigus contains antibodies which bind to the intercellular areas of normal epidermis, so that indirect immuno-fluorescence (p. 42) can also be used to confirm the diagnosis. The titre of these antibodies correlates loosely with clinical activity and may guide changes in the dose of systemic steroids.

Treatment

Because of the severity of this disease, and the difficulty in controlling it, patients should be treated by a dermatologist. Huge doses of systemic steroids, such as prednisolone (Formulary, p. 304) 80–320 mg/day, may be needed at first, and the dose is dropped only when new blisters stop appearing. Immuno-suppressive agents, such as azathioprine and cyclophosphamide, are often used as steroid-sparing agents. Intramuscular or oral gold can also help. Treatment and regular follow-up is usually prolonged.

LEARNING POINT
Pemphigus is more attacking than pemphigoid and needs higher doses of steroids to control it.

Subepidermal bullous diseases

Pemphigoid (bullous pemphigoid)

Cause

Pemphigoid is also an autoimmune disease. IgG antibodies bind to bind to bullous pemphigoid antigen (molecular weight 230 kDa) in the lamina lucida (p. 18) where they activate complement (Fig. 11.5). Serum from about 70% of patients contains antibodies which bind *in vitro* to normal skin at the basement membrane zone. The titre does not correlate with clinical disease activity. The blister is formed by enzymes released from inflammatory cells drawn to the area by chemotactic complement components.

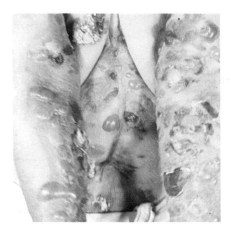

Fig. 11.6 Numerous large tense blisters in an elderly person suggest pemphigoid.

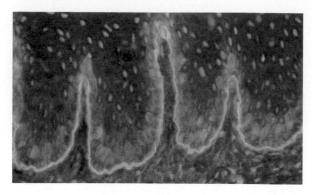

Fig. 11.7 Indirect immunofluorescence using serum from a patient with pemphigoid.

Presentation

Pemphigoid is a chronic, sometimes itchy, blistering disease of elderly patients. Many tense bullae arise from normal skin or from large urticarial plaques (Fig. 11.6). The flexures are often affected; the mucous membranes usually are not. The Nikolsky test is negative.

Course

Pemphigoid is usually self-limiting and treatment can often be stopped after one to two years.

Complications

Untreated, the disease causes much discomfort and the loss of fluid from ruptured bullae. Systemic steroids and immunosuppressive agents carry their usual complications if used for long (Formulary, p. 304 and p. 303 respectively).

Differential diagnosis

It may look like other bullous diseases, especially bullous lupus erythematosus, dermatitis herpetiformis, pemphigoid gestationis, bullous erythema multiforme, and linear IgA bullous disease. Immunofluorescence helps to separate it from these disorders (Fig. 11.5).

Investigations

The histology is that of a subepidermal blister, often filled with eosinophils. Direct immunofluorescence demonstrates a linear band of IgG and C3 along the basement membrane zone. Indirect immunofluorescence, using serum from the patient, identifies IgG antibodies which react with the basement membrane zone in 70% of patients (Fig. 11.7).

Treatment

In the acute phase, prednisolone or prednisone (Formulary, p. 304) at the dose of 40–60 mg/day is needed to control the eruption. Immunosuppressive agents may also be required. The doses are reduced as soon as possible, with the aim of ending up with a low maintenance dose of systemic steroids, taken on alternate days until treatment is stopped.

LEARNING POINTS
1 Death is uncommon and the disease is self-limiting.
2 Some old people get fatal side effects from their systemic steroids.

Pemphigoid gestationis (herpes gestationis)

This is pemphigoid occurring in pregnancy. As in pemphigoid, most patients have linear deposits of C3 along the basement membrane zone (Fig. 11.5), although IgG is detected less often. The condition usually remits after the birth but may return in future pregnancies. It is not caused by a herpes virus; the name herpes gestationis should be discarded so that the disease is not confused with herpes genitalis. Treatment is with systemic steroids. Oral contraceptives should be avoided.

Cicatricial pemphigoid

Like pemphigoid itself, cicatricial pemphigoid is an autoimmune skin disease characterized by deposition of IgG and C3 at the basement membrane zone (Fig. 11.5). It differs from pemphigoid as its blisters and ulcers occur mainly on mucous membranes such as the conjunctivae, the mouth and genital tract. Bullae on the skin itself are uncommon. Lesions heal with scarring; around the eyes this may cause blindness, especially when the palpebral conjunctivae are affected. Treatment is rather ineffective, but systemic steroids and immunosuppressive agents have been used. Good eye hygiene and the removal of ingrowing eyelashes are important.

Linear IgA bullous disease

This is similar to pemphigoid too, but affects children as well as adults. Blisters arise on urticarial plaques, and are more often grouped and on extensor surfaces than in pemphigoid. Children have most bullae near the groin. The conjunctivae may be involved. Linear IgA bullous disease is, as its name implies, associated with linear deposits of IgA and C3 at the basement membrane zone (Fig. 11.5). IgG is sometimes also found. The disorder responds well to oral dapsone (Formulary, p. 307).

Dermatitis herpetiformis

Dermatitis herpetiformis is a chronic, subepidermal, vesicular disease in which the vesicles erupt in groups as in herpes simplex.

Cause

Gluten-sensitive enteropathy, demonstrable by small bowel biopsy, is always present, but most patients do not suffer from diarrhoea, constipation, or malnutrition as this enteropathy is mild, patchy, and involves only the proximal small intestine. Absorption of gluten, or another dietary antigen, may form circulating immune complexes which lodge in the skin. Granular deposits of IgA and C3, in the superficial dermis underneath the basement membrane zone (Fig. 11.5), induce inflammation and separation of epidermis from dermis.

Presentation

The extremely itchy, grouped vesicles develop particularly over the elbows and knees, buttocks, and shoulders (Fig. 11.8). Often, before a vesicle reaches any size, it is broken by scratching. A typical patient, therefore, shows only grouped excoriations, sometimes with added eczematous changes from scratching (Fig. 11.9).

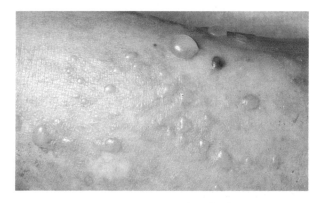

Fig. 11.8 The small, tense, grouped, itchy blisters of dermatitis herpetiformis.

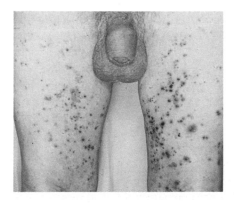

Fig. 11.9 The itchy blisters of dermatitis herpetiformis are quickly destroyed by scratching.

Course

The condition typically lasts for decades.

Complications

Treatment may cause side effects. The complications of gluten-sensitive enteropathy include diarrhoea, abdominal pain, and malabsorption; rarely, small bowel lymphomas have been reported.

Differential diagnosis

The disorder masquerades as scabies, an excoriated eczema, insect bites or neurodermatitis.

Investigations

If a vesicle can be biopsied before it is scratched away, its histology will be that of a subepidermal blister, with neutrophils packing the adjacent dermal papillae. Direct immunofluorescence of uninvolved skin shows granular deposits of IgA, and usually C3, in the dermal papillae and superficial dermis (Fig. 11.5). Small bowel biopsy is recommended as a routine by some centres but not by others unless bowel symptoms are present. The level of antibodies to the endomysium of muscle can be used to monitor severity of the enteropathy as it heals with gluten restriction.

Treatment

The disorder responds to a gluten-free diet: the bowel reverts quickly to normal but the IgA deposits remain in the skin, and the skin disease drags on for many months. Because of this, and because a gluten-free diet is hard to follow and enjoy, many patients prefer to take dapsone (Formulary, p. 307) or sulpha-pyridine. Both can cause severe rashes, haemolytic anaemia, leucopenia, thrombocytopenia, methaemo-globinaemia, and peripheral neuropathy. Regular blood checks are therefore necessary.

Bullous erythema multiforme

Bullous erythema multiforme in the form of Stevens–Johnson syndrome is discussed in Chapter 10.

LEARNING POINTS
*1 Biopsy **non**-involved skin to demonstrate the diagnostic granular deposits of IgA in the dermal papillae.*
2 The gluten enteropathy of dermatitis herpeti-formis seldom causes frank malabsorption.
3 Dapsone works quickly and a gluten-free diet only very slowly. Combine the two at the start and slowly reduce the dapsone.

Toxic epidermal necrolysis (Lyell's disease)

Cause

Toxic epidermal necrolysis is usually due to drug hypersensitivity or toxicity (Chapter 23), but can also be a manifestation of graft-versus-host disease. Sometimes it is unexplained.

Presentation

The skin becomes red and intensely painful, and then begins to come off in sheets like a scald. This leaves an eroded, painful, glistening surface. Nikol-sky's sign is positive (p. 118). The mucous membranes may be affected, including the mouth, eyes, and even the bronchial tree.

Course

The condition usually clears if the offending drug is stopped. New epidermis grows out from hair follicles so that skin grafts are not usually needed. The disorder may come back if the drug is taken again.

Complications

Toxic epidermal necrolysis is a skin emergency and may be fatal. Infection, and the loss of fluids and electrolytes, are life-threatening, and the painful denuded skin surfaces make life a misery.

Differential diagnosis

The epidermolysis in the staphylococcal scalded skin syndrome (p. 163), looks like toxic epidermal necrolysis, but in it only the stratum corneum comes off. Whereas toxic epidermal necrolysis affects adults, the staphylococcal scalded skin syndrome is seen in infancy or early childhood. Histology differentiates the two. Pemphigus may also look similar, but starts more slowly and is more localized. Severe graft-versus-host reactions can also cause this syndrome. Some believe that toxic epidermal necrolysis can evolve from Stevens—Johnson syndrome because some patients have the clinical features of both.

Investigations

Biopsy helps to confirm the diagnosis. The split is subepidermal in toxic epidermal necrolysis, and the entire epidermis may be necrotic. A frozen section may provide a quick answer if there is genuine difficulty in separating toxic epidermal necrolysis from the scalded skin syndrome (p. 163). There are no tests to tell which drug, if any, caused the disease.

Treatment

If toxic epidermal necrolysis is caused by a drug, this must be stopped (Chapter 23). Intensive nursing care and medical support are necessary, including the use of central venous lines, intravenous fluids, and electrolytes. Many patients are treated in units designed to deal with extensive thermal burns. Air suspension beds may increase comfort. The decision to use systemic steroids is becoming controversial, but if they are given it should be for short periods, at the start.

Porphyria cutanea tarda (p. 251)

The bullae and erosions occur on the backs of the hands and on other areas exposed to sunlight.

Epidermolysis bullosa (Chapter 22)

The conditions known as epidermolysis bullosa are inherited diseases, present from birth. There are many forms, but the most severe are due to abnormalities of the structures anchoring the epidermis to the dermis. Poor anchoring allows blisters to develop too easily at sites of trauma.

Epidermolysis bullosa acquisita

In contrast to inherited epidermolysis bullosa, this affects adults. As in pemphigoid, linear deposits of IgG are found at the basement membrane zone, but unlike those of pemphigoid, bullae tend to occur on otherwise normal skin at the site of the trauma (Fig. 11.5). When inflamed plaques are also present the disease may resemble pemphigoid. However, the IgG in patients binds to the anchoring fibrils attached to the lamina densa (see Fig. 2.13). Treatment is unsatisfactory.

Bullous lupus erythematosus

Vesicles and bullae may be seen in severe active systemic lupus erythematosus (p. 124). This disorder is uncommon and carries a high risk of kidney disease. Non-cutaneous manifestations of systemic lupus erythematosus do not respond to dapsone; the bullae, however, do.

CHAPTER 12

Connective tissue disorders

The cardinal feature of these conditions is inflammation in the connective tissue which leads to dermal atrophy or sclerosis, to arthritis, and sometimes to abnormalities in other organs. In addition, antibodies form against normal tissues and cellular components; these disorders are therefore classed as autoimmune. Many have difficulty in remembering which antibody features in which condition: Table 12.1 should help here.

The main connective tissue disorders present as a spectrum ranging from the benign cutaneous variants to severe multisystem diseases (Table 12.2).

Lupus erythematosus

Lupus erythematosus (LE) is a good example of this spectrum, ranging from the purely cutaneous type (discoid LE), through patterns associated with some internal problems (disseminated discoid LE and subacute cutaneous LE), to a severe, multisystem disease (systemic LE) (Table 12.2).

Acute systemic lupus erythematosus

Cause

This is unknown, but hereditary factors, for example complement deficiency, increase susceptibility. Particles looking like viruses have been seen in endothelial cells, and in other tissues, but their role is not clear. Patients with LE have auto-antibodies to DNA, nuclear proteins, and to other normal antigens, and this points to an autoimmune cause.

Presentation

The classic rash of acute systemic LE is an erythema of the cheeks and nose in the rough shape of a butterfly (Figs 12.1 & 12.2). Typically this appears suddenly, with facial swelling. Skin lesions may also be seen in other areas. Some patients develop widespread discoid papulosquamous plaques very like those of discoid LE; others have no skin disease at all.

Other features include peri-ungual telangiectasia (see Fig. 12.7), erythema over the digits, hair fall (especially at the frontal margin of the scalp), and photosensitivity. Severe sunburn may trigger the skin disease and worsen the systemic disease. Mouth ulcers may occur.

Course

The skin changes may be transient, continuous, or recurrent; they correlate well with the activity of the systemic disease. Acute systemic LE may be associated with fever, nephritis, polyarteritis, leucopenia, pleurisy, pneumonitis, pericarditis, myocarditis, and involvement of the central nervous system. Internal involvement may be fatal.

Complications

The skin disease may cause scarring or hyperpigmentation, but the main dangers lie with damage to other organs and the side effects of treatment, especially systemic steroids.

Differential diagnosis

Systemic LE is a great imitator. Its malar rash can be confused with sunburn, polymorphic light eruption, (p. 207), and rosacea (p. 156). The discoid lesions are distinctive, but are also seen in discoid LE and in subacute cutaneous LE. Occasionally they look like psoriasis (p. 55). The hair fall suggests telogen effluvium (p. 77). Plaques on the scalp may cause a

Table 12.1 Some important associations with non-organ specific autoantibodies

Antibody directed against	Nucleoprotein (ANA or ANF) (IF pattern in brackets)	Double stranded DNA	Ro (SSA) and La (SSB)	Sm (ENA)	Cardiolipin	Nuclear RNP	Centromere	Histones	Jo-1	Topoisomerase (Scl-70)
Discoid LE	+ive up to 35% (homogenous and speckled)		Rarely +ive							
Subacute LE	+ive up to 80% (homogenous and speckled)		+ive in 60%							
Systemic LE	+ive up to 100% (homogenous and speckled)	+ive in 50–70% (esp with nephritis)	May be +ive (e.g. 20%) if ANF –ive	+ive in 30%	+ive in subset with recurrent abortions, thrombosis, livedo and skin necrosis		+ive in 6%	+ive in drug-induced cases		
Dermatomyositis	Occasionally +ive (speckled)					Occasionally +ive			+ive in 20%	
Systemic sclerosis	+ive up to 90% (speckled and nucleolar)						+ive in up to 50%			+ive in 20%
Mixed connective tissue disorder	+ive in 100% (speckled)			+ive in high titre – up to 100%		High titre is diagnostic	+ive in 6%			

Table 12.2 Classification of connective tissue disease

Localized disease	Intermediate type	Aggressive multisystem disease
Discoid lupus erythematosus	Subacute lupus erythematosus	Systemic lupus erythematosus
	Juvenile dermatomyositis	Adult dermatomyositis
Morphoea	CREST syndrome	Systemic sclerosis

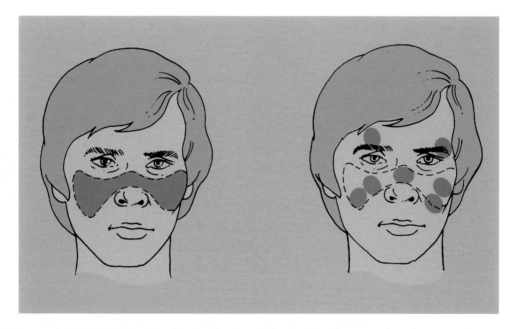

Fig. 12.1 In systemic LE (left) the eruption is often just an erythema, sometimes transient, but occupying most of the 'butterfly' area. In discoid LE (right) the fixed scaling and scarring plaques may occur in the butterfly area (dotted line), but can occur outside it too.

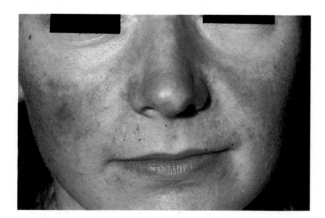

Fig. 12.2 Ill-defined erythema in the butterfly area is suggestive of systemic LE.

scaring alopecia. Systemic LE should be suspected when a characteristic rash is combined with fever, malaise, and internal disease (Table 12.3).

Investigations

Conduct a full physical examination, looking for internal disease. Biopsy of skin lesions is worthwhile because the pathology and immunopathology are distinctive. There is usually some thinning of the epidermis, a vacuolar degeneration of epidermal basal cells, and a mild perivascular mononuclear cell infiltrate. Direct immunofluorescence is helpful: IgG, IgM, IgA, and C3 are found individually or together in a band-like pattern at the dermo-epidermal junction of involved skin and often

Table 12.3 Criteria for the diagnosis of systemic LE (must have at least four)

> Malar rash
> Discoid plaques
> Photosensitivity
> Mouth ulcers
> Arthritis
> Serositis
> Renal disorder
> Neurological disorder
> Haematological disorder
> Immunological disorder
> Antinuclear antibodies (ANA)

Table 12.4 Investigations in systemic LE

Test	Usual findings
Skin biopsy	Degeneration of basal cells, cutaneous atrophy, inflammation around appendages
Skin immunofluorescence	Fibrillar or granular deposits of IgG, IgM, IgA and/or C3 alone in basement membrane zone
Haematology	Anaemia, raised ESR, thrombocytopenia, decreased white cell count
Immunology	Antinuclear antibody, antibodies to double-stranded DNA, false positive tests for syphilis, low total complement level, lupus anticoagulant factor
Urine analysis	Proteinuria or haematuria, often with casts if kidneys involved
Tests for function of other organs	As indicated by history, always test kidney and liver function

uninvolved skin as well. Relevant laboratory tests are listed in Table 12.4.

Treatment

Systemic steroids are the mainstay of treatment. Large doses of prednisolone (Formulary, p. 304) are needed to achieve control, as assessed by symptoms, signs, ESR, total complement level, and tests of organ function. The dose is then reduced to the smallest which suppresses the disease. Immunosuppressive agents, like azathioprine (Formulary,

p. 303) cyclophosphamide, and other drugs, may also be needed (e.g. antihypertensive therapy or anticonvulsants). Intermittent intravenous infusions of gamma globulin show promise. Long-term and regular follow-up is necessary.

LEARNING POINTS

1 Do not wait for the laboratory to confirm that your patient has severe systemic LE: use systemic steroids quickly if indicated by clinical findings.
2 Once committed to systemic steroids adjust their dose on clinical rather than laboratory grounds.

Subacute cutaneous lupus erythematosus

This is less severe than acute systemic LE, but is also often associated with systemic disease. Its cause is unknown, but probably involves an antibody dependent cellular cytotoxic attack on basal cells by K cells bridged by antibody to Ro (SSA) antigen (p. 26).

Presentation

The skin lesions are sharply marginated, scaling, psoriasiform plaques, sometimes annular, lying on the forehead, nose, cheeks, chest, hands, and extensor surfaces of the arms. They tend to be symmetrical and are hard to tell from discoid LE, or systemic LE with widespread discoid lesions. Patients with subacute cutaneous LE are often photosensitive.

Course

As in systemic LE, the course is prolonged. The skin lesions are slow to clear but, in contrast to discoid LE, do so with little or no scarring.

Complications

Systemic disease is frequent. Children born to mothers who have, or have had, this condition are liable to neonatal LE with transient, annular skin lesions and permanent heart block.

Differential diagnosis

The morphology is characteristic, but lesions can be mistaken for psoriasis or widespread discoid LE. Annular lesions may resemble tinea corporis (p. 186) or figurate erythemas (p. 137).

Investigations

Patients with subacute cutaneous LE should be evaluated in the same way as those with acute systemic LE, although deposits of immunoglobulins in the skin and antinuclear antibodies in serum are present less often. Many have antibodies to the cytoplasmic antigen Ro (SSA).

Treatment

Subacute cutaneous LE does better with anti-malarials, such as hydroxychloroquine (Formulary, p. 307), than acute systemic LE. Systemic steroids may be needed too.

Discoid lupus erythematosus

Patients with discoid LE may have one or two plaques only, or many in several areas. The cause is also unknown but UVR is one factor.

Presentation

Plaques show erythema, scaling, follicular plugging (like a nutmeg grater), scarring and atrophy, tel-angiectasia, hypopigmentation, and a peripheral zone of hyperpigmentation. They are well demarcated and lie mostly on sun-exposed skin, of the scalp, face and ears (Figs 12.1 & 12.3).

Course

The disease may spread relentlessly. Scarring is common and hair may be lost permanently if there is scarring in the scalp (Fig. 12.4). Whiteness remains after the inflammation has cleared. It rarely pro-gresses to systemic LE.

Differential diagnosis

Psoriasis is hard to tell from discoid LE when plaques

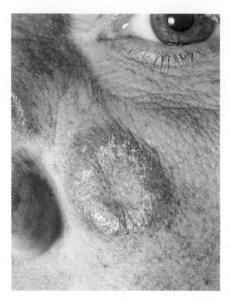

Fig. 12.3 Red, scaly, fixed plaques of discoid LE. This degree of scaling is not uncommon in the active stage.

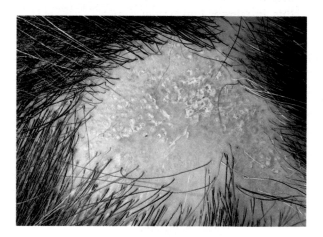

Fig. 12.4 Discoid LE of the scalp leading to permanent hair loss. Note the marked follicular plugging.

first arise but has larger, thicker scales, and later it is usually symmetrical (elbows, knees, scalp, and sacrum). Discoid LE is more common on the face and ears, and in sun-exposed areas. Discoid LE is far more prone than psoriasis to cause hair loss.

Investigations

Most patients with discoid LE remain well. However, screening for systemic LE and internal disease is still worthwhile. A skin biopsy for pathological examination is most helpful if taken from an untreated plaque where appendages are still present (Fig. 12.5). Direct immunofluorescence shows deposits of IgG, IgM, IgA, and C3 at the basement membrane zone of skin. Biopsies for direct immunofluorescence are best taken from older, untreated plaques. Blood tests are usually normal but occasionally serum contains antinuclear antibodies (Table 12.5).

Treatment

Discoid LE needs potent or very potent topical corticosteroids (Formulary, p. 290). In discoid LE, these can even be used on the face, because the risk of scarring is worse than that of atrophy. Topical steroids should be applied twice daily until the lesions disappear or side effects, such as atrophy, develop; weaker preparations can then be used for maintenance. If discoid LE does not respond to this, intralesional injections of triamcinolone (2.5– 5 mg/ml) may help. Stubborn and widespread lesions often do well with oral antimalarials such as hydroxychloroquine (Formulary, p. 307), but rarely these cause irreversible eye damage. The eyes should

Table 12.5 Some factors distinguishing the different types of LE

| | Antinuclear antibodies | Anti Ro (SSA) antibodies | |
		Sun sensitivity	Internal organ involvement
Systemic LE	++++	+++	++
Subacute LE	+	++++	+
Discoid LE	+/−	+	−

therefore be tested before and at intervals during treatment. Sun avoidance and screens are also important.

Dermatomyositis

Dermatomyositis is a subset of polymyositis with distinctive skin changes. When starting after the age of 40, it may signal an internal malignancy.

Presentation

Typical patients have a faint, heliotrope discoloration around their eyes. The lilac colour of the

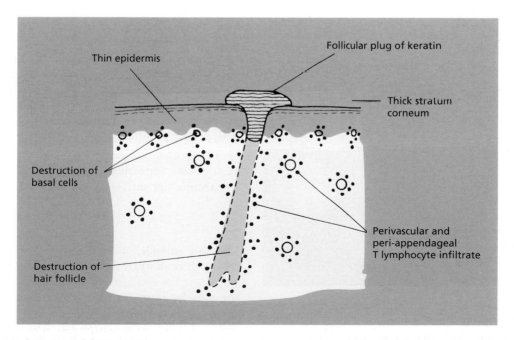

Fig. 12.5 The histology of discoid LE.

heliotrope flower is unique. Some also develop lilac, slightly atrophic papules over the knuckles of their fingers (Gottron's papules), and streaks of erythema over the extensor tendons of the hand. Malar erythema and oedema (Fig. 12.6), peri-ungual telangiectasia (Fig. 12.7), a peculiar mixture of hypo- and hyperpigmentation on light-exposed areas, and the signs of mixed connective tissue disease (see below) may complete the picture.

Course

Many, but not all, patients have weakness of proximal muscles. Climbing stairs, getting up from chairs and combing the hair become difficult. In children the disorder is often self-limiting, but in adults it may be prolonged and progressive. Raynaud's phenomenon, arthralgia, dysphagia, and calcinosis may follow.

Complications

Myositis may lead to permanent weakness and immobility, and inflammation to contractures or cutaneous calcinosis. Some die from their severe myopathy.

Differential diagnosis

Other connective tissue disorders may look similar, particularly mixed connective tissue disease and systemic LE. In LE, finger lesions favour the skin between the knuckles whereas in dermatomyositis the knuckles are preferred. Toxoplasmosis may cause a dermatomyositis-like syndrome. Myopathy may be a side effect of systemic steroids so weakness is not always due to the disease itself.

Investigations

About 30% of adults with dermatomyositis also have an underlying malignancy. Their dermatomyositis coincides with the onset of the tumour and may improve if it is removed. Adult dermatomyositis or polymyositis therefore requires a search for such an underlying malignancy. The levels of muscle enzymes such as aldolase and creatinine phosphokinase (CPK) are often elevated. Electromyography (EMG) detects muscle abnormalities, and biopsy of an affected muscle shows inflammation and destruction. Surprisingly, the ESR is often normal and antinuclear antibodies are usually not detected.

Treatment

Systemic steroids, often in high doses (e.g. prednisolone (Formulary, p. 304) 60 mg/day for an average adult), are the cornerstone of treatment and protect the muscles from destruction. Immunosuppressive agents, such as azathioprine (Formulary, p. 303), also help to control the condition and to reduce the high steroid dose. The rash usually responds too. Main-

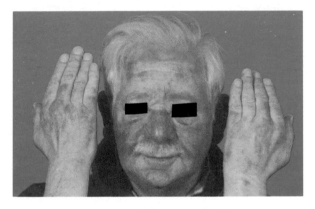

Fig. 12.6 Acute dermatomyositis: oedematous, purple face with erythematous streaks on the backs of the fingers. Severe progressive muscle weakness, but no underlying tumour was found.

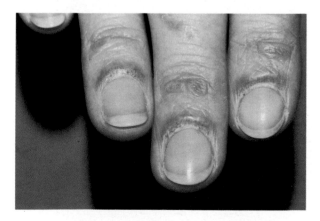

Fig. 12.7 Erythema and telangiectasia of the nail folds are important clues to systemic connective tissue disorders. This patient has dermatomyositis. Note Gottron's papules over the knuckles.

tenance treatment is adjusted according to clinical response and CPK level. As in SLE, intravenous gamma globulin infusions seem promising. Long-term and regular follow-up is necessary.

Systemic sclerosis

In this disorder the skin becomes hard as connective tissues thicken. Its cause is unknown. Changes like those of progressive systemic sclerosis affect workers exposed to polyvinyl chloride monomers or to severe chronic vibration, and are also seen in chronic graft-versus-host reactions after bone marrow transplants.

Presentation

Most patients suffer from Raynaud's phenomenon (p. 139) and sclerodactyly. Their fingers become immobile, hard, and shiny (Fig. 12.8). Some become hyperpigmented and itchy early in their disease. Peri-ungual telangiectasia is common (Fig. 12.7).

Course

As the disease progresses, sclerosis spreads to the face, scalp, and trunk. The nose becomes beak-like, and wrinkles radiate around the mouth (Figs 12.9–12.11). Most have abnormalities of the gut including dysphagia, oesophagitis, constipation, diarrhoea, and malabsorption. Fibrosis of the lungs leads to dyspnoea, and fibrosis of the heart to congestive failure. The kidneys are involved late, but this has a grave prognosis from malignant hypertension.

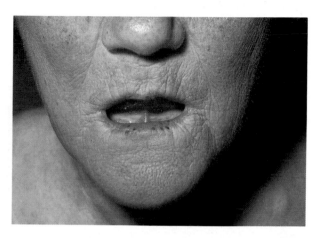

Fig. 12.9 Systemic sclerosis: radial furrowing around the mouth.

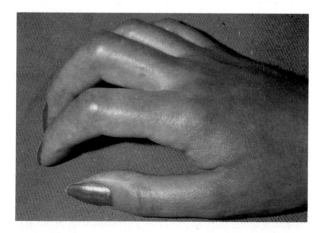

Fig. 12.8 Systemic sclerosis: note the claw deformity due to sclerodactyly.

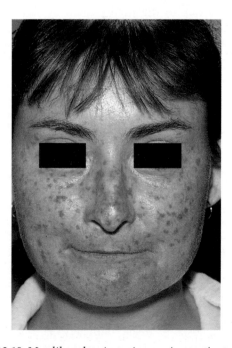

Fig. 12.10 Mat-like telangiectasia seen in a patient with systemic sclerosis.

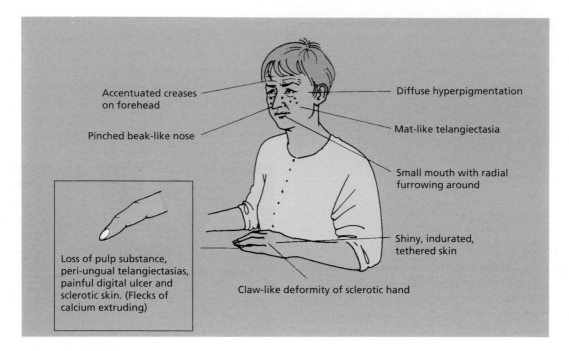

Fig. 12.11 Signs of systemic sclerosis.

Complications

Most are due to the involvement of organs other than the skin, but ulcers of the finger tips and calcinosis are distressing. Hard skin immobilizes the joints and leads to contractures (Fig. 12.8).

Differential diagnosis

Other causes of Raynaud's phenomenon are given in Table 13.5. The differential includes chilblains (p. 136) and erythromelalgia (p. 136). The sclerosis should be distinguished from that of porphyria cutanea tarda, mixed connective tissue disease, the results of exposure to polyvinyl chloride monomers, eosinophilic fasciitis, diabetic sclerodactyly, and an acute arthritis with swollen fingers. Rarely the disease is mimicked by progeria, scleromyxoedema, amyloidosis or carcinoid syndrome.

Investigations

The diagnosis is made clinically as histological abnormalities are seldom present until the physical signs are well established. Laboratory tests should include a fluorescent antinuclear antibody test and the evaluation of the heart, kidney, lungs, joints, and muscles. Barium studies are best avoided as obstruction may follow poor evacuation. Other contrast media are available. X-rays of the hands, measurement of muscle enzymes and immunoglobulin levels, and a blood count, ESR and test for the scleroderma-associated antibody Scl-70 are also worthwhile.

Treatment

This is unsatisfactory. The calcium channel blocker nifedipine may help Raynaud's phenomenon (p. 139). Systemic steroids, salicylates, and antimalarials are often used, but are not of proven value. D-penicillamine has many side effects, especially on renal function. Physiotherapy is helpful. Photopheresis is experimental.

CREST syndrome

This is a variant of systemic sclerosis with a relatively good prognosis associated often with serum antibodies to nuclear centromeres. The mnemonic stands for *C*alcinosis, *R*aynaud's phenomenon, *E*sophageal dysmotility, *S*clerodactyly, and *T*elangiectasia. Telangiectasia is peri-ungual on the fingers and flat, mat-like, or rectangular on the face. Many patients with this syndrome develop a diffuse, progressive, systemic sclerosis after months or years.

Eosinophilic fasciitis

Localized areas of skin become indurated, sometimes after an upper respiratory tract infection or prolonged, severe exercise. Hypergammaglobulinaemia and eosinophilia are present, and a deep skin biopsy, which includes muscle, shows that the fascia overlying the muscle is thickened. Despite its name, and despite a profound eosinophilia in the peripheral blood, the fascia is not eosinophilic or permeated by eosinophils. The disease responds promptly to systemic steroids; the prognosis is good.

Morphoea

Morphoea is a localized form of scleroderma with pale indurated plaques on the skin but no internal sclerosis (Fig. 12.12). Many plaques may be surrounded by a violaceous halo. Its prognosis is usually good and the fibrosis slowly clears leaving slight depression and hyperpigmentation. A rare type may lead to arrest of growth of the underlying bones causing, for example, facial hemi-atrophy or shortening of a limb.

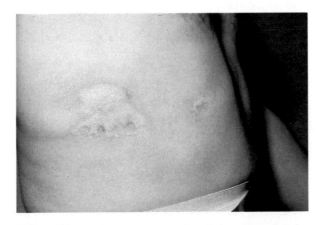

Fig. 12.12 Morphoea. Pale, indurated plaque on the chest; the scalloped lower margin is unusual.

Lichen sclerosus

Many think that this condition is related to morphoea with which it may co-exist. However, its patches are non-indurated, white shiny macules, sometimes with obvious plugging in the follicular openings. Women are affected far more often than men and, though any area of skin may be involved, the classical ivory-coloured lesions often surround the vulva and anus. Intractable itching is common in these areas and the development of vulval carcinoma is a risk. In men the condition may cause stenosis of the urethral meatus and adhesions between the fore-skin and glans of the penis.

Mixed connective tissue disease

This is an overlap between systemic LE and either scleroderma or polymyositis.

Presentation

As in LE, women are affected more often than men. Many develop swollen hands and sclerodactyly, and skin lesions like those of cutaneous LE may also be present. Alopecia is mild and the hair fall mimics telogen effluvium. Peri-ungual telangiectasia and pigmentary disturbances are common. About 25% of patients have a small vessel vasculitis with palpable purpura, leg ulcers, and painful dermal nodules on the hands or elbows. Many show Raynaud's phenomenon, arthritis, serositis, and myositis. Headaches, weakness, fatigue, lymph node enlargement, or hoarseness occur in about one in three patients; renal and CNS disease are less common.

Course

The disorder is chronic, and usually turns into either systemic LE or systemic sclerosis.

Differential diagnosis

The disorder can be confused with systemic LE, dermatomyositis, polymyositis, systemic sclerosis, and other sclerosing processes such as porphyria cutanea tarda (p. 251).

Investigations

Patients with mixed connective tissue disease have antibodies in high titre directed against one or more extractable nuclear antigens. These give a speckled pattern when serum is reacted against nuclei and detected by indirect immunofluorescence. Direct immunofluorescence of involved and uninvolved skin shows IgG within the epidermal nuclei, also in a speckled pattern. Only a third of patients have subepidermal immunoglobulin deposits in involved skin. Most have hypergammaglobulinaemia, a high ESR, oesophageal dysmotility, abnormal pulmonary function tests, and a positive rheumatoid factor. Hypocomplementaemia, leucopenia, anaemia, cryoglobulinaemia, and false positive biological tests for syphilis occur in a few patients.

Treatment

Treatment depends upon which organs are involved, but systemic steroids are usually needed, in the same dosages as for systemic LE. Immunosuppressive agents reduce the dose of systemic steroids, and non-steroidal anti-inflammatory agents help with arthralgia, myalgia, and swelling of the hands.

Other connective tissue diseases

Rheumatoid arthritis

Most patients with rheumatoid arthritis have no skin disease, but some have tiny finger tip infarcts, purpura, ulcers, palmar or peri-ungual erythema, or pyoderma gangrenosum. The commonest skin manifestations are marble-like nodules near joints. These are always associated with the presence of rheumatoid factor. Some patients with rheumatoid arthritis have a vasculitis of larger blood vessels with deep 'pinched out' ulcers on the legs (see Fig. 13.11).

Reiter's syndrome

Reiter's syndrome, precipitated by non-specific urethritis or dysentery, combines skin lesions, arthropathy, conjunctivitis, balanitis, mucositis, and spondylitis. Arthritis is the most severe element. The skin lesions (keratoderma blenorrhagicum) are psoriasis-like, red, scaling plaques, often studded with vesicles and pustules, seen most often on the feet. The toes are red and swollen, and the nails thicken. Psoriasiform plaques may also occur on the penis and scrotum, with redness near the penile meatus. Topical steroids and systemic non-steroidal anti-inflammatory drugs help, but many patients need methotrexate (Formulary, p. 304) or systemic steroids too.

Relapsing polychondritis

This process can affect any cartilage as the disorder is apparently caused by autoimmunity to collagen. The ears are the usual target. The overlying skin becomes red, swollen, and tender. The cartilage in joints, the nose, and the tracheobronchial tree may be involved, so that patients develop floppy ears, a saddle nose, hoarseness, stridor, and respiratory insufficiency. Aortic aneurysms are also seen. Treatment is with systemic steroids and non-steroidal anti-inflammatory drugs. Tracheostomy may be necessary.

Behçet's syndrome

Behçet's syndrome is uncommon and its cause is not known.

Presentation

The two main components are mouth ulcers (often multiple, large and persistent) and genital ulcers, but extracutaneous manifestations are also important. In the eye, hypopyon is characteristic, with anterior and posterior uveitis. Arthritis, meningoencephalitis, vasculitis, and intestinal ulceration may also be features. Other skin lesions include erythema nodosum, superficial thrombophlebitis, and pustules or ulcers at sites of trauma, such as venepuncture (pathergy).

Course

The course is long but the mucocutaneous lesions have a good prognosis.

Complications

Death, blindness, and neurological damage may occur.

Differential diagnosis

The disorder is difficult to diagnose when the full syndrome is not present. Mouth ulcers must be distinguished from aphthae, the ulcers of bullous diseases and nutritional deficiency.

Treatment

It may be treated symptomatically or with systemic steroids or oral colchicine. Immunosuppressive agents including cyclophosphamide, azathioprine, and chlorambucil have also been tried.

Polyarteritis nodosa

This is discussed in Chapter 10 but is considered by some to be a connective tissue disorder.

Panniculitis

Panniculitis is an inflammation of the subcutaneous fat: it includes a number of diseases with different causes but a similar appearance. Some are listed in Table 12.6.

Presentation

Most patients have tender, ill-defined, red, nodules on the lower legs, thighs, and buttocks.

Course

This depends upon the cause. Migratory thrombophlebitis may be associated with underlying

Table 12.6 Causes of panniculitis

Erythema nodosum (p. 111)
Erythema nodosum leprosum (leprosy)
Nodular vasculitis (p. 112)
Weber–Christian type (unknown cause)
Polyarteritis nodosa (p. 114)
Associated with pancreatitis
Associated with systemic LE (lupus profundus)
Cold-induced
Withdrawal of systemic steroids
Superficial thrombophlebitis
Deficiency of α_1-antitrypsin
Factitial (e.g. from injection of milk)

malignancy. In lupus profundus, a panniculitis is associated with discoid or systemic LE. Causes of erythema nodosum are discussed in Chapter 10. Erythema induratum may be caused by tuberculosis. Erythema nodosum leprosum is a reactional state in leprosy. Patients with pancreatitis may liberate enough lipase into the systemic circulation to cause fat in the skin to liquefy and discharge through the overlying skin. The Weber–Christian variant is associated with fever, but its cause is unknown.

Investigations

The type of panniculitis can sometimes be identified by skin biopsy, which must include subcutaneous fat. A complete blood count, ESR, chest X-ray, serum lipase, serum α_1-antitrypsin and tests for antinuclear antibodies are needed.

Treatment

This depends upon the cause. Rest, elevation of affected extremities, and local heat often help symptoms. Non-steroidal anti-inflammatory agents may also bring help in the absence of specific therapy.

CHAPTER 13

Disorders of blood vessels and lymphatics

This chapter includes only those diseases in which the primary abnormality is in a blood or lymphatic vessel. In functional disease, abnormalities of flow are reversible, and there is no vessel wall damage, e.g. in urticaria (discussed in Chapter 10). The diseases of structure include the many types of vasculitis, some of which, with an immunological basis, are also covered in Chapter 10. For convenience, disorders of the blood vessels are grouped according to the size and type of the vessels affected.

Disorders involving small blood vessels

Acrocyanosis

This type of 'poor circulation', often familial, is more common in females than males. The hands, feet, nose, ears, and cheeks become blue-red and cold. The palms are often cold and clammy. The condition is due to arteriolar constriction dilatation of the subpapillary venous plexus, and to cold-induced increases in blood viscosity. The best answer is warm clothes and avoidance of cold.

Erythrocyanosis

This occurs in fat, often young, women. Purple-red mottled discoloration is seen over the buttocks, thighs, and lower legs. Cold provokes it and causes an unpleasant burning sensation. An area of acrocyanosis or erythrocyanosis may be the site where other disorders will settle in the future, e.g. perniosis, erythema induratum, lupus erythematosus, sarcoidosis, cutaneous tuberculosis, and leprosy.

Perniosis (chilblains)

In this common, sometimes familial, condition, inflamed purple-pink swellings appear on the fingers, toes, and rarely ears (Fig. 13.1). They arrive with winter and are induced by cold. They are painful, and itchy or burning on rewarming. Occasionally they ulcerate. Chilblains are due to a combination of arteriolar and venular constriction, the latter predominating on rewarming with exudation of fluid into the tissues. Warm housing and clothing help. Topical remedies rarely work, but oral nifedipidine may be useful (p. 139). The blood pressure should be monitored at the start of treatment and at return visits. Nicotinamide (500 mg three times daily) may be helpful alone or in addition to calcium channel blockers. Sympathectomy may be advised in severe cases.

Erythromelalgia

This is a rare condition in which the hands become red, hot, and painful when they or their owner are exposed to heat. The condition may be idiopathic,

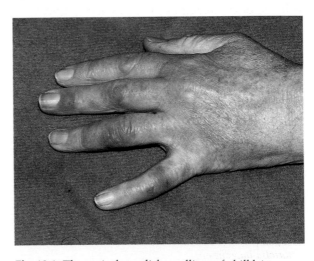

Fig. 13.1 The typical purplish swellings of chilblains.

or due to a myeloproliferative disease (e.g. poly-cythaemia rubra vera or thrombocythaemia), lupus erythematosus, rheumatoid arthritis, diabetes, or hypertension. Small doses of aspirin give sympto-matic relief.

Erythema

Erythema accompanies all inflammatory skin con-ditions. Discrete areas of erythema without scaling are seen in some bacterial and viral infections, and when erythema is associated with oedema ('urticated erythema') it becomes palpable. Drugs (Chapter 23) are another common cause. If no cause is obvious, the rash is often called a 'toxic' or 'reactive' erythema (Table 13.1).

Figurate erythemas

These are chronic eruptions, made up of bizarre serpiginous and erythematous rings. In the past most carried Latin labels; happily, the eruptions are now grouped under the general term of 'figurate erythemas'. Underlying malignancy, a connective tissue disorder, a bacterial, fungal, or yeast infection, worm infestation, drug sensitivity, and rheumatic heart disease should be excluded, but usually the cause remains obscure.

Palmar erythema

This may be an isolated finding in a normal person or be familial. Sometimes it is seen in pregnancy,

Table 13.1 Classification of erythemas

Widespread

Due to infection (bacterial or viral)
Drug reactions
Connective tissue diseases
Underlying malignancy (e.g. figurate erythema)
Idiopathic

Localized

Pregnancy, liver disease, rheumatoid arthritis (causing palmar erythema)
Drug reaction (fixed drug eruption)
Infection (e.g. erythema chronicum migrans due to *Borrelia burgdorferi*)

liver disease or rheumatoid arthritis. Often associ-ated with spider telangiectases (see below), it may be due to increased circulating oestrogens.

Erythema migrans (p. 168)

These annular erythematous lesions are usually solitary, and occur most often on exposed skin after a tick bite. They expand slowly and may become very large.

Telangiectases

This term refers to permanently dilated and visible small vessels in the skin. They appear as linear, punctate or stellate, crimson-purple markings. The common causes are given in Table 13.2.

Spider naevi

These stellate telangiectases do look rather like spiders, with legs radiating from a central, often palpable, feeding vessel. They are seen frequently on the faces of normal children, and may erupt in pregnancy or be the presenting sign of liver disease, with many lesions on the upper trunk. Liver func-tion should be checked in those with many spider naevi. The central vessel can be destroyed by electro-desiccation without local anaesthesia or with a pulsed tunable dye laser (p. 285).

Livedo reticularis

This cyanosis of the skin is net-like or marbled and due to stasis in the capillaries furthest from their arterial supply, i.e. at the periphery of the inverted cone supplied by a dermal arteriole (see Fig. 2.15). 'Cutis marmorata' is the name given to the mottled skin seen in many normal children. It is physiologi-cal and disappears on warming, whereas true livedo reticularis remains.

The causes of livedo reticularis are listed in Table 13.3. Livedo vasculitis and cutaneous polyarteritis are forms of vasculitis associated with livedo reticu-laris (Chapter 10). Some patients with an apparently idiopathic livedo reticularis develop progressive disease in peripheral, cerebral, coronary and renal arteries. Others, usually women, have multiple thrombotic episodes accompanying livedo reticu-

Table 13.2 Causes of telangiectasia

Primary telangiectasia

Hereditary haemorrhagic telangiectasia	Autosomal dominant Nose and GI bleeds Lesions on face
Ataxia telangiectasia	Autosomal recessive Telangiectases develop between the ages of three and five years Cerebellar ataxia Recurrent respiratory infections Immunological abnormalities
Generalized essential telangiectasia	Runs benign course No other associations
Unilateral naevoid telangiectasia	May occur in pregnancy or in females on oral contraceptive

Secondary telangiectasia

Atrophy	Seen on exposed skin of elderly, after topical steroid applications, after X-irradiation and with poikiloderma
Connective tissue disorders	Always worth inspecting nail folds. Mat-like on the face in systemic sclerosis
Prolonged vasodilatation	For example, with rosacea and with venous hypertension
Mastocytosis	Accompanying a rare and diffuse variant
Liver disease	Spider telangiectases are common
Drugs	Nifedipine

Table 13.3 Causes of livedo reticularis

Physiological	Cutis marmorata
Vessel wall disease	Atherosclerosis Connective tissue disorders (especially polyarteritis and systemic LE) Syphilis Tuberculosis
Hyperviscosity states	Polycythaemia/thrombo-cythaemia Macroglobulinaemia
Cryopathies	Cryoglobulinaemia Cold agglutininaemia
Autoimmune	Antiphospholipid syndrome
Congenital	
Idiopathic	

laris. The presence of antiphospholipid antibodies (including anticardiolipin antibody and lupus anti-coagulant) helps to identify this group with the antiphospholipid syndrome.

Erythema ab igne

The appearance of this disorder is also determined by the underlying vascular network. Its reticulate, pigmented erythema, with variable scaling, is due to damage from long-term exposure to local heat — usually from an open fire, hot water bottle, or heating pad (Fig. 13.2). If on one side of the leg it gives a clue to the side of the fire on which granny likes to sit. The condition is common in northern Europe ('tinker's tartan'), but rare in the USA, where central heating is the rule.

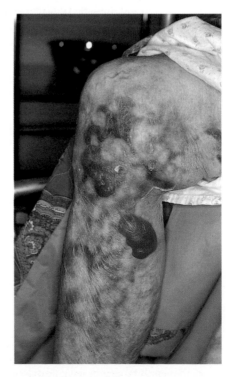

Fig. 13.2 Erythema ab igne: this patient persisted in sitting too close to an open fire and burned herself.

Flushing

This transient vasodilatation of the face may spread to the neck, upper chest and, more rarely, other parts of the body. There is no sharp distinction between flushing and blushing apart from the emotional provocation of the latter. The mechanism varies with the many causes which are listed in Table 13.4. Paroxysmal flushing ('hot flushes'), common at the menopause, is associated with the pulsatile release of luteinizing hormone from the pituitary, as a consequence of low circulating oestrogens and failure of normal negative feedback. However, luteinizing hormone itself cannot be responsible for flushing as this can occur after hypophysectomy. It is possible that menopausal flushing is mediated by central mechanisms involving encephalins. Hot flushes can usually be helped by oestrogen replacement.

Alcohol-induced flushing is most commonly seen in Orientals. Ethanol is broken down to acetaldehyde by alcohol dehydrogenase and acetaldehyde metabolised to acetic acid by aldehyde dehydrogenase (Fig. 13.3). Acetaldehyde accumulation is in part responsible for flushing. Orientals not only may have a high activity variant of alcohol dehydrogenase but also defective aldehyde dehydrogenase. Disulfuram (Antabuse) and, to a lesser extent, chlorpropamide inhibit aldehyde dehydrogenase so that some individuals taking these drugs may flush.

Table 13.4 Causes of flushing

Physiological	Emotional Menopausal
Foods	Hot drinks Spicy foods Additives (monosodium glutamate) Alcohol (especially in Orientals)
Drugs	Vasodilators including nicotinic acid Bromocriptine Calcium channel blockers including nifedipine Chlorpropamide + alcohol (diabetics)

Pathological	Rosacea (p. 156)
	Carcinoid tumours — with asthma and
	    diarrhoea
	Phaeochromocytoma (type producing
	    adrenaline) — with episodic headaches
	    (due to transient hypertension) and
	    palpitations

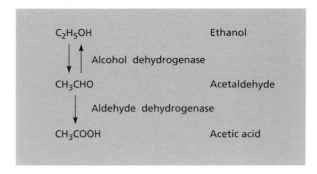

Fig. 13.3 The metabolism of ethanol.

Arterial disease

Raynaud's phenomenon

This is a paroxysmal pallor of the digits provoked by cold or, rarely, emotional stress. At first the top of one or more fingers becomes white. A few minutes later a painful cyanosis appears and the area turns red before the hands return to their normal colour. In severe disease the fingers lose pulp substance, ulcerate, or become gangrenous. Some causes are listed in Table 13.5. Raynaud's disease, often familial, is the name given when no cause can be found. However, some patients with what seems to be Raynaud's disease will later develop a connective tissue disease.

The main treatment is to protect the vulnerable digits from cold. Smoking should be banned. Calcium channel blockers (e.g. nifedipine 10–30 mg three times daily) are the most effective agents though they appear to be most beneficial in patients with primary Raynaud's disease. Patients should be warned about dizziness due to postural hypotension. Initially it is worth giving nifedipine as a 5 mg test dose with monitoring of the blood pressure in the clinic. If this is tolerated satisfactorily the starting dose should be 5 mg daily increasing by 5 mg every five days until a therapeutic dose is achieved (e.g. 5–20 mg three times daily) or until intolerable side effects occur. The blood pressure should be monitored before each incremental increase in the dose. Diltiazem (30–60 mg three times daily) is less effective than nifedipine but has fewer side effects. Systemic vasodilators

Table 13.5 Causes of Raynaud's phenomenon

Familial	Raynaud's disease
Connective tissue diseases	Systemic sclerosis Lupus erythematosus Mixed connective tissue disease
Arterial occlusion	Thoracic outlet syndrome Atherosclerosis Endarteritis obliterans

Repeated trauma	Pneumatic hammer/drill
	  operators ('vibration
	  white finger')

Hyperviscosity	Polycythaemia Macroglobulinaemia
Cryopathies	Cryoglobulinaemia Cryofibrinogenaemia Cold agglutinaemia
Neurological disease	Peripheral neuropathy Syringomyelia
Toxins	Ergot Vinyl-chloride

such as naftidrofuryl oxalate, nicotinic acid and thymoxamine are also worth trying. Glycerol trinitrate ointment, applied once daily may reduce the severity and frequency of attacks and may allow reduction in the dose of calcium channel blockers and vasodilators. Infusions with reserpine or prostacyclin help some severe cases though occasionally sympathectomy is needed.

Polyarteritis nodosa

This is discussed in Chapter 10.

Temporal arteritis

Here the brunt is borne by the larger vessels of the head and neck. The condition affects elderly people and may be associated with polymyalgia rheumatica. The classical site is the temporal arteries which become tender and pulseless, in association with severe headaches. Rarely necrotic ulcers appear on the scalp. Blindness may follow if the ophthalmic arteries are involved, and to reduce this risk systemic steroids should be given as soon as the diagnosis has

been made. In active phases the ESR is high and its level can be used to guide treatment, which is often prolonged.

Atherosclerosis

This occlusive disease, most common in the developed countries, will not be discussed in detail here but involvement of the large arteries of the legs is of concern to dermatologists. It may cause intermittent claudication, nocturnal cramp, ulcers or gangrene. These may develop slowly over the years, or within minutes if a thrombus forms on an atheromatous plaque. The feet are cold and pale, the skin is often atrophic, with little hair, and peripheral pulses are diminished or absent.

Investigations should include urine testing to exclude diabetes mellitus. Fasting plasma lipids (cholesterol, triglycerides and lipoproteins) should be checked in the young, especially if there is a family history of vascular disease. Doppler ultrasound measurements help to distinguish atherosclerotic from venous leg ulcers in the elderly (p. 146). Complete assessment is best carried out by a specialist in peripheral vascular disease or a vascular surgeon.

Arterial emboli

Emboli may lodge in arteries supplying the skin and cause gangrene, ulcers or necrotic papules, depending on the size of the vessel obstructed. Causes include dislodged thrombi (usually from areas of atherosclerosis), fat emboli (after major trauma), infected emboli (e.g. gonococcal septicaemia, or subacute bacterial endocarditis) and tumour emboli.

Pressure sores

Sustained or repeated pressure on skin over bony prominences may cause ischaemia and pressure sores. These are common in patients over 70 years old who are confined to hospital, especially those with a fractured neck or femur. The morbidity and mortality of those with deep ulcers is high.

Cause

The main factors responsible for pressure sores are:

1 Prolonged immobility and recumbency e.g. due to paraplegia, arthritis or apathy.
2 Vascular disease e.g. atherosclerosis.
3 Neurological disease causing diminished sensation.
4 Malnutrition, severe systemic disease and general debility.

Clinical features

The sore begins as a local area of erythema which progresses to a superficial blister or erosion. If pressure continues, deeper damage occurs with the development of a black eschar which, when removed or shed, reveals a deep ulcer, often colonized by pseudomonas aeruginosa. The skin overlying the sacrum, greater trochanter, ischial tuberosity, tuberosity of calcaneus and lateral malleolus is especially susceptible.

Management

The following are important:
1 Prevention by regular turning of recumbent patients and the use of anti-pressure mattresses in susceptible patients.
2 Treatment of malnutrition and the general condition.
3 Debridement. Regular cleansing with normal saline or 0.5% aqueous silver nitrate. Antibacterial preparations locally. Absorbent dressings (see Formulary, p. 296). Semipermeable dressings such as Opsite. Appropriate systemic antibiotic if spreading infection.
4 Plastic surgical reconstruction may be indicated in the young when the ulcer is clean.

Venous disease

Deep vein thrombosis

The common causes are listed in Table 13.6.

The onset may be 'silent' or heralded by pain in the calf, often about 10 days after immobilization for surgery, parturition or an infection. The leg becomes swollen and cyanotic distal to the thrombus. The calf may hurt when handled or if the foot is dorsiflexed (Homan's sign). Sometimes a pulmonary

Table 13.6 Some causes of deep vein thrombosis

Abnormalities of the vein wall	Trauma (operations and injuries)
	Chemicals (intravenous infusions)
	Neighbouring infection (e.g. in leg ulcer)
	Tumour (local invasion)
Abnormalities of blood flow	Stasis (immobility, pressure, pregnancy, heart failure, incompetent valves)
	Impaired venous return
Abnormalities of clotting	Platelets increased or sticky (thrombocythaemia, polycythaemia vera, leukaemia, trauma, splenectomy)
	Decreased fibrinolysis (postoperative)
	Alteration in clotting factors (infection, leukaemia, pregnancy, shock and haemorrhage)
Unknown mechanisms	Malignancy (thrombophlebitis migrans)
	Smoking
	Behçet's syndrome

embolus is the first sign of a silent deep vein thrombosis.

Suitable investigations include Doppler ultrasonography, ^{125}I-fibrinogen isotope leg-scanning, and, rarely, venography.

Treatment is anticoagulation with heparin and later with a coumarin. The value of thrombolytic regimens has yet to be assessed properly. Prevention is important. Deep vein thrombosis after a surgical operation is less frequent now with early postoperative mobilization, regular leg exercises, the use of elastic stockings over the operative period, and prophylaxis with low dose heparin.

Thrombophlebitis

This is thrombosis in an inflamed vein. If the affected vein is varicose or superficial it will be red and feel like a tender cord. The leg may be diffusely inflamed, making a distinction from cellulitis (p. 165) difficult. There may be fever, leucocytosis, and a high ESR. *Migratory superficial thrombophlebitis* should arouse suspicion of an underlying malignancy or pancreatic disease.

Treatment is based on rest, local heat, and non-steroidal anti-inflammatory drugs. Antibiotics or anticoagulants rarely help.

The gravitational syndrome, lipodermatosclerosis and venous leg ulceration

Ulcers of the lower leg, secondary to venous insufficiency, are commoner in women than in men and account for some 85% of all leg ulcers seen in the UK and USA.

Cause

The proper venous drainage of a leg requires three sets of veins: the deep veins surrounded by muscles; the superficial veins; and the veins connecting these two — the perforating or communicating veins (Fig. 13.4). When the leg muscles contract, blood in the deep veins is squeezed back, against gravity, to the heart (the calf muscle pump); reflux is prevented by valves. When the muscles relax, with the help of gravity blood from the superficial veins passes into the deep veins via the communicating vessels. If the valves in the deep and communicating veins are incompetent, hypertension develops in the deep veins. The calf muscle pump now pushes blood into the superficial veins, where the pressure remains high ('venous hypertension') instead of dropping during exercise. This persisting venous hypertension enlarges the capillary bed, and forces fibrinogen out through the capillary walls. Patients with these changes develop 'lipodermatosclerosis' (see below) and have a high serum fibrinogen and reduced blood fibrinolytic activity. The pericapillary fibrin cuff blocks the diffusion of oxygen and nutrients, and the overlying skin becomes hypoxic. As a result, minor trauma leads to ulcers which are slow to heal. Figure 13.5 shows the factors causing venous ulceration.

Clinical features

Venous incompetence is heralded by a feeling of heaviness in the legs and by oedema. Other signs include a red or bluish discoloration, loss of hair,

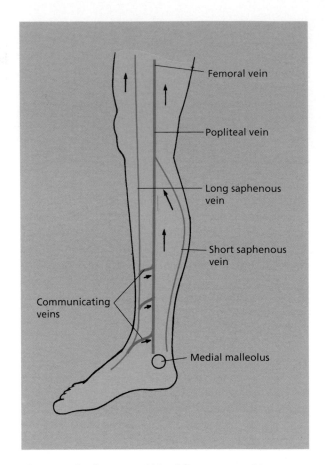

Fig. 13.4 The direction of blood flow in normal leg veins.

induration, pigmentation (mainly haemosiderin from the breakdown of extravasated red blood cells), and atrophie blanche (ivory white scarring with dilated capillary loops) (Fig. 13.6). This combination of signs is sometimes called lipodermatosclerosis. Ulceration is most common near the medial malleolus (Fig. 13.7). Venous ulcers are often large, vary in depth, are sharply demarcated, and are frequently indolent. Incompetent perforating branches (blow-outs) between the superficial and deep veins are best felt with the patient standing.

Under favourable conditions the exudative phase gives way to a granulating and healing phase, signalled by a blurring of the ulcer margin, ingrowth of skin from it, and the appearance of scattered small grey epithelial islands over the base. Prolonged ulceration, with lipodermatosclerosis, gives the leg the look of an inverted champagne bottle.

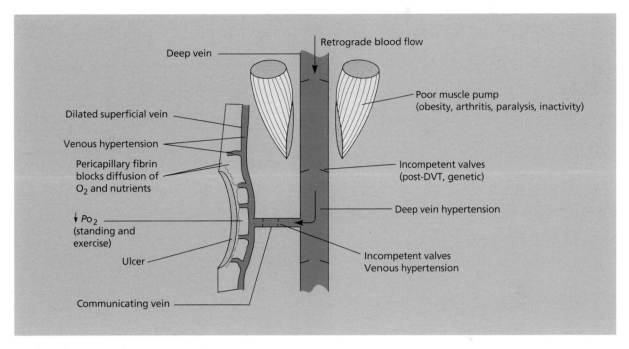

Fig. 13.5 Factors causing venous leg ulceration.

Complications

Bacterial superinfection is inevitable in a long-standing ulcer, but needs systemic antibiotics only if there is a purulent discharge, rapid extension, cellulitis, lymphangitis, or septicaemia.

Eczema (p. 101) is common around venous ulcers (Fig. 13.8). Allergic contact dermatitis (p. 91) is a possibility if the rash worsens or fails to improve with local treatment. Lanolin, parabens (a preservative) and neomycin are the most common sensitizers.

Malignant change can occur. If an ulcer has a hyperplastic base or rolled edge, biopsy may be needed to rule out a squamous cell carcinoma (Fig. 13.9).

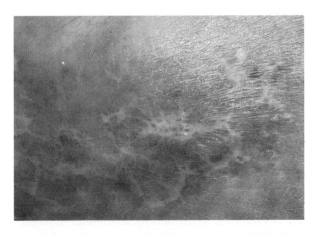

Fig. 13.6 Irregular areas of whitish scarring and dilated capillary loops — the changes of atrophie blanche.

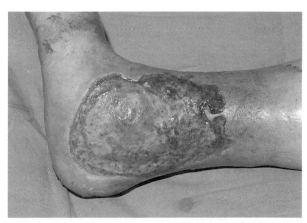

Fig. 13.7 Large venous ulcer overlying the medial malleolus.

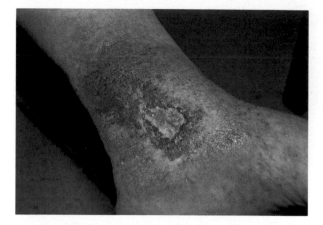

Fig. 13.8 Eczema surrounding a small crusted venous ulcer.

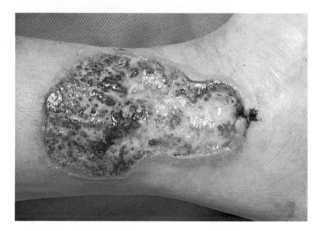

Fig. 13.9 Chronic ulcer failing to respond to treatment. Biopsy, taken from rolled edge, excluded malignant change.

Differential diagnosis

The main causes of leg ulceration are given in Table 13.7. The most important differences between venous and other leg ulcers are:

Atherosclerotic. These ulcers are more common on the toes, dorsum of foot, heel, calf, and shin, and are unrelated to perforating veins. Their edges are often sharply defined, their outline may be polycyclic and the ulcers may be deep and gangrenous. Islands of intact skin are characteristically seen within the ulcer. Claudication may be present and peripheral pulses absent.

Table 13.7 Causes of leg ulceration

Venous hypertension	
Arterial disease	Atherosclerosis
	Buerger's disease
	Giant cell arteritis
	Polyarteritis nodosa
	Systemic sclerosis
Small vessel disease	Diabetes mellitus
	Systemic lupus erythematosus
	Rheumatoid arthritis
	Systemic sclerosis
	Allergic vasculitis
Abnormalities of blood	Immune complex disease
	Sickle cell anaemia
	Cryoglobulinaemia
Neuropathy	Diabetes mellitus
	Leprosy
	Syphilis
	Syringomyelia
	Peripheral neuropathy
Infection	'Tropical ulcer'
	Tuberculosis
	Deep fungal infections
Tumour	Squamous cell carcinoma
	Malignant melanoma
	Kaposi's sarcoma
	Basal cell carcinoma
Trauma	Injury
	Artefact
	Iatrogenic

Vasculitic. These ulcers start as painful palpable purpuric lesions turning into small punched-out ulcers (Fig. 13.10). The involvement of larger vessels is heralded by painful nodules which may ulcerate. The intractable, deep, sharply demarcated ulcers of rheumatoid arthritis are due to an underlying vasculitis (Fig. 13.11).

Thrombotic ulcers. Skin infarction (Fig. 13.12), leading to ulceration, may be due to embolism or to the increased coagulability of polycythaemia or cryoglobulinaemia.

Infective ulcers. Infection is now a rare cause of leg ulcers in the UK but ulcers due to tuberculosis, leprosy, atypical mycobacteria, diphtheria, and deep fungal infections, such as sporotrichosis or chromoblastomycosis, are still seen in the tropics.

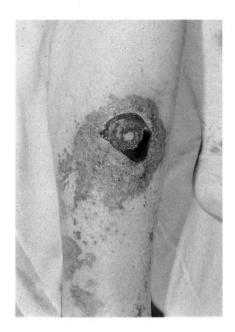

Fig. 13.10 Not all leg ulcers are due to venous hypertension. Surrounding palpable purpura indicates vasculitic cause of this ulcer.

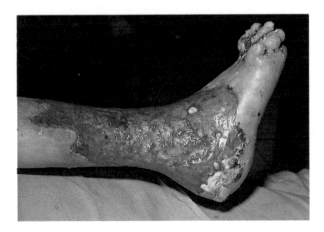

Fig. 13.11 Large, shallow and recalcitrant ulcer complicating rheumatoid arthritis.

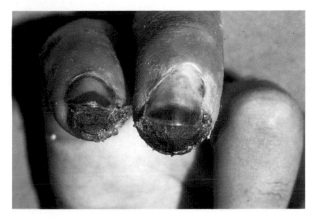

Fig. 13.12 In this case gangrene was due to frostbite. No cryoglobulins were detected.

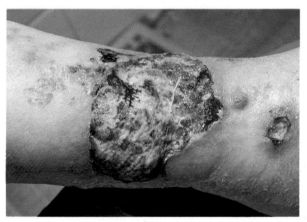

Fig. 13.13 Patient referred with a 'venous ulcer' but biopsy of hyperplastic granulating base confirmed diagnosis of poorly differentiated squamous cell carcinoma.

Malignant ulcers. Squamous cell carcinoma (p. 232) (Fig. 13.13) is the most common, but malignant melanoma (p. 233) and basal cell carcinoma (p. 230) can both present as flat lesions which expand, crust and ulcerate.

Pyoderma gangrenosum (p. 249). This is characterized by large and rapidly spreading ulcers which may be circular or polycyclic and have a blue, indurated, undermined, or pustular margin. Pyoderma gangrenosum may complicate rheumatoid arthritis, ulcerative colitis, or blood dyscrasias.

Investigations

Most chronic leg ulcers are venous, but other causes should be considered, if the signs are atypical. A search for contributory factors, such as obesity, peripheral artery disease, cardiac failure or arthritis, is always worthwhile. Investigations should include:
- Urine test for sugar.
- Full blood count to detect anaemia, which will delay healing.

- Swabbing for pathogens — see Bacterial super-infection above.
- Venography helps to detect surgically remediable causes of venous incompetence.
- Döppler ultrasound may help to assess arterial circulation when atherosclerosis is likely. It seldom helps if the peripheral pulses can easily be felt. If the maximal systolic ankle pressure divided by the systolic brachial pressure ('ankle brachial pressure index') is greater than 0.8 the ulcer is unlikely to be due to arterial disease.

Treatment

Venous ulcers will not heal if the leg remains swollen and the patient chair-bound. Pressure bandages take priority over other measures but not for athero-sclerotic ulcers with an already precarious arterial supply. A common error is to use local treatment which is too elaborate. As a last resort, admission to hospital, for elevation and intensive treatment, may be needed, but the results are not encouraging; patients may stay in the ward for many months but their apparently well-healed ulcers may break down rapidly when they go home.

The list of therapies is extensive. They can be divided into the following categories: physical, local, oral, and surgical.

Physical measures

Compression bandages and stockings. Compression bandaging is vital for most venous ulcers; it reduces oedema and aids venous return. The bandages are applied over the ulcer dressing, from the forefoot to just below the knee. Self-adhesive bandages (e.g. Lestreflex) are convenient and have largely replaced elasticated bandages. Bandages stay on for 2–7 days at a time and are left on at night. One four-layer compression bandaging system includes a layer of orthopaedic wool (Velband), a standard crepe, an Elset elasticated bandage and an elasticated cohesive bandage (e.g. Coban): it requires changing only once a week and is very effective. The combined four layers give 40 mmHg compression at the ankle. Once an ulcer has healed, a graduated compression stocking (e.g. Duomed, Medi Strumpf, or Venosan 2502/2003 [UK] or Jobst or Teds [USA]) from toes to knee (or preferably thigh), should be prescribed. A foam or felt pad may be worn under the stockings to protect vulnerable areas against minor trauma. The stocking should be put on *before* rising from bed.

Elevation of the affected limb, preferably above the hips, aids venous drainage, decreases oedema, and raises oxygen tension in the limb. Patients should rest with their legs up for at least two hours every afternoon. The foot of the bed should be raised by at least six inches; it is not enough just to put a pillow under the feet.

Walking, in moderation, is beneficial, but pro-longed standing or sitting with dependent legs is not.

Physiotherapy. Some physiotherapists are good at persuading venous ulcers to heal. Their secret lies in a combination of the following: leg exercises, elevation, gentle massage, ultrasound treatment to the skin around the ulcers, and graduated com-pression bandaging.

Diet. Many patients are obese and should lose weight.

Local therapy

There are many preparations to choose from; those we have found most useful are listed in the Formulary (p. 295).

Clean ulcers (Fig. 13.14). Dressings need be changed only once or twice a week. Paraffin tulle dressings, plain or impregnated with 0.5% chorhexidine, 0.25% silver proteinate in compound calamine cream spread on a non-stick dressing, 0.5% brilliant green, 1% silver sulphadiazine cream, and simple zinc and castor oil ointment, are all helpful and easy to apply. The area should be gently cleaned with arachis oil, 5% hydrogen peroxide or saline before the next dressing is applied. Sometimes immersing the whole ulcer in a tub of warm water is best, and will loosen or dissolve adherent crusts.

Many dressings have absorbent and protective properties (Formulary, p. 296). These include Granu-flex (which has the advantage of sticking to the surrounding skin), Geliperm and Sorbsan in the UK and Duoderm, Opsite and Tegaderm in the USA.

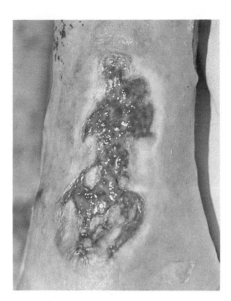

Fig. 13.14 Clean healing ulcer. Weekly dressing would be suitable.

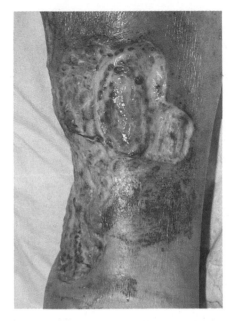

Fig. 13.15 Infected ulcer with sloughing. Tendon visible at bottom of figure. Hospital admission and frequent dressings needed to save leg.

Actisorb (UK) is a useful charcoal dressing which absorbs exudate and minimizes odour.

Medicated bandages (Formulary, p. 296) based on zinc paste, with ichthammol, or with calamine and clioquinol, are useful when there is much surrounding eczema, and can be used for all types of ulcers, even infected, exuding ones. The bandage is applied in strips from the foot to below the knee. Worsening of eczema under a medicated bandage may signal the development of allergic contact dermatitis to a component of the paste, most often parabens (a preservative) or cetylstearyl alcohols.

Infected ulcers (Fig. 13.15). These have to be cleaned and dressed more often than clean ulcers, sometimes even twice daily. Useful preparations include 0.5% silver nitrate, 0.25% sodium hypochlorite, 0.25% acetic acid, potassium permanganate (1 in 10000 dilution) and 5% hydrogen peroxide, all made up in aqueous solution, and applied as compresses with or without occlusion. Helpful creams and lotions include 1.5% hydrogen peroxide, 20% benzoyl peroxide, 1% silver sulphadiazine, 10% povidone-iodine and 0.5% brilliant green (Formulary, p. 295). Dextran polymer beads, and starch polymer beads within cadexomer iodine, are preparations whose main function is to absorb exudate. Although antibiotic tulles are easy to apply and are well tolerated, they

should not be used for long periods as they may induce bacterial resistance or sensitize. Resistance is not such a problem with povidone-iodine, and a readily applied non-adherent dressing impregnated with this antiseptic may be useful. Surrounding eczema is helped by weak or moderate strength local steroids, which must never be put on the ulcer itself. Lassar's paste, zinc cream or paste bandages (see above) are suitable alternatives.

Oral treatment

The following may be helpful.
- *Diuretics.* Pressure bandaging is more important as the oedema associated with venous ulceration is largely mechanical. Diuretics will combat the oedema of cardiac failure.
- *Analgesics.* Adequate analgesia is important. Aspirin may not be well tolerated by the elderly. Paracetamol (not available in the USA), or acetaminophen is often adequate but dihydrocodeine may be required. Analgesia may be needed only when the dressing is changed.
- *Antibiotics.* Ulcers need not be 'sterilized' by local or systemic antibiotics. Short courses of

systemic antibiotics should be reserved for spreading infection (see under Complications above) but are sometimes tried for pain or even odour. Bacteriological guidance is needed and the drugs used include erythromycin and flucloxacillin (streptococcal or staphylococcal cellulitis), metronidazole (*Bacteroides* infection) and ciprofloxacin (*Pseudomonas aeruginosa* infection).

• *Ferrous sulphate* and *folic acid*. For anaemia.

• *Zinc sulphate*. May help to promote healing, especially if the plasma zinc level is low.

• *Oxypentifylline* (pentoxyfylline, USA) is fibrinolytic, increases the deformability of red and white blood cells, decreases blood viscosity and diminishes platelet adhesiveness. It increases the rate of healing of venous ulcers when used with compression bandages.

• *Stanozolol*. This anabolic steroid may not heal an existing ulcer more quickly, but may prevent ulceration in lipodermatosclerosis and may protect against recurrences. The manufacturer's advice on contraindications, e.g. prostatic cancer and abnormal liver function, and on monitoring treatment, must not be overlooked.

• *Oxerutins*. These may help the oedema and symptoms of venous insufficiency and are said to reduce leakage from capillaries by acting on the endothelial cells.

Surgery

Autologous pinch or split-thickness grafts have a place. Lyophilized pig dermis, and synthetic films similar to skin, may also be tried. The day may soon come when more patients can be treated with sheets of human epidermis grown in tissue culture. In general these work best on clean ulcers.

Venous surgery on younger patients with varicose veins may prevent recurrences, those with atherosclerotic ulcers should see a vascular surgeon for assessment. Some blockages are surgically remediable.

Purpura

Purpura, petechiae and ecchymoses may be due to a coagulation or platelet disorder, or to an abnormal vessel wall or surrounding dermis. Some common causes are listed in Table 13.8. In general, coagulation

---

LEARNING POINTS

1 Whatever you put on an ulcer it will never heal if the ankle is oedematous.
2 Watch out for allergy to local applications.
3 Never put topical steroids on ulcers.
4 Most ulcers, despite positive bacteriology, are not much helped by systemic antibiotics.

Table 13.8 Causes of intracutaneous bleeding

Coagulation defects
Inherited defects, e.g. haemophilia, Christmas disease
Connective tissue disorders
Disseminated intravascular coagulation
Paraproteinaemias (e.g. macroglobulinaemia)
Acquired defects (e.g. liver disease, anticoagulant therapy, vitamin K deficiency, drugs)

Platelet defects
Thrombocytopenia
  idiopathic
  connective tissue disorders, especially LE
  disseminated intravascular coagulation
  haemolytic anaemia
  hypersplenism
  giant haemangiomas (Kasabach–Merritt syndrome)
  bone marrow damage (cytostatic drugs, leukaemia, carcinoma)
  drugs (quinine, aspirin, thiazides and sulphonamides)
Abnormal function
  von Willebrand's disease

Vascular defect
Raised intravascular pressure (coughing, vomiting, venous hypertension, gravitational)
Vasculitis (including Henoch–Schönlein purpura)
Infections (e.g. meningococcal septicaemia, Rocky Mountain spotted fever)
Drugs (carbromal, aspirin, sulphonamides, quinine, phenylbutazone and gold salts)
Painful bruising syndrome
Idiopathic (progressive pigmented dermatoses)

Lack of support from surrounding dermis
Senile purpura
Corticosteroid therapy
Scurvy (perifollicular purpura)
Lichen sclerosus et atrophicus
Systemic amyloidosis

defects give rise to ecchymoses and external bleeding. Platelet defects present more often as purpura, though bleeding and ecchymoses may still occur. Vasculitis of small vessels causes purpura, often palpable and painful, but not bleeding; this is discussed in Chapter 10. Purpura from vasodilatation and gravity is seen in many diseases of the legs, especially in the elderly (defective dermis around the blood vessels), and seldom requires extensive investigation.

Cryoglobulinaemia is a rare cause of purpura, which is most prominent on exposed parts. It may also cause cold urticaria (p. 105) and livedo reticularis (p. 137). The condition may be idiopathic, or secondary to myeloma, leukaemia or an autoimmune disease.

Investigations

These must include a platelet count, prothrombin time, and a full blood count and biochemical screen. Electrophoresis is needed to exclude hypergammaglobulinaemia and paraproteinaemia. Cryoglobulinaemia should also be excluded. A coagulation screen, including measurement of fibrin degradation products, is often necessary. The bleeding time, and a Hess tourniquet test for capillary fragility, help less often. Skin biopsy will confirm a small vessel vasculitis.

Treatment

Treat the underlying condition. Replacement of relevant blood fractions may be needed initially. Systemic steroids are usually effective in vasculitis (Chapter 10).

Disorders of the lymphatics

Lymphoedema

Lymphoedema is firm and pits poorly. Long-standing lymphoedema may lead to gross hyperkeratosis, as in the so-called 'mossy foot'.

Cause

Lymphoedema may be primary or secondary. The primary forms are developmental defects though signs may only appear in early puberty, or even in adulthood. Sometimes lymphoedema involves only one leg. Secondary causes are listed in Table 13.9.

Treatment

Elevation, graduated compression bandages (e.g. Duomed and Medi Strumpf), diuretics and the early treatment of lymphangitis or erysipelas are the cornerstones of treatment. If erysipelas recurs, long-term penicillin should be given. Surgery occasionally helps to remove an obstruction or restore drainage.

Lymphangitis

This streptococcal infection of the lymphatics may occur without any lymphoedema. A tender red line extends proximally. Flucloxacillin or erythromycin is usually effective.

Table 13.9 Causes of secondary lymphoedema

Recurrent lymphangitis	Erysipelas, infected pompholyx
Lymphatic obstruction	Filariasis, granuloma inguinale, tuberculosis, tumour
Lymphatic destruction	Surgery, radiation therapy, tumour
Uncertain aetiology	Rosacea Melkersson—Rosenthal syndrome (facial nerve palsy, fissuring of tongue and lymphoedema of lip) Yellow nail syndrome

CHAPTER 14

Sebaceous and sweat gland disorders

Disorders of the sebaceous glands

Acne vulgaris

Acne is a disorder of the pilosebaceous apparatus, peaking in adolescence, and characterized by comedones, papules, pustules, cysts and scars.

Prevalence

Nearly all teenagers have some acne. Most try at some time anti-acne preparations which they buy straight from their pharmacist.

Acne affects the sexes equally. Its age of onset is usually between 12 and 14 years, tending to be earlier in females. The peak age and severity in females is 16–17 years and in males 17–19.

Cause

Many factors combine to cause acne (Fig. 14.1):
- *Sebum*. Sebum excretion is increased. However, this alone need not cause acne; patients with acromegaly, or with Parkinson's disease, have high sebum excretion rates but no acne. Furthermore, sebum excretion often remains high long after acne has gone away.

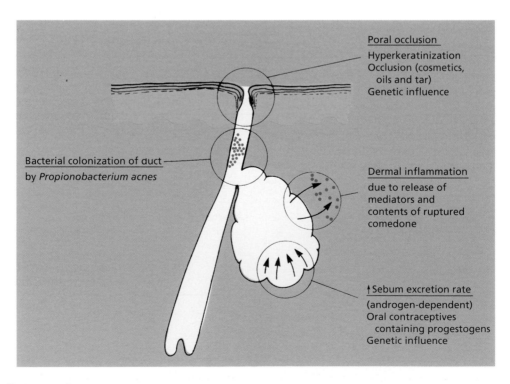

Poral occlusion
Hyperkeratinization
Occlusion (cosmetics, oils and tar)
Genetic influence

Bacterial colonization of duct by *Propionobacterium acnes*

Dermal inflammation due to release of mediators and contents of ruptured comedone

↑Sebum excretion rate (androgen-dependent)
Oral contraceptives containing progestogens
Genetic influence

Fig. 14.1 Factors causing acne.

- *Hormonal.* Androgens (from the testes, ovaries and adrenals) are the main hormones to stimulate sebum excretion, though other hormones have minor effects too (e.g. thyroid hormones and growth hormone). Those castrated before puberty never develop acne. In acne the sebaceous glands respond excessively to what are usually normal levels of these hormones (increased sensitivity of the target organ). This may be due to 5α reductase activity being higher in the target sebaceous glands than in other parts of the body. This enzyme converts testosterone into a more active metabolite, 5α-dihydrotestosterone, which in turn binds to specific receptors in sebaceous glands, increasing sebum excretion. Fifty per cent of females with acne have slightly raised free testosterone levels (usually due to a low level of sex hormone binding globulin rather than a high total testosterone) but this is still only a fraction of the concentration in males and its relevance is debatable. Infantile acne may follow transplacental stimulation of a child's adrenals.
- *Poral occlusion.* Oil, cosmetics, or other factors cause the epithelium to overgrow the follicular surface. This causes the follicle to retain sebum and increases the concentration of bacteria and free fatty acids within the follicle. Rupture of the follicle is associated with intense inflammation.
- *Mechanical.* Excessive scrubbing or the rubbing of chin straps or a fiddle (see Fig. 14.6) can rupture occluded follicles.
- *Bacterial.* *Propionobacterium acnes*, a normal skin commensal, plays a pathogenic role. It colonizes the pilosebaceous ducts, breaks down triglycerides releasing free fatty acids, produces substances chemotactic for inflammatory cells and induces the ductal epithelium to secrete pro-inflammatory cytokines, including IL-1, IL-2 and TNF-α (p. 29). The inflammatory reaction is kept going by type III and type IV immune reactions (p. 31).
- *Genetic.* The condition is familial but its mode of inheritance is debatable.

Presentation: common type

Lesions are confined to the face, shoulders, upper chest and back. Seborrhoea (greasy skin) (Fig. 14.2), is often present. Open comedones (blackheads), due to the plugging by keratin and sebum of the pilosebaceous orifice, or closed comedones (whiteheads),

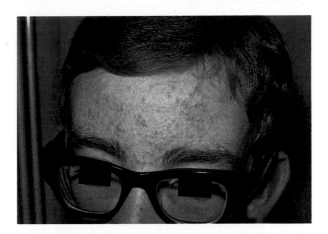

Fig. 14.2 The seborrhoea, comedones and scattered inflammatory papules of teenage acne.

due to accretions of keratin and sebum deeper in the pilosebaceous duct, are always seen. Inflammatory papules, nodules and cysts occur, with one or two types of lesion predominating. Depressed or hypertrophic scarring may follow.

Presentation: variants

Conglobate. Conglobate means gathered into balls (Latin: *globus*, ball). This severe form of acne consists of abscesses or cysts, with intercommunicating sinuses, which contain thick serosanguinous fluid or pus. On resolution, it leaves deeply pitted or hypertrophic scars, sometimes joined by keloidal bridges (Fig. 14.3).

Fulminans. Acne fulminans is a rare variant in which conglobate acne is accompanied by fever, joint pains and a high ESR.

Exogenous. Tars, chlorinated hydrocarbons, oils, and oily cosmetics may cause or exacerbate acne. Suspicion should be raised if the distribution is odd or if comedones predominate (Figs 14.4–14.6).

Excoriated. This is seen most often in young girls. Obsessional picking or rubbing leaves discrete denuded areas (Fig. 14.7).

Late onset. This type too occurs mainly in women and is often limited to the chin (Fig. 14.8). Nodular

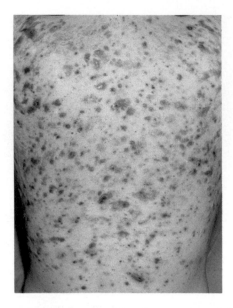

Fig. 14.3 Conglobate acne with inflammatory nodules, pustulocystic lesions and depressed scars.

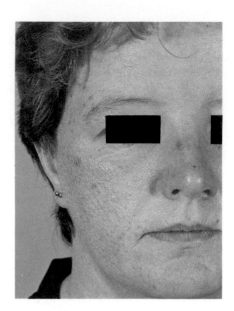

Fig. 14.5 Acne with numerous closed comedones. Caused by frequent use of a sunscreen oil.

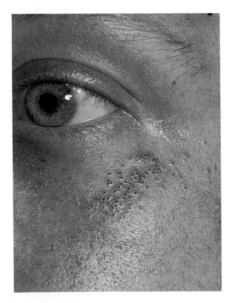

Fig. 14.4 A group of open comedones (blackheads) following the use of a greasy cosmetic.

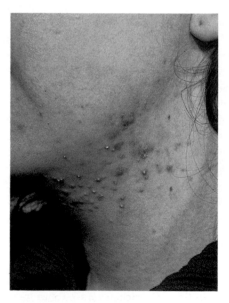

Fig. 14.6 Papulopustular lesions in an odd distribution. The patient played the violin ('fiddler's neck').

and cystic lesions predominate. It is stubborn and persistent.

Infantile. This rare type is present at birth and is presumed to occur from maternal hormones. It is

more common in males, and may last for up to three years. Its morphology is like that of common acne (Fig. 14.9). Unfortunately it may be the forerunner of severe acne in adolescence.

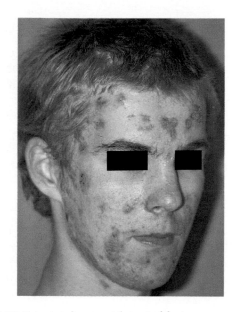

Fig. 14.7 Excoriated acne with typical lesions.

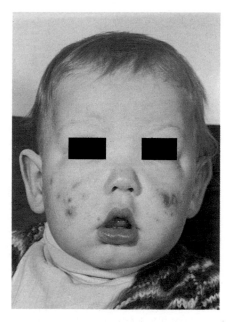

Fig. 14.9 Infantile acne. Pustulocystic lesions on the cheeks.

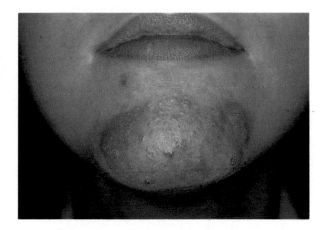

Fig. 14.8 Late onset acne in a woman. Often localized to the chin.

Drug-induced. Corticosteroids, androgenic and anabolic steroids, gonadotrophins, oral contraceptives, lithium, iodides, bromides, anti-tuberculosis and anticonvulsant therapy may cause an acneiform rash (Fig. 14.10).

Tropical. This affects Caucasoids in hot, humid climates. It occurs mainly on the trunk, and responds poorly to any treatment other than return to a temperate climate.

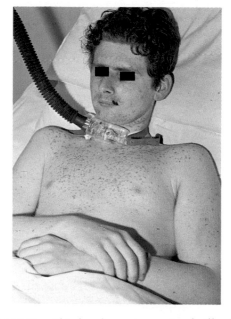

Fig. 14.10 Steroid-induced acne in a seriously ill patient.

Course

Although acne clears by the age of 23–25 years in 90% of patients, some 5% of women and 1% of men still need treatment in their thirties or even forties.

Investigations

None are usually necessary. Cultures are occasionally needed to exclude a pyogenic infection, an anaerobic infection, or Gram-negative folliculitis. Only a few laboratories routinely culture propionobacterium acnes and test its sensitivity to antibiotics. Any acne, including infantile acne, which is associated with virilization needs investigation to exclude an androgen-secreting tumour of the adrenals or ovaries. Tests should then include the measurement of plasma testosterone, sex hormone binding globulin, dehydroepiandrosterone sulphate, androstenedione and, depending on the results, ultrasound examination of the ovaries and adrenals.

Differential diagnosis

Rosacea (p. 156) affects older individuals: comedones are absent, lesions occur only on the face, and the rash has an erythematous background. Pyogenic folliculitis can be excluded by culture. Hidradenitis suppurativa (p. 160) is associated with acne conglobata, but attacks the axillae and groin.

Treatment

Local treatment is enough for most patients with comedo-papular acne. Both local and systemic treatment are needed for pustular–cystic–scarring acne (Fig. 14.11).

Local treatment (Formulary, p. 294).

1 *Regular gentle cleansing* with soap and water should be encouraged, to remove surface sebum. Antibacterial cleansers are also useful — e.g. chlorhexidine.

2 *Benzoyl peroxide*. This is applied only at night initially, but can be used twice daily in the absence of excessive dryness and irritation. It is wise to start with a 2.5% or 5% preparation, moving up to 10% if necessary. Benzoyl peroxide bleaches coloured materials.

3 *Retinoids*. Tretinoin. This vitamin A analogue normalizes follicular keratinization, and is especially effective against comedones. Patients should be warned about skin irritation and photosensitivity. It can be prescribed as a lotion, cream or gel. The

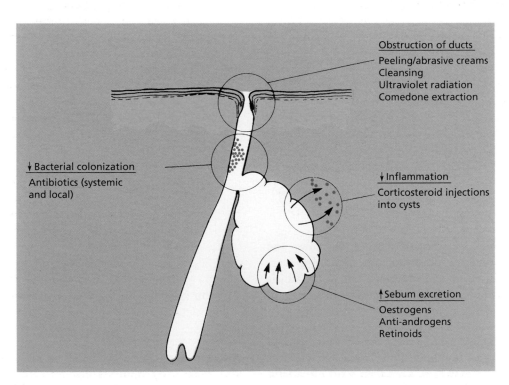

Fig. 14.11 Therapeutic approaches to acne.

weakest preparation should be used first, and applied overnight on alternate nights. Sometimes, after a week or two, it has to be stopped temporarily because of irritation. As with benzoyl peroxide it may be worth increasing the strength of tretinoin after six weeks if it is tolerated well. The combination of benzoyl peroxide in the morning and tretinoin at night has many advocates.

Isotretinoin 0.05% is made up in a gel base (not available in USA) and applied once or twice daily. Isotretinoin irritates less than the same concentration of tretinoin.

The prudent physician often avoids prescribing topical retinoids to a pregnant woman with acne.

4 *Azelaic acid* (not available in USA) has a bacteriocidal effect on *P. acnes* and *Staph. epidermis*: it is anti-inflammatory and inhibits the formation of comedones by reducing proliferation of keratinocytes. It is applied twice daily but should not be used for more than six months at a time.

5 *Abrasive pastes* containing aluminium oxide may also help with comedones, but aggressive scrubbing should be discouraged.

6 *Sulphur*. A number of time-honoured preparations containing sulphur are available on both sides of the Atlantic. Some are included in the Formulary (p. 294).

7 *Local antibiotics*. These include topical tetracycline, sulphacetamide, clindamycin, and erythromycin (Formulary, p. 294) and are alternatives to benzoyl peroxide or tretinoin.

8 *Aluminium chloride*. Alcoholic solutions of aluminium chloride act as antiperspirants, and may help tropical acne.

9 *Cosmetic camouflage*. Cover-ups are useful in some patients, especially females, whose scarring is unsightly. They also help to obscure post-inflammatory pigmentation. A range of make-ups is available in the UK and USA (Formulary, p. 289).

Systemic treatment

Antibiotics:

● *Tetracyclines*. Oxytetracycline and tetracycline. An average dose for an adult is 250 mg up to four times daily, but up to 1.5 g/day may be needed in resistant cases. It should not be used for less than four months and may be needed for a year or two, or even longer. It should be taken on an empty stomach, one hour before meals or four hours after food as the absorption of tetracyclines is decreased by milk, antacids and calcium, iron and magnesium salts. The dose should be tapered in line with clinical improvement, an average maintenance dose being 250–500 mg/day. Even with long courses serious side effects are rare, though candidal vulvovaginitis may force a change to a narrower spectrum antibiotic such as erythromycin.

● Minocycline, 50 mg twice daily or 100 mg once daily (in modified release preparation) is now preferred by many dermatologists, although it is much more expensive. Its absorption is not significantly affected by food or drink. It is much more lipophilic than oxytetracycline and so probably concentrates in the sebaceous glands. It is bacteriologically more effective than oxytetracycline and tetracycline and, unlike erythromycin, no appreciable resistance by proprionobacteria to minocycline has been recorded. It is effective even when oxytetracycline has failed.

Doxycycline, 100 mg once or twice daily is a cheaper alternative to minocin, but is more frequently associated with phototoxic skin reactions.

Tetracyclines should not be taken in pregnancy or be given to children under 12 as they are deposited in growing bone and developing teeth, causing stained teeth and dental hypoplasia. Rarely longterm administration of minocycline may cause greyish pigmentation; this is more common in those with actinic facial damage.

● Erythromycin (dosage as for oxytetracycline) is the next antibiotic of choice but is preferable to a tetracycline in women who might become pregnant. Its major drawback is the development of resistant proprionobacteria which leads to therapeutic failure.

● Trimethoprim is used by some as a third-line antibiotic for acne, when a tetracycline and erythromycin have not helped. White blood cell counts should be monitored.

Hormonal. A combined antiandrogen/oestrogen treatment (Dianette: 2 mg cyproterone acetate and 0.035 mg ethinyloestradiol) is available in many countries and may help with persistent acne in women. Monitoring is as for any patient on an oral contraceptive and further contraceptive measures are unnecessary. Courses last for eight to twelve months and the drug is then replaced by a low oestrogen/low progestogen oral contraceptive. These drugs must not be used for males.

For women with acne who also require oral contraception, a combined oestrogen progestogen preparation or a triphasic pill is best. Women taking antibiotics should be warned of their possible interaction with oral contraceptives; they should use other contraceptive precautions, especially if the antibiotics induce diarrhoea.

13-Cis-retinoic acid (isotretinoin). Ro-Accutane (Accutane, USA; Formulary, p. 306) is an oral retinoid which inhibits sebum excretion, the growth of *P. acnes*, and acute inflammatory processes. The drug is reserved for severe acne, unresponsive to the measures outlined above. It is routinely given for 4 months only, in a dose of 0.5−1 mg/kg body weight per day; young men with truncal acne usually require the higher dose. A full blood count, liver function and fasting lipid levels should be checked and routine urine analysis performed before the start of the course, and then at four weeks after starting the drug. Some physicians also monitor at ten and sixteen weeks and perform a final check one month after completing the course. The drug seldom has to be stopped. Isotretinoin is highly teratogenic: women should sign a form confirming that they have been warned about this, and should take an oral contraceptive or Dianette for two months before starting isotretinoin, throughout treatment and for three months thereafter. A test for pregnancy should usually be done before starting treatment and at follow-up visits. Other side effects of isotretinoin include dry skin, dry and inflamed lips and eyes, nosebleeds, muscle aches, changes in night-time vision and hair loss; these are often tolerated, especially if the acne is doing well. Occasionally isotretinoin flares acne at first, but this effect is usually short lived and the drug may be continued.

Diet. It is sensible for patients to avoid foods (e.g. nuts, chocolates, dairy products and wine) which they think make their acne worse, but there is little evidence that any dietary constituent, except iodine, causes acne.

Physical

Ultraviolet B radiation therapy often helps with exacerbations. Two-month courses, during which the patient attends two or three times weekly, are usually adequate.

Cysts can be incised and drained with or without local anaesthetic.

Intralesional injections of 0.1 ml of triamcinolone acetonide (2.5−10 mg/ml) hasten the resolution of stubborn cysts, but may leave atrophy.

Dermabrasion. This may be useful to smooth out facial scars. A high-speed rotating wire brush planes down to a bleeding dermis. It should not be carried out if there are any active lesions and does not help depressed 'ice-pick' scars. Unsightly hyperpigmentation may follow in darker skins.

Collagen injections. Bovine collagen may be injected into depressed scars to improve their appearance. Patients with a history of any autoimmune disorder are excluded from this treatment. Shallow atrophic lesions do better than discrete 'ice-pick' scars. The procedure is expensive and has to be repeated every six months as the collagen is resorbed.

LEARNING POINTS
1 Do not prescribe short courses of many different antibiotics.
2 Avoid tetracyclines in children and pregnant women.
3 Make sure that females with acne are not pregnant before you put them on isotretinoin, and that they do not become pregnant during the course and for three months after it.

Rosacea

Rosacea affects the face of adults, usually women. Although its peak incidences is in the thirties and forties, it may also be seen in the young or old. It may co-exist with acne but is distinct from it.

Cause and histopathology

The cause is still unknown. The condition is often seen in those who flush easily, in response to warmth, spicy food, alcohol or embarrassment. Any psychological abnormalities, including neuroticism and depression, are secondary to the skin condition. No pharmacological defect has been found which explains these flushing attacks. Sebum excretion rate and skin microbiology are normal. A pathogenic role for the tiny hair follicle mite, *Demodex folliculorum*, has not been proved.

Clinical course and complications

The cheeks, nose, centre of forehead, and chin are most commonly affected; the peri-orbital and peri-oral areas are spared (Fig. 14.12). Intermittent flushing is followed by a fixed erythema and telangiectases. Discrete, domed, inflamed papules, papulopustules and, rarely, nodules develop later. Rosacea, unlike acne, has no comedones or seborrhoea. It is usually symmetrical. Its course is prolonged, with exacerbations and remissions. Complications include blepharitis, conjunctivitis and, occasionally, keratitis. Rhinophyma, due to hyperplasia of the sebaceous glands and connective tissue on the nose, is a striking complication (Fig. 14.13) which is more common in males. Lymphoedema, below the eyes and on the forehead, is a tiresome feature in a few cases. Patients treated with potent topical steroids

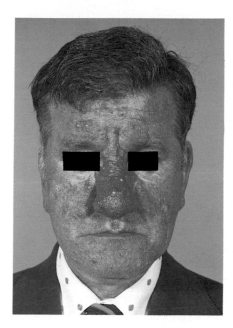

Fig. 14.13 Severe rosacea and rhinophyma.

may develop a rebound flare of pustules, worse than the original rosacea, when treatment is stopped.

Differential diagnosis

Acne has already been mentioned. Rosacea can be distinguished from it by the background of erythema and telangiectases, and by the absence of comedones. The distribution of lesions is different and it develops later in life. Seborrhoeic eczema (p. 98), systemic lupus erythematosus (p. 124) and photo-dermatitis should be considered, but the papulopustules of rosacea are not seen. The flushing of rosacea may be confused with menopausal symptoms and, rarely, with the carcinoid syndrome. Superior vena caval obstruction may be mistaken for lymphoedematous rosacea.

Treatment

Tetracyclines, prescribed as for acne (p. 155), are the traditional treatment and are usually effective. Erythromycin is the antibiotic of second choice. Courses should last for at least 10 weeks, and, after gaining control with 500–1000 mg daily, the dose may be cut to 250 mg daily. The condition recurs in about half of the patients within two years but

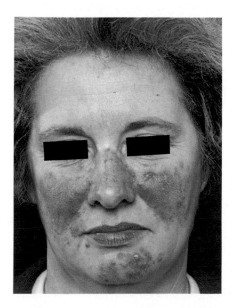

Fig. 14.12 Typical rosacea of a middle-aged woman, with papules and pustules on a background of erythema.

repeated antibiotic courses, rather than prolonged maintenance, are generally recommended. Topical 0.75% metronidazole gel (Formulary p. 294). It is applied sparingly twice daily and is nearly as effective as oral tetracycline. It may be tried before systemic treatment and is especially useful in treating 'stuttering' recurrent lesions which do not then need repeated systemic courses of antibiotics. Rarely systemic metronidazole or 13-*cis*-retinoic acid (p. 306) is needed for stubborn rosacea. Rosacea and topical steroids go badly together (Fig. 14.14); if possible patients should use traditional applications such as 2% sulphur in aqueous cream or 1% ichthammol in zinc cream. Sunscreens may help if sun exposure is an aggravating factor. Changes in diet or drinking habits seldom help.

LEARNING POINT
Never put strong topical steroids on rosacea. If you do, skin addiction, rebound flares, and a cross dermatologist will all figure in your nightmares.

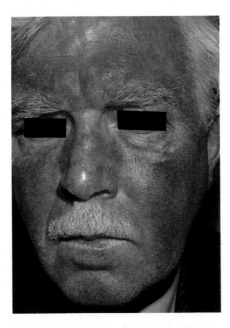

Fig. 14.14 The result of the prolonged use of potent topical steroids for rosacea. Note the extreme telangiectasia, but absence of papules and pustules.

The sweat glands

Eccrine and apocrine glands have been discussed in Chapter 2. Disorders may follow increased or decreased sweating, or blockage of their ducts.

Disorders of eccrine sweat apparatus

Generalized hyperhidrosis

Thermal hyperhidrosis

The 'thermostat' for sweating lies in the the preoptic area of the hypothalamus. Sweating follows any rise in body temperature whether it is due to exercise, environmental heat or an illness. The sweating in acute infections, and in some chronic illnesses (e.g. Hodgkin's disease), may be due to a lowering of the 'set' of this thermostat.

Other causes of general hyperhidrosis

• Emotional stimuli, hypoglycaemia, opiate withdrawal, and shock cause sweating by a direct or reflex stimulation of the sympathetic system at hypothalamic or higher centres. When sweating is accompanied by a general sympathetic discharge it occurs on cold, pale skin.
• Lesions of the central nervous system (e.g. a cerebral tumour or cerebrovascular accident) may cause generalized sweating, presumably by interfering directly with the hypothalamic centre.
• Phaeochromocytoma, the carcinoid syndrome, diabetes mellitus, thyrotoxicosis, Cushing's syndrome, and the hot flushes of menopausal women, have all been associated with general sweating. The mechanisms are not clear.

Local hyperhidrosis

Local hyperhidrosis mainly plagues young adults. The commonest areas are the palms, soles and axillae. Too much sweating there is embarrassing, if not socially crippling. A sodden shirt in contact with a dripping armpit, a wet handshake, and stinking feet, are hard crosses to bear. Seldom is any cause found, but organic disease, especially thyrotoxicosis, acromegaly, tuberculosis and Hodgkin's disease, should be considered. A blatant anxiety state is occasionally present, but more often an otherwise normal person is understandably concerned about his or her antisocial condition. A vicious circle emerges in which increased anxiety drives further sweating.

The problem may be no more than one end of the normal physiological range. How many students sitting exams have to dry their hands before putting pen to paper? It is only when the sweating is gross, or continuous, that medical advice is sought. Such sweating is often precipitated by emotional stimuli and stops during sleep.

Treatment

Topical applications. The most useful preparation for axillary hyperhidrosis is 20% aluminium chloride hexahydrate in an alcohol base (Formulary, p. 289). It is applied to the dry axillae every night at first. Soon the interval can be increased, and many need to use the preparation only once or twice a week. The frequency of application may have to be cut down if the preparation irritates the skin; this is most likely if it is applied soon after shaving or when the skin is wet. Aluminium chloride also helps hyperhidrosis of the palms and soles, but it is less effective there.

Potassium permanganate soaks (1 : 10 000 aqueous solution) combat the bacterial superinfection of sweaty feet which is responsible for their foul smell. The patient should soak the feet for 15 minutes twice a day until the smell has improved and be warned that potassium permanganate stains the skin and everything else brown. Occasionally glutaraldehyde solutions are used instead, but allergy and yellow-stained skin are potential complications.

Iontophoresis is the passage of a low-voltage direct current across the skin. Iontophoresis with tap water or with the anticholinergic drug glycopyrronium bromide may help palmar or plantar hyperhidrosis. Patients attend two to three times a week for treatment until the condition improves. Repeated courses or maintenance therapy may be required.

Systemic treatment. The side effects of anticholinergic therapies often limit their usefulness.

Surgery is seldom used now, as the above measures are usually effective. However, recalcitrant axillary hyperhidrosis may be treated by removing the vault of the axilla which bears most of the sweat glands; these can be identified preoperatively by applying starch and iodine which interact with sweat to colour the starch blue. Cervical sympathectomy is the last resort in palmar hyperhidrosis; the gains seldom outweigh the drawbacks.

> **LEARNING POINT**
> *20% aluminium chloride hexahydrate in an alcohol base has now taken over from anticholinergic drugs and surgery for those with sweaty armpits and hands.*

Hypohidrosis and anhidrosis

Anhidrosis due to abnormality of the sweat glands

Heat stroke

Heat stroke, due to sweat gland exhaustion, is a medical emergency seen most often in an elderly person moving to a hot climate. It may also occur in the young, during or after prolonged exercise. Patients present with hyperthermia, dry skin, weakness, headache, cramps and confusion leading to vomiting, hypotension, oliguria, metabolic acidosis, hyperkalaemia, delirium and death. They should be cooled down immediately with cold water, and fluids and electrolytes must be replaced.

Hypohidrotic ectodermal dysplasia

This rare disorder is inherited as an X-linked recessive trait, in which the sweat glands are either absent or decreased. Affected boys have a characteristic facial appearance, with poor hair and teeth (Figs 8.11 & 8.12), and are intolerant of heat.

Prematurity

The sweat glands function poorly in premature babies nursed in incubators and hot nurseries.

Anhidrosis due to abnormalities of the nervous system

Anhidrosis may follow abnormalities anywhere in the sympathetic tract, from the hypothalamus to the peripheral nerves. It may therefore be a feature of multiple sclerosis, a cerebral tumour, trauma, Horner's syndrome, or peripheral neuropathy (e.g. leprosy, alcoholic neuropathy and diabetes). Patients with widespread anhidrosis are heat-intolerant, developing nausea, dizziness, tachycardia and hyperthermia in hot surroundings.

Anhidrosis or hypohidrosis due to skin disease

Local hypohidrosis has been reported in many skin diseases, especially in those which scar (e.g. lupus erythematosus and morphoea). It may be a feature of Sjogren's syndrome, ichthyosis, psoriasis and miliaria profunda (see below).

Interference with sweat delivery

Miliaria

This is the result of plugging or rupture of sweat ducts. It occurs in hot, humid climates, at any age, and is common in overclothed infants in hot nurseries. The physical signs depend on where the ducts are blocked.

Miliaria crystallina
Tiny clear, non-inflammed vesicles which look like dew. The most superficial type.

Miliaria rubra (prickly heat)
Tiny erythematous and very itchy papules.

Miliaria profunda
Larger erythematous papules or pustules. The deepest type.

Treatment

The best treatment is to move to a cooler climate or into air conditioning. Clothing which prevents the evaporation of sweat (e.g. nylon shirts) should be avoided; cotton is best. Claims have been made for ascorbic acid by mouth, but in our hands it rarely if ever helps. Topical steroids reduce irritation but should only be used briefly. Calamine lotion cools and soothes.

Disorders of the apocrine sweat glands

Suppurative hidradenitis (apocrine acne)

This is a severe, chronic, suppurative disease of the apocrine glands. Many papules, pustules, cysts, sinuses and scars occur in the axillae, groin and perianal areas. It may co-exist with conglobate acne. Its cause is unknown but slightly raised androgen levels are found in some affected females. It is probably not a primary infection of the apocrine glands, though *Staphylococcus aureus*, anaerobic streptococci and *Bacterioides* spp. are frequently present, and one group of workers has implicated *Streptococcus milleri* as the main pathogen. Treatment is unsatisfactory but should be as for acne vulgaris in the first instance. Incision and drainage of abscesses, and injections of intralesional triamcinolone 5–10 mg/ml may reduce the incidence of deforming scars and sinus formation. Systemic anti-androgens may be useful in women. Severe cases need plastic surgery to remove large areas of affected skin.

Fox–Fordyce disease

This rare disease of the apocrine ducts is comparable to miliaria rubra of the eccrine duct. It occurs in women after puberty. Itchy skin-coloured or light brown papules appear in the axillae and other areas where apocrine glands are found, such as the breasts and vulva. Treatment is not usually necessary but removal of the affected skin, or electrodesiccation of the most irritable lesions may be considered.

CHAPTER 15

Infections

Bacterial infections

Skin flora

The surface of the skin teems with harmless micro-organisms. These, the resident flora, are most numerous in moist hairy areas, rich in sebaceous glands. Organisms are found, in clusters, in irregularities in the stratum corneum and within the hair follicles. The skin bacteria are a mixture of harmless and poorly classified micrococci and diphtheroids. *Staphylococcus epidermidis* predominates on the surface and anaerobic diphtheroids deep in the hair follicles. The proportion of the different types varies from person to person; but, once established, an individual's skin flora tends to remain stable and may help to defend the skin against outside pathogens by bacterial interference or antibiotic production. Nevertheless, overgrowth of skin diphtheroids can itself lead to three clinical problems:

Trichomycosis axillaris

The axillary hairs become beaded with concretions, usually yellow, made up of colonies of commensal diphtheroids. Clothing may become stained in the armpits. Topical antibiotic ointments, or shaving, will clear the condition.

Pitted keratolysis

The combination of unusually sweaty feet and occlusive shoes encourages the growth of organisms which can digest keratin. The result is a cribriform pattern of fine, punched-out depressions on the soles, coupled with an unpleasant smell. Four per cent formalin soaks or 20% aluminium chloride hexahydrate in alcohol are helpful.

Erythrasma

Some diphtheroid members of the skin flora can produce porphyrins when grown in a suitable medium: as a result their colonies fluoresce coral pink under Wood's light. Overgrowth of these strains is sometimes the cause of symptom-free macular, wrinkled, slightly scaly, pink, brown or macerated white areas, most often found in the armpits or groins, or between the toes. These areas also fluoresce coral pink with Wood's light. Topical fusidic acid or miconazole will clear the condition.

Staphylococcal infections

Staphylococcus aureus is not part of the resident flora of the skin other than in a minority who carry it in their nostrils, perineum or armpits. Carriage rates vary with age. Nasal carriage is almost invariable in babies born in hospital, becomes less frequent during infancy, and rises again during the school years to the adult level of roughly 20%. Rather fewer carry the organism elsewhere (Fig. 15.1). Staphylococci can also grow, without causing obvious sepsis, on areas of diseased skin such as eczema. A minor breach in the skin's defences is probably necessary for a frank staphylococcal infection to establish itself: some strains seem particularly likely to cause skin sepsis.

Impetigo

Cause

This condition can be caused by staphylococci, streptococci, or by both together. As a useful rule of thumb, the bullous type is usually caused by *S. aureus*, whereas the crusted ulcer type is caused

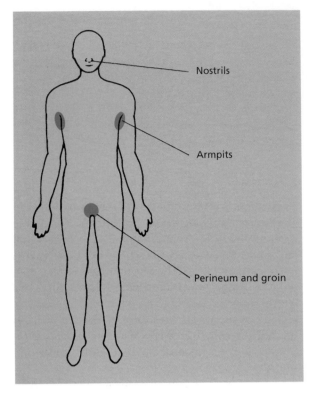

Fig. 15.1 Sites of possible staphylococcal carriage.

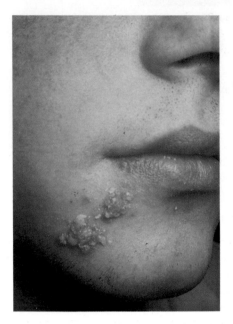

Fig. 15.2 Impetigo on a common site showing the typical honey-coloured crusting.

by beta-haemolytic strains of streptococci. It is highly contagious.

Presentation

A thin-walled blister forms, but ruptures rapidly, leaving an extending area of exudation and yellowish crusting (Fig. 15.2). Multiple lesions often occur, particularly around the face. The lesions may be more obviously bullous in infants. A follicular type of impetigo (superficial folliculitis) is also common.

Course

The condition may spread rapidly through a family or class. It tends to clear slowly even without treatment.

Complications

Streptococcal impetigo may trigger an acute glomerulonephritis.

Differential diagnosis

Herpes simplex may become impetiginized, as may eczema. Always think of a possible underlying cause such as this. For example, recurrent impetigo of the head and neck should prompt a search for scalp lice.

Investigation and treatment

The diagnosis is usually made on clinical grounds. Swabs should be taken and sent to the laboratory for culture, but treatment should not be held up until the results are available. Systemic antibiotics are needed for severe cases (flucloxacillin or erythro-mycin), or if a nephritogenic strain of streptococcus is suspected (penicillin V). For minor cases the removal of crusts and a topical antibiotic such as neomycin, fusidic acid, mupirocin, or bacitracin will suffice (Formulary, p. 292).

Ecthyma

This is the term used to describe ulcers forming under a crusted surface infection. The site may have been that of an insect bite or of neglected minor trauma. The bacterial pathogens and their treatment are similar to those of impetigo; however, in contrast to impetigo, ecthyma heals with scarring.

Furunculosis (boils)

Cause

A boil is an acute pustular infection of a hair follicle, usually with *Staphylococcus aureus*. Adolescent boys are especially susceptible to them.

Presentation and course

A tender red nodule (Fig. 15.3) enlarges and later may discharge pus and its central 'core', before healing to leave a scar. Fever and enlarged draining nodes complete the picture. Most patients have one or two boils only and then clear; a few patients suffer from a tiresome sequence of boils (chronic furunculosis).

Complications

Cavernous sinus thrombosis is an unusual complication of boils on the central face. Septicaemia may occur but is rare.

Differential diagnosis

The diagnosis is straightforward but hidradenitis suppurativa (p. 160) should be considered if only the groin and axillae are involved.

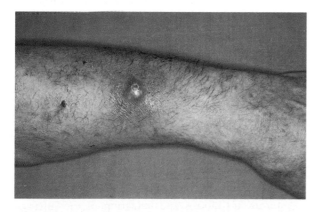

Fig. 15.3 A single furuncle on the forearm.

Investigations in chronic furunculosis

- General examination: look for underlying skin disease, e.g. scabies, pediculosis, eczema.
- Test the urine for sugar. Full blood count.
- Culture swabs from lesions, and carrier sites (nostrils, perineum) of patient and immediate family.
- Immunological evaluation only if the patient has recurrent or unusual internal infections too.

Treatment

Acute episodes will respond to an appropriate antibiotic; sometimes incision speeds healing.

In chronic furunculosis (Fig. 15.4):
- Treat carrier sites such as the nose and groin twice daily for six weeks with an appropriate antiseptic or antibiotic cream (e.g. mupirocin). Treat family carriers similarly.
- Treat lesions with a local antibiotic cream. In stubborn cases add six weeks of a systemic antibiotic chosen to cover organism's proven sensitivities.
- Daily bath using an antiseptic soap.
- Improve hygiene and nutritional state, if faulty.

Carbuncle

A group of adjacent hair follicles becomes deeply infected with *Staphylococcus aureus*, leading to a swollen, painful, suppurating area discharging pus from several points. The pain and systemic upset are greater than those of a boil. Diabetes must be excluded; treatment needs both topical and systemic antibiotics. The multiple deep, pus-filled pockets are not easy to drain surgically. Consider the possibility of a fungal kerion (p. 186) in unresponsive carbuncles.

Scalded skin syndrome

In this condition the skin changes resemble a scald. Erythema and tenderness are followed by the loosening of large areas of overlying epidermis (Fig. 15.5). In children the condition is usually staphylococcal in origin. Organisms in what may be only a minor local infection, such as impetigo, release a toxin (exfoliatin) which causes a split to occur high in the epidermis. With systemic antibiotics the outlook is good.

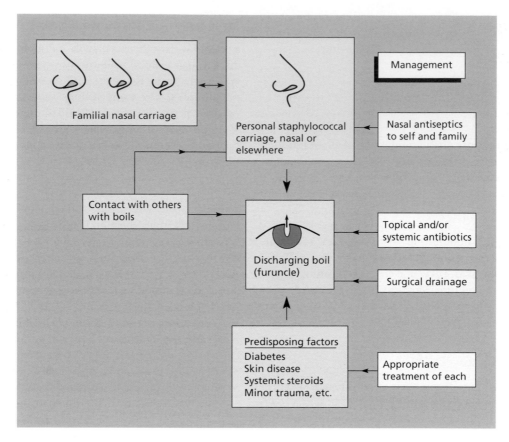

Fig. 15.4 Chronic furunculosis.

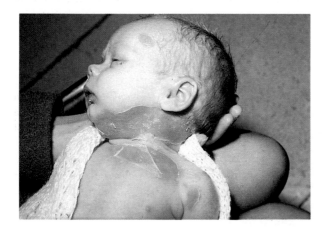

Fig. 15.5 Staphylococcal scalded skin syndrome in a child. The overlying epidermis is loosening in the red areas.

This is in contrast to toxic epidermal necrolysis which is usually drug-induced; the damage to the epidermis in TEN is full thickness, and skin biopsy will distinguish it from the scalded skin syndrome (p. 123).

Toxic shock syndrome

A staphylococcal toxin is responsible for this condition in which fever, a rash, usually a widespread erythema, and sometimes circulatory collapse, are followed a week or two later by characteristic desquamation most marked on the fingers and hands. Many cases have followed staphylococcal overgrowth in the vagina of women using tampons. Systemic antibiotics and irrigation of the infected site are needed.

Streptococcal infections

Erysipelas

The first warning of an attack is often malaise, shivering and a fever. After a few hours the affected area of skin becomes red, and the eruption spreads with a well-defined advancing edge. Blisters may develop on the red plaques (Fig. 15.6). Untreated, the condition may even be fatal, but it responds rapidly to systemic penicillin. The causative streptococci may gain their entry through a split in the skin, for example between the toes or under an ear lobe.

Episodes may repeatedly affect the same area and lead to persistent lymphoedema. Low dosage long-term oral penicillin V will usually cut down the frequency of recurrences. The cause of the original skin split, perhaps a minor tinea pedis, should be treated too.

LEARNING POINTS

1 Unlike lightning, erysipelas often strikes in the same place twice.
2 Shivering and malaise precede the rash but that is when the penicillin should be given.
3 Recurrent bouts may need long-term prophylactic penicillin.

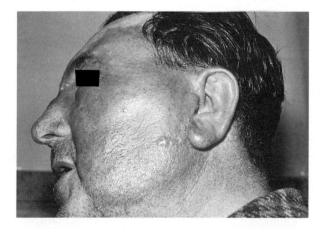

Fig. 15.6 Erysipelas — note sharp demarcation and gross oedema. The portal of entry here was in the external ear.

Cellulitis

This refers to an inflammation of the skin occurring at a deeper level than erysipelas. The subcutaneous tissues are involved and the area is more raised and swollen; the erythema is less marginated than in erysipelas. The condition often follows an injury and favours areas of hypostatic oedema. Streptococci, staphylococci, or other organisms may be the cause. Treatment is elevation, rest and systemic antibiotics.

Necrotizing fasciitis

A mixture of pathogens, usually including streptococci and anaerobes, is responsible for this rare condition which requires emergency treatment. At first the infection resembles a dusky, often painful, cellulitis, but it quickly turns into an extending necrosis of the skin and subcutaneous tissues. The prognosis is often poor despite early surgical debridement and systemic antibiotics.

Erysipeloid

It is convenient to mention this here, but the causative organism is *Erysipelothrix insidiosa* and not a streptococcus. It infects a wide range of animals, birds and fish. In humans, infections are most common in butchers, fish-mongers and cooks, the organism penetrating the skin after a prick from an infected bone. Usually such infections are mild, and localized to the area around the inoculation site. The swollen purple area spreads slowly with a clear-cut advancing edge. With penicillin the condition clears quickly; without it, resolution may take several weeks.

Cat-scratch disease

The infective agent is the bacillus, *Rochalimaea henselae*. A few days after a cat bite or scratch, a reddish granulomatous papule appears at the site of inoculation. Tender regional lymphadenopathy follows some weeks later, and lasts for several weeks, often being accompanied by a mild fever. The glands may discharge before settling spontaneously. There is no specific treatment.

Spirochaetal infections

Syphilis

Cause

Infection with the causative organism, *Treponema pallidum*, may be congenital, or acquired through transfusion with contaminated blood, or by accidental inoculation. The most important route, however, is through sexual contact with an infected partner.

Presentation

Congenital syphilis. A high standard of antenatal care ensures that syphilis in the mother is detected and treated during pregnancy — congenital syphilis is then rare. Otherwise, stillbirth is a common outcome, though some children with congenital syphilis may develop the stigmata of the disease only in late childhood. Some features of early and late congenital syphilis are listed in Fig. 15.7.

Acquired syphilis. The features of the different stages are given in Fig. 15.8. After an incubation period (9–90 days), a primary chancre develops at the site

of inoculation. Often this is genital, but oral and anal chancres are not uncommon. A typical chancre is an ulcerated, though not painful, button-like lesion of up to 1 cm in diameter accompanied by local

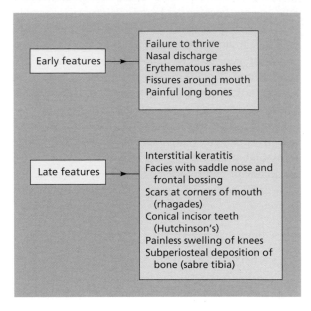

Fig. 15.7 The early and late features of congenital syphilis.

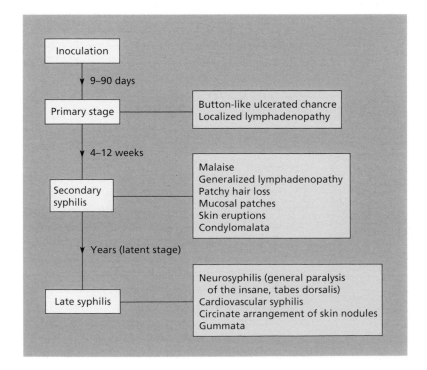

Fig. 15.8 The stages of syphilis.

lymphadenopathy. Untreated it lasts about six weeks and then clears leaving an inconspicuous scar.

The secondary stage may be reached while the chancre is still subsiding. Systemic symptoms and a generalized lymphadenopathy usher in eruptions which at first are macular and inconspicuous, and later papular and more obvious. Lesions are distributed symmetrically and are of a coppery, ham colour. Classically there are obvious lesions on the palms and soles. Annular lesions are also not uncommon. Condyloma lata are moist papules in the genital and anal areas. Other signs include 'moth-eaten' alopecia and mucus patches in the mouth.

The skin lesions of late syphilis may be nodules which spread peripherally and clear centrally, leaving a serpiginous outline. Gummas are granulomatous areas; in the skin they quickly form punched-out ulcers which heal poorly to leave papery white scars.

Clinical course

Even if left untreated, most of those who contract syphilis have no further problems after the secondary stage has passed. Others develop cutaneous or systemic manifestations of late syphilis.

Differential diagnosis

The skin changes of syphilis may mimic many other skin diseases. Always consider the following:
- *Chancre.* Chancroid (multiple and painful), herpes simplex, anal fissure, cervical erosions.
- *Secondary syphilis*:
  Eruption — measles, german measles, drug eruptions, pityriasis rosea, lichen planus, psoriasis.
  Condylomas — genital warts, piles.
  Oral lesions — aphthous ulcers.
- *Late syphilis.* Bromide and iodide reactions, other granulomas, erythema induratum.

Investigations

The diagnosis of syphilis in its infectious (primary and secondary) stages can be confirmed using dark-field microscopy to show up spirochaetes in smears from a chancre, an oral lesion, or a moist area in a secondary eruption.

Serological tests for syphilis become positive only some five to six weeks after infection (usually a week or two after the appearance of the chancre). The traditional tests (WR and VDRL) have now largely been replaced by more specific ones (e.g. the *Treponema pallidum* haemagglutination test and the fluorescent treponemal antibody/absorption test). These more sensitive tests tend not to become negative after treatment if an infection has been present for more than a few months.

Treatment

Penicillin is still the treatment of choice (e.g. for early syphilis benzathine penicillin 1.2 mega units given intramuscularly into each buttock at a single session, or procaine penicillin, 600 000 units intramuscularly, daily for 10 days), with erythromycin and tetracycline effective alternatives for those with penicillin allergy. The use of long-acting penicillin injections overcomes the ever-present danger of poor compliance with oral treatment. Every effort must be made to trace and treat infected contacts.

LEARNING POINTS
1 Syphilis is still around and today's general was yesterday's lieutenant.
2 It is still worthwhile checking for syphilis in perplexing rashes.

Yaws

Yaws is distributed widely across the poorer parts of the tropics. The spirochaete, *Treponema pallidum* subsp. *pertenue*, gains its entry through skin abrasions. After an incubation period of up to six months, the primary lesion, a crusting and ulcerated papule known as the 'mother yaw', develops at the site of inoculation; later it may enlarge to an exuberant raspberry-like swelling which lasts for several months before healing to leave an atrophic pale scar. In the secondary stage, other lesions may develop in any area but do so especially around the orifices. They are not unlike the primary lesion but are smaller and more numerous ('daughter yaws'). Hyperkeratotic plaques may appear on the palms and soles. The tertiary stage is characterized by ulcerated gummatous skin lesions, hyperkeratosis of the palms and soles, and a painful periostitis which distorts the long bones. Serological tests for syphilis are positive. Treatment is with penicillin.

Lyme disease

The spirochaete *Borrelia burgdorferi* is responsible for this condition, named after the town in the USA where it was first recognized. It is transmitted to humans by ticks of the genus *Ixodes* commonly harboured by deer. The site of the tick bite becomes the centre of a slowly expanding erythematous ring ('erythema migrans', Fig. 15.9). Later, many annular, non-scaly plaques may develop. In the USA about half of those affected develop arthritis and heart disease; both seem less common in European cases. Other internal complications include meningitis and cranial nerve palsies. Treated early the condition clears well with oral amoxycillin or doxycycline: patients affected systemically need longer courses of parenteral antibiotics. Confirmation of infection is by serology, though this is usually negative in the first few weeks after innoculation.

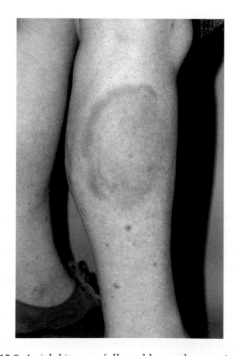

Fig. 15.9 A tick bite was followed by erythema migrans.

Other infections

Chronic gonococcal septicaemia

Skin lesions are important as a clue to the diagnosis of this condition, in which the symptoms and signs of classical gonorrhoea are usually absent. A patient with recurring fever and joint pains develops sparse crops of skin lesions, usually around the hands and feet. The grey, often haemorrhagic, vesicopustules are characteristic. Rather similar lesions may occur in chronic meningococcal septicaemia.

Mycobacterial infections

Tuberculosis

The steady decline of tuberculosis in developed countries has been reversed in some areas where AIDS is especially prevalent, but tuberculosis of the skin is still uncommon.

Inoculation tuberculosis

Lupus vulgaris follows the inoculation of tubercle bacilli into the skin of a person with a high degree of immunity. Lesions occur most often around the head and neck. A reddish-brown scaly plaque slowly enlarges, and may damage deeper tissues such as cartilage, leading to ugly mutilation. Scarring and contractures may follow.

Diascopy (p. 39) shows up the characteristic brownish 'apple jelly' nodules and the clinical diagnosis should be confirmed by a biopsy. A warty variant exists.

Scrofuloderma

The skin overlying a tuberculous lymph node or joint may become involved in the process. The subsequent mixture of lesions (irregular puckered scars, fistulae and abscesses) is most commonly seen in the neck.

Tuberculides

A number of skin eruptions have been, in the past, attributed to a reaction to internal foci of tuberculosis. Of these the best authenticated are the 'papulonecrotic tuberculides', recurring crops of firm dusky papules, which may ulcerate, and which favour the points of the knees and elbows.

Erythema induratum (Bazin's disease)

Erythema induratum is the presence of deep purplish ulcerating nodules on the backs of the lower legs, usually in women with a poor, 'chilblain' type of circulation. Sometimes this is associated with a tuberculous focus elsewhere. Erythema nodosum (p. 111) may also develop as the result of tuberculosis elsewhere.

Treatment

The treatment of all types of cutaneous tuberculosis should be with a full course of a standard antituberculosis regimen. There is no longer any excuse for the use of one drug alone.

Leprosy

Cause

Mycobacterium leprae was discovered by Hansen in 1874, but has still not been cultured *in vitro*, though it can be made to grow in some animals (armadillos, mouse foot-pads, etc.). In humans the route of infection is through nasal droplets from cases of lepromatous leprosy.

Epidemiology

Some 15 million people suffer from leprosy. Most live in the tropics and subtropics, but the ease of modern travel means that some cases are seen in northern Europe and the USA.

Presentation

The range of clinical manifestations and complications depends upon the immune response of the patient (Fig. 15.10). Those with a high resistance tend to develop a paucibacillary tuberculoid type and those with low resistance a multibacillary lepromatous type. Between the extremes lies a spectrum of reactions, classified as 'borderline'. Those most like the tuberculoid type are known as borderline

tuberculoid (BT) and those nearest to the lepromatous type as borderline lepromatous (BL). The clinical differences between the two polar types are given in Fig. 15.11.

Differential diagnosis

Tuberculoid leprosy. Consider the following — in none of which is there any loss of sensation:
- Vitiligo (p. 213) — loss of pigment is usually complete.
- Pityriasis versicolor (p. 191) — scrapings show mycelia and spores.
- Pityriasis alba — a common cause of fine scaly and hypopigmented areas on the cheeks of children.
- Post-inflammatory depigmentation of any cause.
- Sarcoidosis, granuloma annulare, necrobiosis lipoidica.

Lepromatous leprosy. Widespread leishmaniasis may closely simulate lepromatous leprosy. The nodules seen in neurofibromatosis and mycosis fungoides and multiple sebaceous cysts may cause confusion, as may the acral deformities seen in yaws and systemic sclerosis. Leprosy is a great imitator.

Investigations

- Biopsy of skin or sensory nerve.
- Skin or nasal smears, with Ziehl–Nielsen or Fité stains, will show up the large number of organisms seen in the lepromatous type.
- Lepromin test. This is of no use in the diagnosis of leprosy, but once the diagnosis has been made it will help in deciding on the type of disease present (positive in tuberculoid type).

Treatment

The emergence of resistant strains of *M. leprae* means that it is no longer wise to treat leprosy with dapsone alone. It should now be used in combination, usually with rifampicin, and also with clofazimine for lepromatous leprosy. A brief period of isolation is needed only for patients with infectious lepromatous leprosy; with treatment they quickly become non-infectious and can return to the community. However, their management should remain in the hands of physicians with a special interest in the disease.

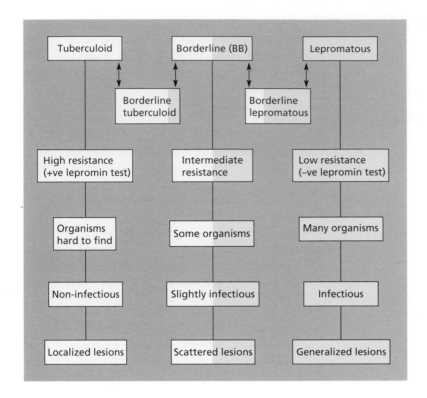

Fig. 15.10 The spectrum of leprosy: tuberculoid to lepromatous.

Tuberculoid forms are usually treated for six to twelve months; multibacillary leprosy needs treatment for at least two years.

Special care is needed with the two types of lepra reaction which may occur during treatment:
- Type 1 (reversal) reactions are seen mainly in tuberculoid disease — lesions become red and angry, and pain and paralysis may follow neural inflammation. They are usually treated with salicylates, chloroquine, non-steroidal and steroidal anti-inflammatory drugs.
- Type 2 reactions are common in lepromatous leprosy and include erythema nodosum, nerve palsies, lymphadenopathy, arthritis, iridocyclitis, epididymo-orchitis and proteinuria. They are treated with the same drugs which are used for type 1 reactions, and also with thalidomide.

The household contacts of lepromatous patients are at risk of developing leprosy and should be followed up. Child contacts may benefit from prophylactic therapy and BCG innoculation.

Other mycobacterial infections

Mycobacteria are widespread in nature, living as environmental saprophytes. Some can infect humans.

Mycobacterium marinum lives in water. Human infections have occurred in epidemics centred on infected swimming pools. Another route of infection is through minor skin breaches in those who clean out tropical fish tanks. After a three-week incubation period an indolent abscess or ulcerated nodule forms at the site of inoculation; later nodules may develop along the draining lymphatics (sporotrichoid spread) (p. 193). The lesions heal spontaneously, but slowly. Resolution may be speeded by an eight-week course of trimethoprim/sulphamethoxazole or minocycline.

Mycobacterium ulcerans. Infections are confined to certain humid tropical areas where the organism lives on the vegetation, and are most common in Uganda (Buruli ulcers). The necrotic spreading ulcers, with their undermined edges, are usually found on the legs. Drug therapy is disappointing and

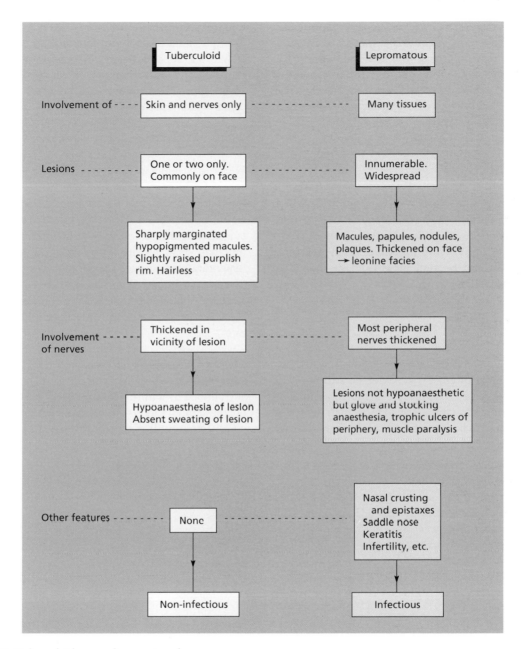

Fig. 15.11 Tuberculoid versus lepromatous leprosy.

the treatment of choice is probably surgical removal of infected tissue.

Leishmaniasis

Leishmania organisms are protozoa whose life cycle includes stages in phlebotomus flies, from which they are transmitted to humans. Different species, in different geographical areas, cause different clinical pictures.

- *Leishmania tropica* is found around the Mediterranean coast and in southern Asia; it causes chronically discharging skin nodules (oriental sores).
- *Leishmania donovani* is the cause of kala-azar, a

disease characterized by fever, hepatosplenomegaly and anaemia. The skin may show an irregular darkening, particularly on the face and hands.

Antimony compounds are still the treatment of choice in most types of leishmaniasis. Destructive measures, including cryotherapy, are sometimes used for localized skin lesions.

Viral infections

The viral infections dealt with here are those which commonly present at dermatology clinics. A textbook of infectious diseases should be consulted for details of systemic viral infections, many of which, like measles and german measles, have their own specific rashes.

Viral warts

Cause

The human papilloma virus (HPV) has still not been cultured *in vitro*. Nevertheless the technique of DNA hybridization has allowed more than 60 'types' of the virus to be recognized, each with its own range of clinical manifestations. HPV-1, 2, and 4, for example, tend to be found in common warts, while HPV-6, 11, 16, and 18 are most commonly found in genital warts. Infections occur when infected skin scales come into contact with breaches in the skin or mucous membranes.

Presentation

Warts may adopt a variety of patterns (Fig. 15.12), some of which are described below.

Common warts (Figs 15.13 & 15.14). The first sign is a smooth skin-coloured papule, often more easily felt than seen. As the lesion enlarges, an irregular hyperkeratotic surface develops with the classic 'warty' appearance. Common warts usually occur on the hands but are also often on the face and genitals. They are more often multiple than single. Pain is rare.

Plantar warts. These are characterized by a rough surface, protruding only slightly from the skin and surrounded by a horny collar (Fig. 15.15). On paring, oozing capillary loops distinguish plantar warts from corns. Often multiple, plantar warts may be painful.

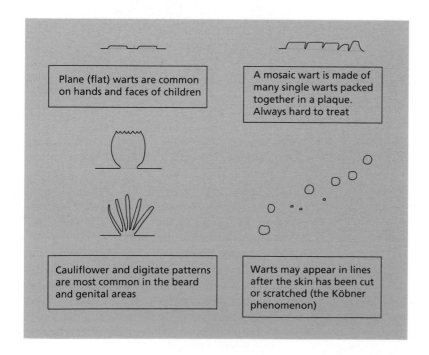

Fig. 15.12 Viral warts — variations on the theme.

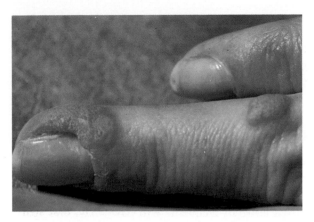

Fig. 15.13 Typical common warts on the fingers.

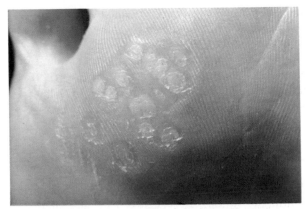

Fig. 15.16 Group of warts under the forefoot pared to show mosaic pattern.

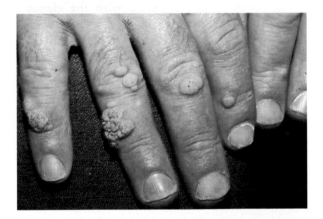

Fig. 15.14 Multiple hand warts in a fishmonger.

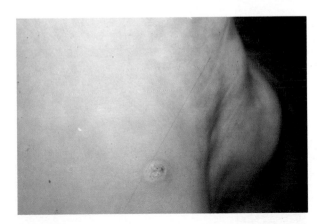

Fig. 15.15 Solitary plantar wart on the heel.

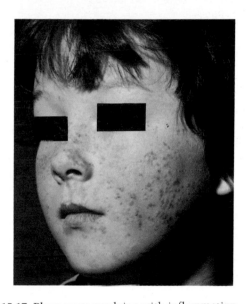

Fig. 15.17 Plane warts resolving with inflammation.

vidual warts. They are most common on the soles but are also seen on palms and around finger nails. They are usually not painful.

Plane warts (Fig. 15.17). These smooth, flat-topped papules are most commonly seen on the face and brow and on the backs of the hands. Usually skin-coloured or light brown, they become inflamed as they resolve spontaneously. Lesions are multiple, painless, and, as with common warts, sometimes arranged along a scratch line.

Facial warts. These are most common in the beard

Mosaic warts (Fig. 15.16). These plaque-like hyperkeratotic lesions, often extensive, are made up of multiple, small, tightly packed but discrete indi-

area of the adult male and are liable to be spread by shaving. A digitate appearance is common. Lesions may be ugly but are painless.

Anogenital warts (condyloma acuminata) (Figs 15.18 & 15.19). Papillomatous cauliflower-like lesions, with a moist macerated vascular surface, may appear anywhere in this area. They may coalesce to form huge lesions causing discomfort and irritation. The vaginal and anorectal mucosae may be affected. The presence of anogenital warts in children raises the possibility of sexual abuse, but most often is due to autoinoculation from common warts elsewhere.

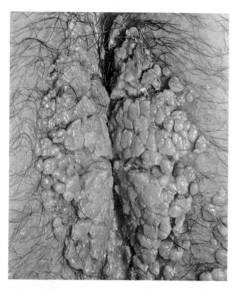

Fig. 15.18 Exuberant peri-anal warts.

Course

Warts resolve spontaneously in the healthy as their immune response overcomes the infection: this happens within six months in 30% of patients. Spontaneous resolution, sometimes heralded by punctate blackening due to capillary thrombosis (Fig. 15.20), leaves no trace. Mosaic warts are notoriously slow to resolve and often resist all treatment. Warts persist and spread in immunocompromised patients, e.g. those on immunosuppressive therapy or with lymphoreticular disease. Seventy per cent of renal allograft recipients will have warts five years after transplantation.

Complications

1 Some plantar warts are very painful.
2 Epidermodysplasia verruciformis is a rare inherited disorder in which there is universal wart infection, usually with HPV of unusual types. An impairment of cell-mediated immunity (p. 32) is commonly found and ensuing carcinomatous change frequently occurs.
3 Malignant change is otherwise rare though infections with HPV of certain genital strains may predispose to cervical carcinoma. HPV infections in immunocompromised patients (e.g. renal allograft recipients) have also been linked with skin cancer most commonly on light-exposed areas.

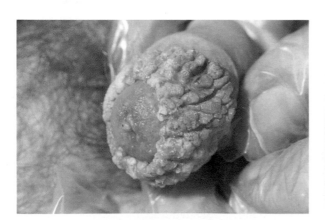

Fig. 15.19 Massive penile warts in an immunosuppressed patient.

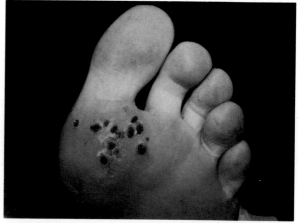

Fig. 15.20 Spontaneous resolution of a group of plantar warts. The blackness is due to capillary thrombosis.

Differential diagnosis

Most warts are easily recognized. The following must be ruled out:

• *Molluscum contagiosum* (p. 180) — smooth dome-shaped and pearly, with central umbilication. Caused by a pox virus.

• *Plantar corns* — on pressure areas, no capillary bleeding on paring. Have a central keratotic core and are painful.

• *Granuloma annulare* (p. 247) — surface is smooth, the lesions dermal, and the outline often annular.

• *Condyloma lata* — seen in syphilis. Rare but should not be confused with condyloma acuminata (warts). Lesions are flatter, greyer and less well defined. In doubt, other signs of secondary syphilis (p. 167) should be looked for, and serological tests carried out.

• *Amelanotic melanomas and other epithelial malignancies* — verrucose nodules in patients over the age of 40 should be examined with special care. Mistakes have been made in the past.

Treatment

Palmoplantar warts. Home treatment is best and can be carried out with one of the many wart paints now available (Formulary, p. 293). Most contain salicylic acid (12–20%). The success rate is good if the patient is prepared to persist with regular treatment. Paints should be applied once daily, after moistening the warts in hot water for at least five minutes. After drying, dead tissue and old paint are removed with an emery board or pumice stone. Enough paint to cover the surface of the wart, but not the surrounding skin, is applied and allowed to dry. Warts on the plantar surface should be covered with plasters though this is not necessary elsewhere. Side effects are rare if these instructions are followed. Wart paints should not be applied to facial or anogenital skin, or to patients with adjacent eczema.

If no progress is being made after regular and correct use of the salicylic acid wart paint for 12 weeks, then a paint containing formaldehyde or glutaraldehyde is worth trying. A useful way of dealing with multiple small plantar warts is for the area to be soaked for 10 minutes each night in a 4% formalin solution. A few patients may become allergic to this.

Cryotherapy, with carbon dioxide or liquid nitrogen, is effective. However, it is painful and should perhaps remain, after wart paints, the second line of treatment for most patients. A cotton-tipped applicator dipped into liquid nitrogen, or a CO_2 stick, is applied to the wart until a small frozen halo appears in the surrounding normal skin (Fig. 15.21). If further treatment is necessary the optimal interval is three weeks. A few minutes tuition from a dermatologist will help a practitioner wishing to start cryotherapy. Blisters should not be provoked intentionally, but occur from time to time, and should not alarm patients who have been forewarned.

Anogenital warts. Women with anogenital warts, or who are the partners of men with anogenital warts, should have regular tests of cervical cytology since the wart virus can cause cervical cancer.

Cryotherapy is suitable for treating anogenital warts. Some prefer to use podophyllin paint (Formulary, p. 293) which should be applied carefully to the warts and allowed to dry before powdering with talc. On the first occasion it should be washed off with soap and water after two hours but if there has been little discomfort this may be increased stepwise to six hours. Treatment is best carried out weekly by a doctor or nurse and not by the patient. Podophyllin must not be used in pregnancy.

Facial common warts. These are best treated with electrocautery or a hyfrecator but also surrender to careful cryotherapy. Shaving, if essential, should be with a brushless foam and a disposable razor.

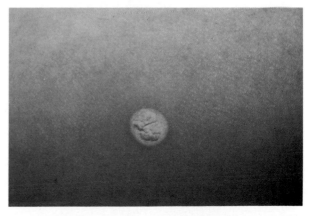

Fig. 15.21 A wart treated with cryotherapy: area includes a small frozen halo of normal surrounding skin.

Plane warts. On the face these are best left untreated and the patient or parent can be reasonably assured that spontaneous resolution will occur. When treatment is demanded, careful freezing is the best method.

Solitary, stubborn, or painful warts. These may be removed under local anaesthetic with a curette, though cure is not assured with this or any other method and a scar often follows. Surgical excision is never justifiable (Fig. 15.22). Bleomycin can also be injected into such warts with success but this treatment should only be carried out by a specialist.

LEARNING POINTS
1 Do not hurt children with cryotherapy without a good trial of a wart paint first.
2 Treat most warts with a wart paint for 12 weeks before referring.
3 Do not leave scars: nature does not.
4 Avoid podophyllin during pregnancy.
5 Do not miss an amelanotic malignant melanoma.

Varicella (chickenpox)

Cause

The herpes virus varicella-zoster is spread by the respiratory route; its incubation period is about 14 days.

Presentation and course

Slight malaise is followed by the development of papules which turn rapidly into clear vesicles, the contents of which soon become pustular. Over the next few days the lesions crust and then clear, sometimes leaving white depressed scars. Lesions appear in crops, are often itchy and are most profuse on the trunk and least profuse on the periphery of the limbs (centripetal). Second attacks are rare.

Complications

- Pneumonitis, with pulmonary opacities on X-ray.
- Secondary infection of skin lesions.
- Haemorrhagic or lethal chickenpox in the immunocompromised.
- Scarring.

Differential diagnosis

Smallpox, mainly centrifugal anyway, has been universally eradicated now, and the diagnosis is seldom in doubt.

Investigations

None are usually needed.

Treatment

Acyclovir (Formulary, p. 301) should be reserved for severe attacks and for immunocompromised patients; for the latter hyperimmune globulin can also be used to prevent disease if given within a day or two of exposure. For mild attacks calamine lotion topically is all that is required. A live attenuated vaccine is now available and may be used for children who otherwise might have unusually severe chickenpox, for example those with leukaemia in remission.

Herpes zoster

Cause

Shingles is also caused by the herpes virus varicella-

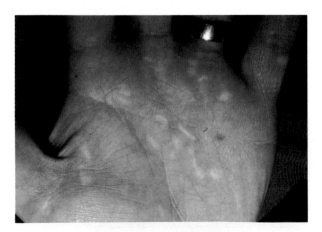

Fig. 15.22 Multiple scars following the injudicious surgical treatment of warts.

zoster. An attack is due to the reactivation, usually for no apparent reason, of virus which has remained dormant in a sensory root ganglion since an earlier episode of chickenpox (varicella). The incidence of shingles is highest in old age, and in conditions such as Hodgkin's disease, AIDS, and leukaemia, which weaken the normal defence mechanisms. Shingles does not occur in epidemics; its clinical manifestations are due to virus acquired in the past; however, patients with zoster may transmit the virus to others in whom it will cause chickenpox (Fig. 15.23).

Presentation and course

Attacks usually start with a burning pain soon followed by erythema and grouped, sometimes blood-filled, vesicles scattered over a dermatome. The clear vesicles quickly become purulent, and over the space of a few days burst and crust. Scabs usually separate in two to three weeks, sometimes leaving depressed depigmented scars.

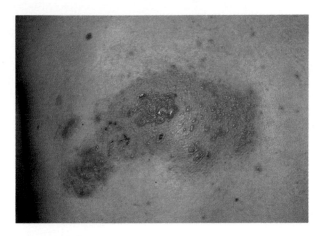

Fig. 15.24 Herpes zoster of a mid-thoracic dermatome.

Zoster is characteristically unilateral (Figs 15.24 & 15.25). It may affect more than one adjacent dermatome. The thoracic segments and the ophthalmic division of the trigeminal nerve are involved disproportionately often.

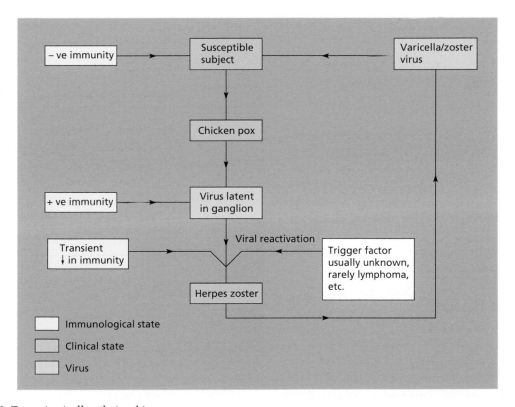

Fig. 15.23 Zoster/varicella relationships.

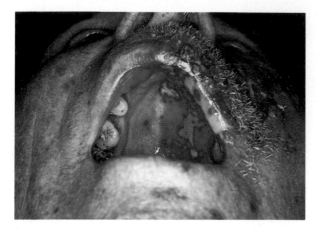

Fig. 15.25 Herpes zoster of the second division of the trigeminal nerve with severe ulceration of one side of the palate.

It is not uncommon for a few pock-like lesions to be found outside the main segment of involvement, but a generalized chickenpox-like eruption accompanying segmental zoster should raise suspicions of an underlying immunocompromised state or malignancy, particularly if the lesions are unusually haemorrhagic or necrotic.

Complications

- Secondary bacterial infection is common.
- Motor nerve involvement is much less common, but has led to paralysis of ocular muscles, the facial muscles, the diaphragm, and the bladder.
- Zoster of the ophthalmic division of the trigeminal nerve may lead to corneal ulcers and scarring. A good clinical clue here is involvement of the nasociliary branch (vesicles grouped on the side of the nose).
- Persistent neuralgic pain, after the acute episode is over, is most common in the elderly.

Differential diagnosis

Occasionally the initial pain, before the rash has appeared, is taken for an emergency such as acute appendicitis or myocardial infarction. Otherwise the dermatomal distribution, and the pain, allow zoster to be distinguished easily from herpes simplex, eczema, and impetigo.

Investigations

Blister fluid can be sent to the laboratory for culture in the few cases when the diagnosis is in doubt. Clinical suspicions about underlying conditions, such as Hodgkin's disease, chronic lymphatic leukaemia, or AIDS, will require further investigation.

Treatment

Mild attacks need only rest, analgesics, and bland applications such as calamine. Secondary bacterial infection should be treated appropriately.

Systemic acyclovir should be used for severe cases, and especially for ophthalmic zoster (Formulary, p. 301). To achieve its maximum effect, treatment has to start within the first two days of an attack. We are among those who think that acyclovir cuts down the incidence of post-herpetic neuralgia. We now prefer it to the tapered course of prednisolone recommended by some to help prevent neuralgia in the elderly. Famciclovir (Formulary, p. 301) is a recently introduced alternative which, like acyclovir, depends on virus-specific thymidine kinase for its antiviral activity. A trial of systemic carbamazepine or four weeks of topical capsaicin cream (Formulary, p. 296) is worthwhile in established post-herpetic neuralgia.

LEARNING POINTS
1 Post-herpetic neuralgia affects the old rather than the young.
2 Systemic acyclovir only works if given within 48 hours of the onset.
3 Look for an underlying cause when there is widespread involvement.

Herpes simplex

Cause

Herpes virus hominis is the cause of herpes simplex. The virus is ubiquitous and carriers may continue to shed virus particles in their saliva or tears. It has been separated into two types. The lesions caused by type II virus occur mainly on the genitals, while those of type I are usually extragenital: this distinction is not absolute however.

The route of infection may be through mucous membranes or abraded skin. After the episode associated with the primary infection, the virus may become latent, possibly within nerve ganglia, but still capable of giving rise to recurrent bouts of vesication (recrudescences).

Presentation

The primary infection. The most common regonizable manifestation of a primary type I infection in children is an acute gingivostomatitis accompanied by malaise, headache, fever, and enlarged cervical nodes. Vesicles, soon turning into ulcers, can be seen scattered over the lips and mucous membranes. The illness lasts about two weeks.

Primary type II virus infections, usually transmitted sexually, cause multiple and painful genital or peri-anal blisters which rapidly ulcerate.

The virus can also be inoculated directly into the skin, for example during wrestling. A herpetic whitlow is one example of this direct inoculation: the uncomfortable pus-filled blisters on a finger tip are seen most often in medical personnel attending patients with unsuspected herpes simplex infections.

Recurrent (recrudescent) infections. These occur in roughly the same place each time: they may be precipitated by respiratory tract infections (cold sores), UVR, menstruation or even stress. Common

sites include the face and lips (type I) (Fig. 15.26) and the genitals (type II) but lesions can occur anywhere. Tingling, burning, or even pain, is followed within a few hours by the development of erythema and clusters of tense vesicles. Crusting occurs within 24–48 hours and the whole episode lasts about twelve days.

Complications

- Herpes encephalitis or meningitis may occur without any cutaneous clues.
- Disseminated herpes simplex: widespread vesicles may be part of a severe illness in newborns, debilitated children or immunosuppressed adults.
- Eczema herpeticum: patients with atopic eczema are particularly susceptible to widespread cutaneous herpes simplex infections. Those looking after patients with atopic eczema should stay away if they develop cold sores.
- Herpes simplex may cause recurrent dendritic ulcers leading to corneal scarring.
- Erythema multiforme (p. 109) may in some patients regularly follow recurrent herpes simplex infections.

Investigations

Nonc are usually needed. Doubts over the diagnosis can be dispelled by culturing the virus from vesicle fluid. Antibody titres rise with primary, but not with recurrent infections.

Treatment

'Old-fashioned' remedies will suffice for occasional mild attacks of recurrent herpes simplex. Dabbing with surgical spirit is helpful and secondary bacterial infection may be reduced with topical framycetin sulphate or sodium fusidate. For more severe and frequent attacks, acyclovir cream, providing it is used at the first sign of the recrudescence, and applied five or six times a day for the first four days of the episode, may cut down the length of attacks and perhaps increase the intervals between them.

Acyclovir tablets (Formulary, p. 301), 200 mg five times daily for five days, will also shorten an attack, and should be prescribed for those with widespread or systemic involvement. Recurrences in the immunocompromised can usually be prevented by long-term treatment at a lower dose.

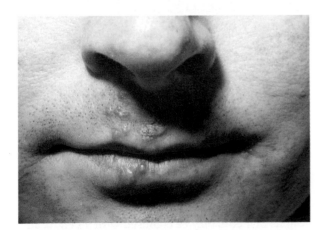

Fig. 15.26 The grouped vesicles of herpes simplex, here provoked by sunlight.

Molluscum contagiosum

Cause

This common pox virus infection can be spread by direct contact, for example sexually, or by towels, clothing, etc.

Presentation and course

The incubation period varies from two to six weeks. Often several members of one family are affected. Individual lesions are shiny, white or pink, and hemispherical; they grow slowly up to 0.5 cm in diameter. A central punctum which may contain a cheesy core, gives the lesions their characteristic umbilicated look.

On close inspection a mosaic appearance may be seen (Fig. 15.27). Multiple lesions are common (Fig. 15.28) and their distribution depends on the mode of infection. Atopic individuals and the immunocompromised are prone to especially extensive infections, spread by scratching and the use of topical steroids (Fig. 15.29).

Untreated lesions usually clear, often after a brief local inflammation, in six to nine months. Large solitary lesions may take longer. Some leave depressed scars.

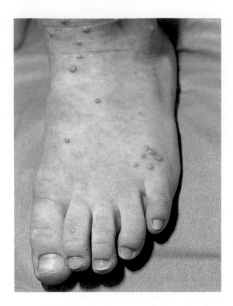

Fig. 15.28 Multiple lesions scattered over the foot of a child: some show the typical punctum.

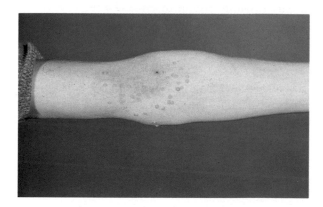

Fig. 15.29 Molluscum lesions concentrated in an area of atopic eczema in the elbow flexures.

Complications

Eczematous patches often appear around mollusca. Traumatized or overtreated lesions may become secondarily infected.

Differential diagnosis

Inflamed lesions may simulate a boil. Large solitary lesions in adults may be confused with a keratocanthoma (p. 227) an intradermal naevus (p. 223), or even a cystic basal cell carcinoma (p. 230). Confusion

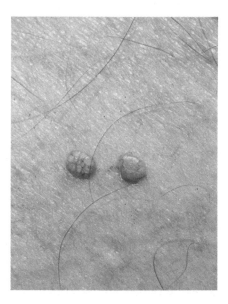

Fig. 15.27 Two typical molluscum lesions, one of which shows a mosaic appearance.

with warts should not arise — these have a rough surface and no central pore.

Investigations

None are usually needed, but the diagnosis can be confirmed by looking under the microscope for large swollen epidermal cells which are easily seen in unstained preparations of debris expressed from a lesion.

Treatment

Many simple destructive measures cause inflammation and then resolution. These include squeezing out the lesions with forceps, piercing them with an orange stick (preferably without phenol), and curettage. Liquid nitrogen is also effective.

These measures are fine in adults, but young children dislike them and it is reasonable to play for time using aureomycin ointment, or instructing the mother carefully how to apply a wart paint once a week to lesions well away from the eyes. Sometimes a local anaesthetic cream (EMLA; see Formulary, p. 296) under polythene occlusion for an hour will help children to tolerate more attacking treatment. Sparse eyelid lesions can be left alone but patients with numerous lesions may need to be referred to an ophthalmologist for curettage. Common sense measures will help to limit spread within the family.

LEARNING POINTS

1 If you cannot tell mollusca from warts buy a lens.
2 Do not hurt young children with mollusca with radical treatment. You will not be able to get near them next time something goes wrong.

Orf

Cause

Contagious pustular dermatitis is a common condition in lambs. Its cause is a parapox virus which can be transmitted to those handling infected animals. The condition is, therefore, most commonly seen on the hands of shepherds, of their wives who bottle-feed lambs, and of butchers, vets and meat porters.

Presentation and course

The incubation period is five to six days. Lesions, which may be single or multiple, start as small firm papules which change into flat-topped apparently pustular nodules with a violaceous and erythematous surround. The condition clears up spontaneously in about a month.

Complications

- Lymphadenitis and malaise are common.
- Erythema multiforme.
- 'Giant' lesions in the immunosuppressed.

Differential diagnosis

Diagnosis is usually simple if contact with sheep is recognized. Milker's nodules, a pox virus infection acquired from cow's udders, may look similar to orf, as may staphylococcal furuncles.

Investigations

None are usually needed. In doubt the diagnosis can be confirmed by the distinctive electron microscopic appearance of the virus obtained from crusts.

Treatment

A topical antibiotic will help prevent secondary infection; otherwise no active therapy is needed.

Acquired immunodeficiency syndrome (AIDS)

The AIDS epidemic was first recognized in the USA in 1981. The early cases were male homosexuals with pneumocystis pneumonia or Kaposi's sarcoma and immunosuppression. Later it became clear that the human immunodeficiency virus (HIV) could be acquired from contaminated body fluids, particularly semen and blood, in many ways, the importance of which varies from country to country. In the UK and the USA, for example, most cases have been homosexual or bisexual men: in parts of Africa, on the other hand, the disease is most often spread heterosexually.

Other groups at high risk are intravenous drug abusers who share contaminated needles and syringes, and haemophiliacs who were given infected blood products. Up to a half of babies born to infected mothers will be infected transplacentally.

It has been estimated that, worldwide, at least half a million people have now had AIDS, and the epidemic is not slackening off.

Pathogenesis

The human immunodeficiency viruses, HIV-1 and HIV-2 (mainly in West Africa), are retroviruses containing reverse transcriptase enzymes which allow the virus to be incorporated into the chromosomes of the host cell. Their main target is a subset of T lymphocytes (helper/inducer cells) which express glycoprotein CD4 molecules on their surface. These bind to the surface envelope of the HIV. Viral replication within the helper/inducer cells kills them, and their depletion leads to the loss of cell-mediated immunity so characteristic of HIV infection. A variety of opportunistic infections may then follow.

Course of the disease

The original infection may be asymptomatic, or be followed by a glandular fever-like illness at the time of seroconversion. After a variable latent phase, which may last several years, a persistent generalized lymphadenopathy develops. The term 'AIDS-related complex' refers to the next stage, in which many of the symptoms of AIDS (e.g. fever, weight-loss, fatigue, or diarrhoea) may be present without the opportunistic infections or tumours characteristic of full-blown AIDS. Not all of those infected with HIV will develop AIDS but for those who do the average time from infection to the onset of AIDS is about 10 years. Once AIDS develops about half will die within one year and three-quarters within four years.

Skin changes in AIDS

Skin conditions are often the first clue to the presence of AIDS. The following are important:
1 *Kaposi's sarcoma* (Figs 15.30–15.32) — is the initial

presentation in up to one-quarter of AIDS patients, being especially common in homosexual men. The lesions of classical Kaposi's sarcoma are multiple, purplish nodules (see Fig. 19.49); in AIDS the lesions may be atypical, sometimes looking like bruises (Fig. 15.31) or pyogenic granulomata (p. 241). The diagnosis can easily be missed.
2 *Seborrhoeic eczema and folliculitis* (Fig. 15.33) — are seen in at least 50% of patients, often starting at an early stage of immunosuppression. The underlying cause may be an overgrowth of pityrosporum yeasts. An itchy folliculitis of the head, neck and trunk, and an eosinophilic folliculitis, possibly due to the multiplication of demodex folliculorum, have also been described.
3 *Skin infections* — florid, unusually extensive or

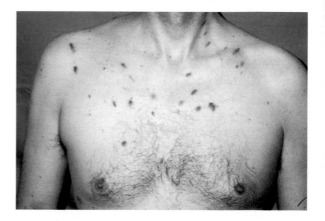

Fig. 15.30 Disseminated Kaposi's sarcoma in AIDS.

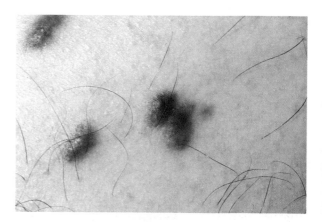

Fig. 15.31 Kaposi's sarcoma in AIDS.

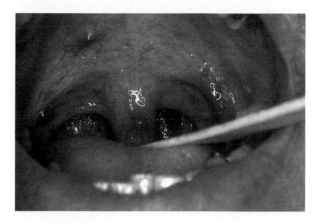

Fig. 15.32 Kaposi's sarcoma of hard palate, anterior fauces and uvula in AIDS.

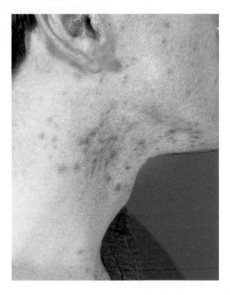

Fig. 15.33 Seborrhoeic dermatitis (otitis externa) and seborrhoeic folliculitis in HIV disease.

atypical examples of common infections may be seen with one or more of the following: herpes simplex, herpes zoster, molluscum contagiosum, candida, tinea, pityriasis versicolor, scabies, and staphylococci. Hairy leukoplakia, often on the sides of the tongue, may be due to proliferation of the Epstein–Barr virus. Bacillary angiomatosis may look like Kaposi's sarcoma and is due to the bacillus which causes cat-scratch fever. Syphilis may co-exist with AIDS as may mycobacterial infections.

4 *Other manifestations* — dry skin is common in AIDS; so is pruritus. Psoriasis may start or worsen with AIDS. Diffuse alopecia is not uncommon.

Management

The clinical diagnosis of HIV infection is confirmed by a positive blood test for antibodies to the virus. Patients should be counselled before and after testing for HIV antibody. Sexual contacts of infected individuals should be traced. No specific treatment for the underlying condition exists, and so the emphasis must be on prevention of infection and on education of the public. Monitoring the level of T helper cells may act as a guide to the progression of the disease. The benefits of zidovudine have to be balanced against its side effects. Otherwise treatment is symptomatic and varies according to the type of infection detected. Prophylactic treatment against a number of life-threatening infections is worthwhile and prolongs life expectancy.

Mucocutaneous lymph node syndrome
(Kawasaki's disease)

The cause may be a recent parvovirus infection. The disease affects young children whose erythema, though often generalized, becomes most marked in a glove and stocking distribution. Peeling around the fingers and toes is one obvious feature but is not seen at the start.

The episode is accompanied by fever and usually resolves within two weeks. Despite its name, not all patients have lymphadenopathy. The danger of this condition lies in the proportion of children who develop myocarditis and coronary artery disease. The pathology is close to that of polyarteritis nodosa. Treatment with aspirin has been recommended as a way of reducing the risk of coronary artery involvement. Gammaglobulin should also be given.

Gianotti–Crosti syndrome

This is a rather uncommon reaction to infection with hepatitis B virus in childhood. Small reddish papules erupt bilaterally over the limbs and face, and fade over the course of a few weeks. Jaundice is uncommon though tests of liver function give abnormal results.

Herpangina

This is an acute infectious illness, caused by group A Coxsackie viruses. The patient is usually a child with a fever, and a severe sore throat covered in many small vesicles which rapidly become superficial ulcers. Episodes resolve in about a week.

Hand, foot and mouth disease

This is usually due to Coxsackie A16. Minor epidemics occur in institutions. The oral vesicles are larger and fewer than those of herpangina. The hand and foot lesions are small greyish vesicles with a narrow rim of redness around. The condition settles within a few days.

Measles

An incubation period of 10 days is followed by fever, conjunctival injection, photophobia, and upper respiratory tract catarrh. Koplik's spots are seen at this stage on the buccal mucosa. The characteristic rash starts after a few days, on the brow and behind the ears, and soon becomes extensive before fading with much desquamation.

German measles (rubella)

Lymphadenopathy occurs a few days before the evanescent pink macular rash which fades, first on the trunk, over the course of a few days. Rubella during the first trimester of pregnancy carries a risk of damage to the unborn child.

Erythema infectiosum (fifth disease)

This is caused by the human parvovirus and occurs in small outbreaks, often in the spring. A slapped-cheek erythema is quickly followed by a reticulate erythema of the shoulders. The affected children feel well, and the rash clears over the course of a few days. Other features, sometimes not accompanied by a rash, include transient anaemia and arthritis.

Fungal infections

Dermatophyte infections (ringworm)

Cause

Three genera of dermatophyte fungi cause tinea infections (ringworm):
- *Trichophyton* (skin, hair and nail infections).
- *Microsporum* (skin and hair).
- *Epidermophyton* (skin and nails).

Dermatophytes invade keratin only, and the inflammation they cause is due to metabolic products of the fungus or to delayed hypersensitivity. In general, zoophilic fungi (those transmitted to man by animals) cause a more severe inflammation than anthropophilic ones (spread from person to person).

Presentation and course

This depends upon the site (Fig. 15.34), and on the strain of fungus involved.

Tinea pedis (athlete's foot). This is the commonest type of fungal infection in man. The sharing of wash places, for example in coal mines, and of swimming pools, predisposes to infection: occlusive footwear encourages relapses.

Most cases are due to one of three organisms: *Trichophyton rubrum* (the most common and the most stubborn), *Trichophyton mentagrophytes* var. *interdigitale* and *Epidermophyton floccosum*.

There are three common clinical patterns:
1 Soggy interdigital scaling, particularly in the fourth and fifth interspace (all three organisms) (Fig. 15.35).
2 A diffuse dry scaling of the soles (usually *T. rubrum*).
3 Recurrent episodes of vesication (usually *T. mentagrophytes* var. *interdigitale* or *E. floccosum*).

Tinea of the nails. Toe nail infection is usually associated with tinea pedis. The initial changes occur at the free edge of the nail which becomes yellow and crumbly (Fig. 15.36). Subungual hyperkeratosis, separation of the nail from its bed, and thickening may then follow. Usually only a few nails are infected

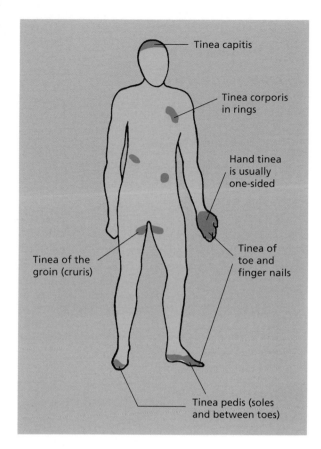

Fig. 15.34 Sites susceptible to dermatophyte infections.

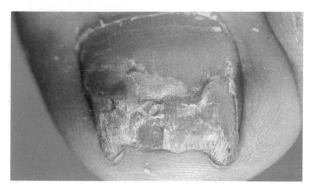

Fig. 15.36 Chronic tinea of the big toe nail. Starting distally, the thickness and discoloration are spreading proximally.

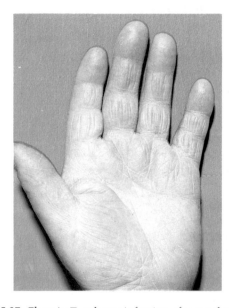

Fig. 15.37 Chronic *T. rubrum* infection of one palm. Minimal erythema, and dry powdery scaling most marked in the skin creases. Always look for similar changes on the feet.

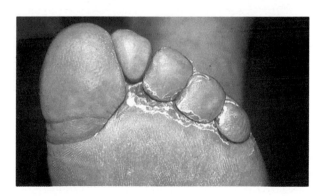

Fig. 15.35 Tinea pedis. Scaly area spreading to the sole from the toe webs.

but rarely all are. Finger nail lesions are similar, but less common, and are seldom seen without a chronic *T. rubrum* infection of the skin of the hands.

Tinea of the hands. This is usually asymmetrical and associated with tinea pedis. *T. rubrum* may cause a barely perceptible erythema of one palm with a characteristic powdery scale in the creases (Fig. 15.37).

Tinea of the groin. This is common and affects men more often than women. The eruption is often unilateral or asymmetrical. The upper inner thigh is involved and lesions expand slowly to form sharply demarcated plaques with peripheral scaling (Fig. 15.38). A few vesicles or pustules may be seen within the lesions. The organisms are the same as those causing tinea pedis.

Tinea of the trunk and limbs. Tinea corporis is characterized by plaques with scaling and erythema most pronounced at the periphery (Fig. 15.39). A few small vesicles and pustules may be seen within them. The lesions expand slowly and healing in the centre leaves a typical ring-like pattern.

Tinea of the scalp (tinea capitis). This is usually a disease of children. The causative organism varies from country to country.

Fungi derived from animal sources (zoophilic fungi) induce a more intense inflammation than do those spread from person to person (anthropophilic fungi). In ringworm acquired from cattle, for example, the boggy swelling, inflammation and pustulation is often so fierce that a bacterial infection may be suspected; such a lesion is called a kerion and the hair loss associated with it may be permanent. Tinea of the beard area is usually due to zoophilic species and shows the same features (Fig. 15.40).

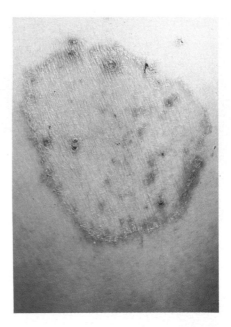

Fig. 15.39 Typical tinea of the trunk showing an active red scaly edge and central clearance.

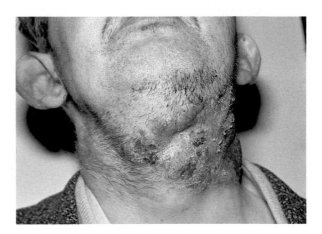

Fig. 15.40 Animal ringworm of the beard area showing boggy inflamed swellings (kerion).

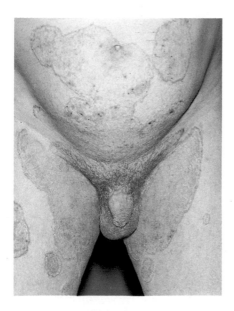

Fig. 15.38 A very gross example of tinea of the groin. The *T. rubrum* infection has spread on to the abdomen and thighs, aided by the use of topical steroids.

Anthropophilic organisms cause bald rather scaly areas, with minimal inflammation, and hairs broken off 3−4 mm from the scalp (Fig. 15.41). In favus, due to *Trichophyton schoenleinii*, the picture is dominated by foul-smelling yellowish crusts surrounding many scalp hairs, and sometimes leading to scarring alopecia.

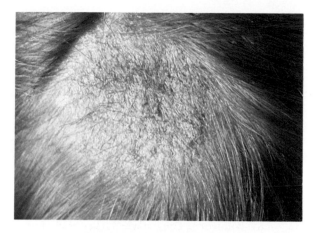

Fig. 15.41 Tinea capitis of the type spread from person to person. Scaly area with broken hairs.

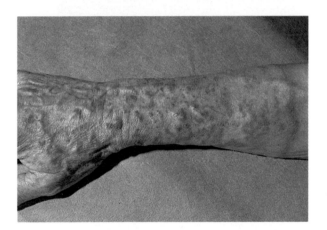

Fig. 15.42 'Tinea incognito'. Topical steroid applications have thinned the skin and altered much of the morphology. A recognizable active spreading edge is still visible.

Complications

1 Fierce animal ringworm of the scalp may lead to permanent scarring alopecia.
2 A florid fungal infection anywhere may induce vesication on the sides of the fingers and palms (trichophytide).
3 Epidemics of ringworm may occur in schools.
4 The usual appearances of a fungal infection may be masked when it is mistreated with topical steroids (tinea incognito) (Fig. 15.42).

Table 15.1 Common problems in the differential diagnosis of dermatophyte infections

Area	Differential diagnosis
Scalp	Alopecia areata, psoriasis, seborrhoeic eczema, carbuncle, trichotillomania
Feet	Erythrasma, interdigital intertrigo, eczema
Trunk	Discoid eczema, psoriasis, candidiasis, pityriasis rosea
Nails	Psoriasis, paronychia
Hand	Chronic eczema, granuloma annulare

Differential diagnosis

This varies with the site. Some of the commoner problems are listed in Table 15.1.

Investigations

Microscopic examination of a skin scraping, nail clipping or plucked hair is a simple procedure. The scraping should be taken from the scaly margin of a lesion with a scalpel blade, and clippings from the most crumbly part of a nail. Broken hairs should be plucked with tweezers. Specimens are cleared in potassium hydroxide (p. 39). Branching hyphae are easily seen (see Fig. 4.4) using a scanning (×10) or low-power (×25) objective lens with the iris diaphragm almost closed and the condenser racked down. Hyphae may also be seen within a cleared hair shaft, or spores may be noted around it.

Cultures should be carried out in a mycology or bacteriology laboratory. Transport medium is not necessary, and specimens should be sent in folded black paper. The report may take as long as a month; microscopy is much quicker.

Wood's light (ultraviolet light) examination of the scalp usually reveals a green fluorescence of the hairs in *Microsporum audouini* and *M. canis* infections. The technique is useful for screening children in institutions where outbreaks of tinea capitis still sometimes occur, but some fungi (e.g. *Trichophyton tonsurans*) do not fluoresce.

Treatment

Local. This is all that is needed for minor infections of the skin. The more recent imidazole preparations, e.g. miconazole and clotrimazole (Formulary, p. 292), have largely superseded time-honoured remedies such as benzoic acid ointment (Whitfield's ointment) and tolnaftate. They should be applied twice daily. Magenta paint (Castellani's paint), although highly coloured, is helpful for exudative or macerated areas in body folds or toe webs. Occasional dusting with an antifungal powder is useful to prevent relapses.

Topical nail preparations. Many patients now prefer to avoid systemic treatment. For them a nail lacquer containing amorolfine is worth a trial. It should be applied once or twice a week for six months; it is effective against stubborn moulds such as Hendersonula and Scopulariopsis. Both amorolfine and tioconazole nail solution (Formulary, p. 292) may be used as adjuncts to systemic therapy (see below).

Systemic. This is needed for tinea of the scalp and of the nails, and for widespread or chronic infections of the skin which have not responded to local measures.

Terbinafine (Formulary, p. 299) is a new drug which seems likely to supercede griseofulvin. It acts by inhibiting fungal squalene epoxidase and does not interact with the cytochrome P-450 system. It is fungicidal and so cures chronic dermatophyte infections more quickly and more reliably than griseofulvin. Cure rates of 80–90% can be expected for infected finger nails after a six week course of terbinafine, and for infected toe nails after a three month course. It is not effective in pityriasis versicolor or Candida infections.

Griseofulvin (Formulary, p. 299) was for many years the drug of choice for chronic dermatophyte infections. It has proved to be a safe drug, but treatment may have to be stopped because of persistent headache, nausea, vomiting, or skin eruptions. The drug should not be given in pregnancy or to patients with liver failure or porphyria. It interacts with coumarin anticoagulants, the dose of which may have to be increased. Its effectiveness falls if barbiturates are being taken at the same time.

Griseofulvin is fungistatic and treatment for infected nails has to be prolonged (average of 12 months for finger nails, and at least 18 months for toe nails). The disappointing results for toe nail infections seen in some 30–40% of cases can be improved by the concomitant use of topical nail preparations (see above).

Itraconazole (Formulary, p. 300) is now preferred to ketoconazole which occasionally damages the liver, and is a reasonable alternative to terbinafine and griseofulvin if these are contraindicated. It is effective in tinea corporis, cruris and pedis; and also in nail infections, though without a licence for this use in many countries. Fungistatic rather than fungicidal, it interferes with the cytochrome P-450 system. Its wide spectrum makes it useful also in pityriasis versicolor and candidiasis.

LEARNING POINTS

1 Do not prescribe griseofulvin or terbinafine for psoriasis of the nails or chronic paronychia. Always get mycological proof first.
2 Think of a dermatophyte infection in asymmetrical 'eczemas' which are worsening with local steroids.
3 Consider tinea in acute inflammatory and purulent reactions of the scalp and beard.

Candidiasis

Cause

Candida albicans is a classic opportunistic pathogen. Even in transient and trivial local infections, in the apparently fit, one or more predisposing factors such as obesity, moisture and maceration, diabetes, pregnancy, the use of broad-spectrum antibiotics, or perhaps the use of the contraceptive pill, will often be found to be playing some part. Opportunism is even more obvious in the overwhelming systemic infections of the immunocompromised (Fig. 15.43).

Presentation

This varies with the site (Fig. 15.44).

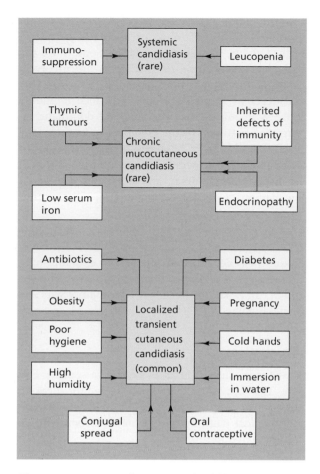

Fig. 15.43 Factors predisposing to the different types of candidiasis.

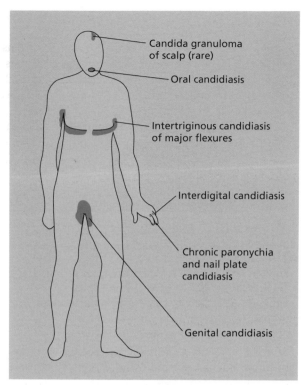

Fig. 15.44 Sites susceptible to *Candida* infection.

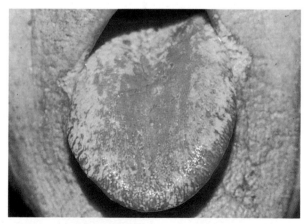

Fig. 15.45 Candidal angular stomatitis associated with severe candidiasis of the tongue.

Oral candidiasis. One or more whitish adherent plaques (like bread sauce) appear on the mucous membranes. If wiped off they show an erythematous base. Under dentures candidiasis will produce sore red areas. Angular stomatitis, usually in denture wearers (Fig. 15.45), may be candidal.

Candida intertrigo. A moist glazed area of erythema and maceration appears in a body fold; the edge shows soggy scaling, and outlying satellite papulopustules. These changes are most common under the breasts, and in the armpits and groin, but can also occur between the fingers of those whose hands are often in water (Fig. 15.46).

Genital candidiasis. Most commonly presents as a sore itchy vulvovaginitis, with white curdy plaques adherent to the inflamed mucous membranes, and a whitish discharge. The eruption may extend to the groin folds. Conjugal spread is common, and in males similar changes may occur under the foreskin.

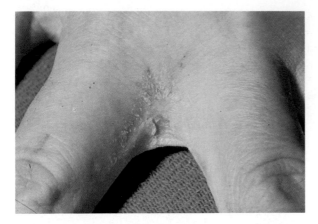

Fig. 15.46 A barmaid whose hands, constantly immersed in water, have developed candidal intertrigo between the middle and index fingers.

Diabetes, pregnancy, and antibiotic therapy are common predisposing factors.

Paronychia. Acute paronychia is usually bacterial, but in chronic paronychia *Candida* may be the sole pathogen or be found with other opportunists such as *Proteus* or *Pseudomonas*. The proximal and sometimes the lateral nail folds of one or more fingers become bolstered and red (Fig. 15.47). The cuticles are lost and small amounts of pus may be expressed. The adjacent nail plate becomes ridged and discoloured. Predisposing factors include wet work, poor peripheral circulation and vulval candidiasis.

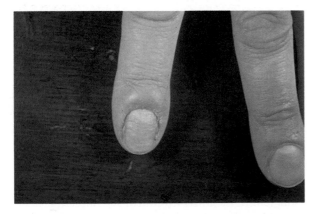

Fig. 15.47 Chronic paronchyia with loss of the cuticle and bolstering of the proximal nail fold. Secondary ridging and discoloration of the nail plate are common.

Chronic mucocutaneous candidiasis. Persistent candidiasis, affecting most or all of the areas described above, may start in infancy. Sometimes the nail plates as well as the nail folds are involved. *Candida* granulomas may appear on the scalp. Several different forms have been described including those with autosomal recessive and dominant inheritance patterns. In the *Candida* endocrinopathy syndrome chronic candidiasis occurs with one or more endocrine defects the most common of which are hypoparathyroidism, and Addison's disease. A few late-onset cases have underlying thymic tumours.

Systemic candidiasis. This is seen against a background of severe illness, leucopenia and immunosuppression. The skin lesions are firm red nodules which can be shown by biopsy to contain yeasts and pseudohyphae.

Investigations

Swabs from suspected areas should be sent for culture. The urine should always be tested for sugar. In chronic mucocutaneous candidiasis a detailed immunological work-up will be needed, focussing on cell-mediated immunity.

Treatment

Underlying predisposing factors should be sought and eliminated. For example, denture hygiene may be important. Infected skin folds should be separated and kept dry. Those with chronic paronychia should keep their hands warm and dry.

Amphotericin, nystatin and the imidazole group of compounds are all effective topically. For the mouth, these are available as oral suspensions, lozenges and oral gels (Formulary, p. 291). False teeth should be removed at night, washed and steeped in a nystatin solution. For other areas of candidiasis, creams, ointment and pessaries are available (Formulary, p. 292). Magenta paint is also a useful but messy remedy for the skin flexures. In chronic paronychia the nail folds can be packed with an imidazole cream or drenched in an imidazole solution several times a day. Both itraconazole and fluconazole (Formulary, p. 300) have now superceded ketoconazole. Genital candidiasis responds well to a single day's treatment with either. Both are also valuable for recurrent oral candidiasis of the immunocompromised, and for the various types of chronic mucocutaneous candidiasis.

LEARNING POINTS
1 Always check the urine for sugar.
2 Remember that griseofulvin has no action against Candida.

Pityriasis versicolor

Cause

The old name, tinea versicolor, should be dropped now as the disorder is caused by commensal yeasts (*Pityrosporum orbiculare*), but not by dermatophyte fungi. It is the overgrowth of these yeasts, particularly in hot humid conditions, which is responsible for the clinical lesions.

Carboxylic acids released by the organisms inhibit the normal increase in pigment production by melanocytes after exposure to sunlight. The term 'versicolor' refers to this process through which the superficial scaly patches, fawn or pink on non-tanned skin (Fig. 15.48), become pale after exposure to sunlight (Fig. 15.49). The condition should be regarded as non-infectious.

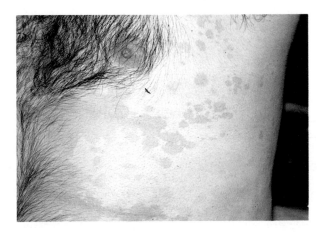

Fig. 15.48 Pityriasis versicolor: fawn areas stand out against the untanned background.

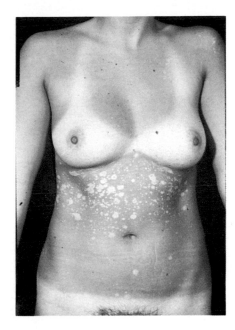

Fig. 15.49 This patient's holiday was spoilt by versicolor ruining her expensive tan.

Presentation and course

The fawn or depigmented areas, with their slightly branny scaling and wrinkling (Fig. 15.50), look ugly. Otherwise they are symptom-free or only slightly itchy. Lesions are most common on the upper trunk but may become widespread. Untreated lesions persist, and depigmented areas, even after adequate treatment, are slow to regain their former colour. Recurrences are common.

Differential diagnosis

In vitiligo (p. 213), the border is clearly defined, scaling is absent, lesions are larger, the limbs and face are often affected, and depigmentation is more complete; however, it may sometimes be hard to distinguish vitiligo from the pale, non-scaly areas of treated versicolor. Seborrhoeic eczema of the trunk tends to be more erythematous, and is often confined to the presternal or interscapular areas. Pityriasis alba often affects the cheeks. Pityriasis rosea, tinea corporis, secondary syphilis, and erythrasma seldom cause real confusion.

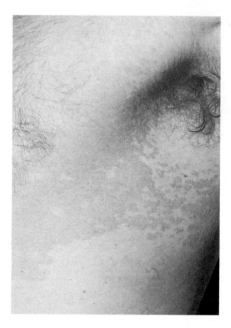

Fig. 15.50 A common site for pityriasis versicolor. The hint of scaling becomes more obvious after gentle scraping with a blade.

Investigations

Scrapings, prepared and examined as for a dermatophyte infection (p. 39), show a mixture of short, branched hyphae and spores (spaghetti and meatballs). Culture is not helpful.

Treatment

A topical preparation of one of the imidazole group of antifungal drugs (Formulary, p. 292) can be applied at night to all affected areas for two to four weeks. Equally effective, but messier and more irritant, is a 2.5% selenium sulphide mixture in a detergent base (Selsun shampoo). This should be lathered on to the patches after an evening bath, and allowed to dry. Next morning it should be washed off. Three applications at weekly intervals are adequate. A shampoo containing ketoconazole is now available (Formulary, p. 288) and is less messy and as effective as selenium ones. Recently, systemic itraconazole (200 mg daily for seven days) has been shown to be curative.

Deep fungal infections

Histoplasmosis

Histoplasma capsulatum is found in soil and in the droppings of some animals, for example bats. Airborne spores are inhaled and cause lung lesions which are in many ways like those of tuberculosis. Later, granulomatous skin lesions may appear, particularly in the immunocompromised. Amphotericin B or itraconazole, given systemically, is often helpful.

Coccidioidomycosis

The causative organism, *Coccidioides immitis*, is present in the soil in arid areas in the USA. Its spores are inhaled, and the pulmonary infection may be accompanied by a fever. At this stage erythema nodosum (p. 111) may be seen. In a few patients the infection becomes disseminated, with ulcers or deep abscesses in the skin. Treatment is with amphotericin B or itraconazole.

Blastomycosis

Infections with *Blastomyces dermatitidis* are virtually confined to rural areas of the USA. Rarely the organism is inoculated into the skin; more often it is inhaled and then spreads systemically from the pulmonary focus to other organs including the skin. There the lesions are ulcerated discharging nodules which spread peripherally with a verrucose edge, while tending to clear and scar centrally. Treatment is with systemic amphotericin B or itraconazole.

Sporotrichosis

The causative fungus, *Sporotrichium schenkii*, lives saprophytically in soil or on wood in warm humid countries.

Infection is through a wound, where later a lesion like an indolent boil arises. Later still nodules appear, in succession, along the draining lymphatics. Potassium iodide or itraconazole are both effective.

Actinomycosis

The causative organism, *Actinomyces israelii*, is bacterial but traditionally considered with the fungi. It has long, branching hyphae and is part of the normal flora of the mouth and bowel. In actinomycosis, a lumpy induration and scarring co-exist with multiple sinuses discharging pus containing 'sulphur granules', made up of tangled filaments. Favourite sites are the jaw, and the chest and abdominal walls. Long-term penicillin is the treatment of choice.

Mycetoma (Madura foot)

Various species of fungus or actinomycetes may be involved. They gain access to the subcutaneous tissues, usually of the feet or legs, via a penetrating wound. The area becomes lumpy and distorted, later enlarging and developing multiple sinuses. Pus exuding from these shows tiny diagnostic granules. Surgery may be a valuable alternative to the often poor results of medical treatment with systemic antibiotics or antifungal drugs depending on the organism isolated.

CHAPTER 16

Infestations

To be infested is to harbour animal parasites on or in the body. Such parasites are common in tropical countries and less so in temperate ones. Infestations fall into two main groups:

1 Those due to arthropods.
2 Those due to worms.

Arthropods

Table 16.1 lists some of the ways in which arthropods can affect the skin. Only a few can be discussed here.

Insect bites

The skin changes are due in part to the pharmacologically active substances injected and in part to a sensitization reaction to injected antigens. A wheal may appear within a few minutes, to be followed by a firm itchy persistent papule, often with a central haemorrhagic punctum. Bullous reactions are common on the legs of children. The diagnosis is usually obvious: when it is not the term papular urticaria may be used.

Papular urticaria

Cause

Papular urticaria is nothing more than an excessive, possibly allergic, reaction to insect bites. The source of the bites may be simple garden pests but more often is a parasite on a domestic pet; sometimes it cannot be traced. Human fleas are now rather uncommon. Perhaps the term 'papular urticaria', with its hint that the condition is a variant of ordinary urticaria, should now be dropped.

Table 16.1 Arthropods and their effects on the skin

	Manifestations
Insects	
Hymenoptera	Bee and wasp stings Ant bites
Lepidoptera	Caterpillar dermatitis
Coleoptera	Blisters from cantharidin
Diptera	Mosquito and midge bites Myiasis
Aphaniptera	Human and animal fleas
Hemiptera	Bed bugs
Anaplura	Lice infestations
Mites	
Demodex folliculorum	Normal inhabitant of facial hair follicles
Sarcoptes scabei	Human and animal scabies
Food mites	Grain itch, grocer's itch, etc.
Harvest mites	Harvest itch
House dust mite	Possible role in atopic eczema
Cheyletiella	Papular urticaria
Ticks	Tick bites
	Vector of rickettsial infections and erythema migrans (p. 137)

Presentation

Lesions are usually most marked on the arms or legs. They consist of recurrent groups or lines of small itchy excoriated urticarial papules which may become bullous and infected (Fig. 16.1). Some clear to leave small scars or pigmented areas.

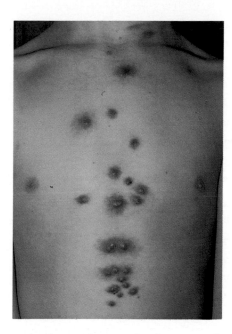

Fig. 16.1 Florid insect bites on the chest. Note the tendency of the now infected lesions to lie in lines and groups.

Course

Surprisingly often only one member of a family is affected. Lesions tend to start after infancy and a child will usually 'grow out' of the problem in a few years even if the source of the bites is not dealt with. Individual lesions last for one or two weeks and recur in distinct crops, especially in the summer — hence the lay term 'heat bumps'. The lesions will disappear with any change of environment, for example on holiday.

Complications

Itching may lead to much discomfort and loss of sleep. Impetiginization is common.

Differential diagnosis

The grouped excoriated papules of papular urticaria are quite distinct from scabies, in which burrows are the diagnostic feature. Atopic prurigo may be more difficult to distinguish but here there is usually a family history of atopy and often frankly eczematous plaques in a typical distribution.

Investigations

The parents should be encouraged to act as detectives in their own environment, but some resist the idea that the lesions are due to bites. This attitude is often supported by veterinarians who, after a superficial look at infested animals, pronounce them clear. In such cases the animal should be brushed vigorously while standing on a polythene sheet. Enough dandruff-like material can then be obtained to send to a reliable veterinary laboratory. Often the cause is a *Cheyletiella* mite infestation.

Treatment

Local treatment with Eurax HC ointment or calamine lotion, and the regular use of insect repellants, may be of some help but the ultimate solution is to trace the source of the bites.

Infested animals should be treated by a veterinarian and insecticidal powders should be used for soft furnishings in the home. Sometimes professional exterminators are needed. It has to be admitted that even these measures sometimes meet with little success.

Bed bugs (hemiptera)

During the day bed bugs hide in crevices in walls and furniture: at night they can travel considerable distances to reach a sleeping human. Burning wheals, turning into firm papules, occur in groups wherever the crawling bugs have easy access to the skin; the face, neck and hands are the most common sites. Treatment should be directed towards the application of insecticides to walls and furniture likely to be harbouring the bugs.

Myiasis

The larvae of several species of fly will develop only if deposited in living flesh: man is one of several possible hosts. The skin lesions may look like boils, but movement may be detected within. The diagnosis is proved by incising the nodule and extracting the larva.

Lice infestations (pediculosis)

Lice are flattened wingless insects which suck blood. Their eggs, attached to hairs or clothing, are known as nits. The main features of all lice infestations are severe itching, followed by scratching and secondary infection.

Two species are obligate parasites in man: *Pediculus humanus* (with its two varieties *P. humanus capitis*, the head louse, and *P. humanus corporis*, the body louse) and *Phthirus pubis* (the pubic louse).

Head lice

Cause

Head lice are still common, affecting up to 10% of children even in the smartest schools. The head louse itself measures some 3–4 mm in length and is greyish, and often rather hard to find. However, its egg cases (nits) can be seen easily enough, firmly stuck to the hair shafts (Fig. 16.2). Spread from person to person is achieved by head-to-head contact, shared combs or hats.

Presentation and course

The main symptom is itching, at first around the sides and back of the scalp and then more generally over it. Scratching and secondary infection soon follow and, in heavy infestations, the hair may

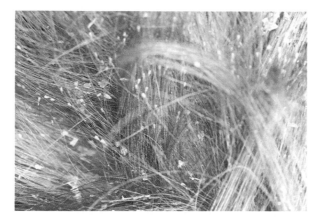

Fig. 16.2 Pediculosis capitis: numerous oval eggs (nits) can be seen scattered throughout the scalp hair, but the adult lice are not seen here.

become matted and smelly. Draining lymph nodes often enlarge.

Complications

Secondary bacterial infection may be severe enough to cause the child to become generally listless and feverish.

Differential diagnosis

All patients with recurrent impetigo or crusted eczema on their scalps should be carefully examined for the presence of nits.

Investigations

None are usually required.

Treatment

Malathion and carbaryl lotions (Formulary, p. 293) are probably the treatments of choice now. Both kill lice and eggs effectively; malathion has the extra value of sticking to the hair and so protects against reinfection for six weeks. Many public health authorities alternate their use every three years to lessen the risk of resistant strains emerging. They should be applied to the scalp and left on for 12 hours — the application should be repeated after one week and other members of the family and school mates should be checked. Lindane (gamma-benzene hexachloride) lotion or permethrin creme rinse (Formulary, p. 293) are reasonable alternatives.

A tooth comb helps to remove nits and occasionally matting is so severe that the hair has to be clipped short. A systemic antibiotic may be needed to deal with severe secondary infection.

Body lice

Cause

Body louse infestations are now uncommon except in the unhygienic and socially deprived. Morphologically the body louse looks just like the head louse, but lays its eggs in the seams of clothing in contact with the skin. Transmission is via infested bedding or clothing.

Presentation and course

Self-neglect is usually obvious: against this background there is severe and widespread itching, especially on the trunk. The bites themselves are soon obscured by excoriations and crusts of dried blood or serum. In chronic untreated cases ('vagabond's disease') the skin becomes generally thickened, eczematized, and pigmented; lymphadenopathy is common.

Differential diagnosis

In scabies characteristic burrows will be seen (p. 198). Other causes of chronic itchy erythroderma include eczema and lymphomas, but these are ruled out by the finding of lice and nits.

Investigations

Clothing should be examined for the presence of eggs in the inner seams.

Treatment

First and foremost treat the infested clothing and bedding. Lice and their eggs are killed by tumble drying, by high temperature laundering, and by dry cleaning. Less competent patients will need help here. Once this has been achieved, 1% lindane lotion or 5% permethrin creme rinse (Formulary, p. 293) may be used on the patient's skin.

Pubic lice

Cause

Pubic lice (crabs) are broader than scalp and body lice, and their second and third pairs of legs are well adapted to cling on to hair. These lice are usually spread by sexual contact, and most commonly infest young adults.

Presentation

Severe itching in the pubic area is followed by eczematization and secondary infection. Among the excoriations will be seen small blue-grey macules of altered blood at the site of bites. The shiny,

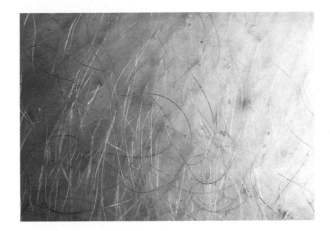

Fig. 16.3 The shiny translucent nits of the pubic louse, together with one or two shy adult lice.

translucent nits are less obvious than those of head lice (Fig. 16.3). Pubic lice spread most extensively in hairy males and may affect the eyelashes.

Differential diagnosis

Eczema of the pubic area may give rise to similar symptoms but lice and nits are not seen.

Investigations

The possibility of other co-existing sexually transmitted diseases should be kept in mind.

Treatment

The pubic hair, and hair on the thighs and around the anus, should be treated with aqueous lindane, malathion solution or permethrin cream, as alcohol-based lotions are too fierce for the scrotum. The same argument applies to the eyelashes, where aqueous solutions are to be preferred. Treatment should be repeated after one week, and infected sexual partners should also be treated. Shaving the area is not necessary.

Scabies

Cause

Scabies is caused by the mite *Sarcoptes scabei* var. *hominis* (Fig. 16.4). Adult mites are 0.3–0.4 mm

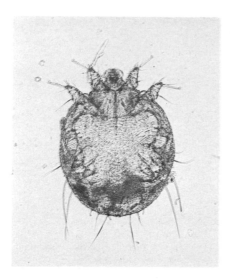

Fig. 16.4 The adult female acarus (scabies mite).

long and therefore just visible, though hard to see except through a lens. It is now well established that the mites are transferred from person to person by close bodily contact and not via inanimate objects.

Once on the skin, fertilized female mites burrow through the stratum corneum at the rate of about 2 mm per day, and produce two or three oval eggs each day. These turn into sexually mature mites in two to three weeks. The number of mites varies from case to case, from less than 10 in a clean adult to many more in an unwashed child.

The generalized eruption of scabies, and its itchiness, are thought to be due to a sensitization to the mites or their products.

Epidemiology

The prevalence of scabies in many populations rises and falls cyclically, peaking every 15 to 20 years. The idea of 'herd immunity' has been put forward to explain this, spread being most easy when a new generation of susceptible individuals has arisen.

Presentation

For the first four to six weeks after infestation there may be no itching; but thereafter pruritus dominates the picture, often affecting several people and being particularly bad at night.

The most dramatic part of the eruption — excoriated, eczematized or urticarial papules — is usually on the trunk, but these changes are non-specific and a burrow has to be identified to confirm the diagnosis (Figs 16.5 & 16.6).

Most burrows lie on the sides of the fingers, finger webs, sides of the hand, and on the flexural aspects of the wrists. Other favourite sites include the elbows, ankles and feet (especially in infants; Fig. 16.7), nipples and genitals (Fig. 16.8). Only in infancy does scabies affect the face. Burrows are easily missed, grey-white, slightly scaly, tortuous lines of up to 1 cm in length. The acarus may be seen through a lens as a small dark dot at the most recent, least scaly end of the burrow. With experience

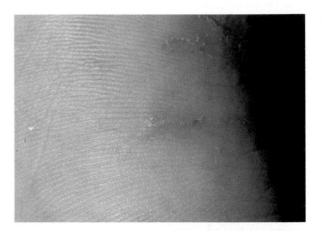

Fig. 16.5 A group of typical burrows on the side of the hand.

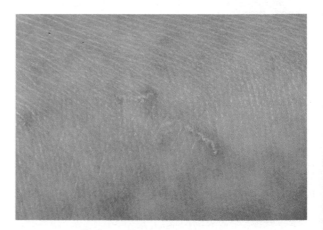

Fig. 16.6 Obvious burrows on the side of a foot.

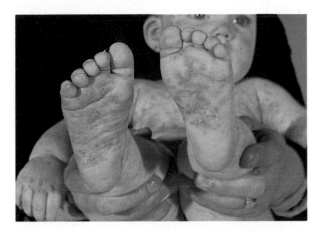

Fig. 16.7 The characteristic plantar lesions of scabies in infancy.

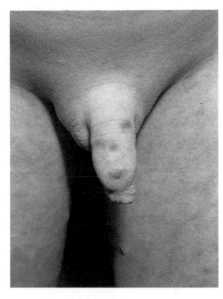

Fig. 16.9 Unmistakable rubbery nodules on the penis — diagnostic of scabies.

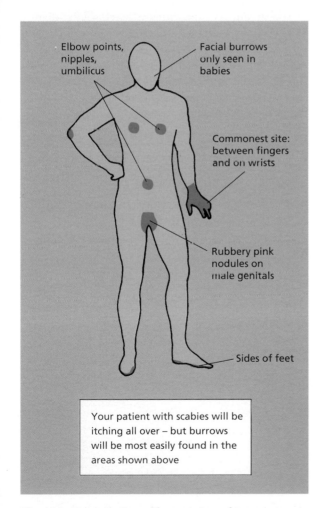

Elbow points, nipples, umbilicus

Facial burrows only seen in babies

Commonest site: between fingers and on wrists

Rubbery pink nodules on male genitals

Sides of feet

Your patient with scabies will be itching all over – but burrows will be most easily found in the areas shown above

Fig. 16.8 Common sites of burrows in scabies.

it can be removed for microscopic confirmation (p. 39). On the genitals, burrows are associated with erythematous, rubbery nodules (Fig. 16.9).

Course

Scabies persists indefinitely unless treated. In the chronic stage, the number of mites may be small and diagnosis is correspondingly difficult. Relapses after apparently adequate treatment are common and can be put down to reinfestation from undetected and untreated contacts.

Complications

● Secondary infection, with pustulation, is common (Fig. 16.10). Rarely glomerulonephritis may follow this.
● Repeated applications of scabicides may cause skin irritation and eczema.
● Persistent itchy red nodules may remain on the genitals or armpits of children for some months after adequate treatment.
● Venereal disease may be acquired at the same time as scabies.
● Crusted (Norwegian) scabies, which may not be itchy, is a widespread crusted eruption in which vast

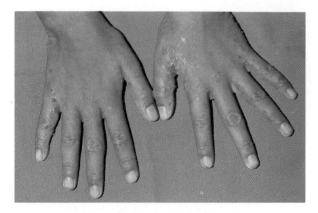

Fig. 16.10 Crusting due to infection of finger web burrows.

numbers of mites are found. It affects mental defectives or the immunosuppressed, and may be the unsuspected source of epidemics of ordinary scabies.

Differential diagnosis

Only scabies shows the characteristic burrow. Animal scabies from pets induces an itchy rash in humans but this lacks burrows. The lesions of papular urticaria (p. 194) are excoriated papules, in groups, mainly on the legs. Late-onset atopic eczema (p. 95), cholinergic urticaria (p. 105), lichen planus (p. 67), and dermatitis herpetiformis (p. 121) have their own distinctive features. Fibreglass can also cause epidemics of itching.

Investigations

With practice an acarus can be picked neatly from the end of its burrow and identified microscopically; failing this, eggs and mites can be seen microscopically in burrow scrapings mounted in potassium hydroxide (p. 198).

Treatment

● Use an effective scabicide: there are many on the market (Formulary p. 293). Five per cent permethrin cream has recently become available in the UK. Lindane passes readily through the skin and settles in the body fat where it is slowly broken down. High blood levels can cause neurological side effects, rarely including convulsions. Lindane is best avoided in those with low body fat (e.g. anorexics and athletes

in training) and in those suffering from epilepsy or other CNS diseases. It should also be avoided in pregnant or lactating women, and probably also in children under five.
● For babies over two months, toddlers and young children we advise permethrin cream, 25% benzyl benzoate diluted with three parts of water or 6% precipitated sulphur in white soft paraffin (petrolatum).
● Do not just treat the patient: treat all members of the family and sexual contacts, whether they are itching or not (Fig. 16.11).
● Have a printed sheet to give to the patient and go through it with them — scabies victims are notoriously confused. The number of applications varies from dermatologist to dermatologist. There is no doubt that some preparations, such as malathion, disappear quickly from the skin, leaving it vulnerable to any mites which hatch out after three days from eggs which have survived. A second application, three days after the first, is then essential. With lindane, which lingers on the skin, and with permethrin, this is less important.

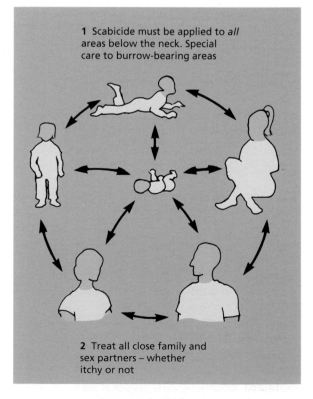

1 Scabicide must be applied to *all* areas below the neck. Special care to burrow-bearing areas

2 Treat all close family and sex partners — whether itchy or not

Fig. 16.11 The treatment of scabies.

• Make sure that patients grasp the fact that scabicides have to be applied to all areas of skin below the jaw line, including the genitals, soles of the feet and skin under the free edge of the nails. If the hands are washed, the scabicide should be reapplied. Perhaps the main reason for recommending a second application is that it will cover areas left out during an inefficient first application. A petrolatum bath before treatment is no longer recommended because it may increase lindane absorption.

• Ordinary laundering deals satisfactorily with clothing and sheets. Mites die in clothing unworn for one week.

• Residual itching may last for several days, or even a few weeks, but this does not need more application of the scabicide. Rely instead on calamine lotion.

LEARNING POINTS
1 Paravenereal diseases hunt in packs: has your patient with scabies also got pubic lice, genital mollusca, or even something worse?
2 Never forget the contacts — itchy or not — as they will reinfect your patient and waste everybody's time.

Parasitic worms

A textbook of tropical medicine should be consulted for more details on this subject.

Onchocerciasis

This is endemic in much of Central America and Africa where it is an important cause of blindness. The buffalo gnat (*Simulium* species) carries the filarial worm to humans. Infested humans become itchy with an excoriated papular eruption. Later the skin may thicken and become hyper- or hypopigmented. Dermal nodules are found, mainly near bony prominences, and contain both mature worms and microfilariae. It is the latter which invade the eye leading to blindness. The diagnosis is confirmed by detecting active microfilariae in skin snips teased out in saline and examined microscopically. Ivermectin (not yet on the market in the UK) is now the treatment of choice. A single dose produces a prolonged reduction of microfilarial levels, and should be repeated every year until the adult worms die out. Diethylcarbamazine and suramin are now obsolete.

Filariasis

This condition is endemic throughout much of the tropics. The adult filarial worms, usually *Wuchereria bancrofti*, inhabit the lymphatics where they excite an inflammatory reaction with episodes of lymphangitis and fever, gradually leading to lymphatic obstruction and lymphoedema, usually of the legs or scrotum. Such swellings may be massive (elephantiasis). Microfilariae are found in the peripheral blood, mainly at night; their vector from human to human is the mosquito in which the larvae mature. Diethylcarbamazine is the treatment of choice.

Larva migrans

The larvae of hookworms, which can go through their full life cycle only in cats or dogs, may penetrate human skin in contact with soil or sand contaminated by the faeces of these animals. The movement of the larvae under the skin causes tortuous red itchy lines to appear, moving forwards at the rate of a few millimetres a day. The larvae eventually die but this can be speeded up by the topical application of 10% thiabendazole (made by grinding two 0.5 g tablets in 10 g of preparation). Recently, systemic albendazole has been shown to be effective when taken over three days.

Other worm infestations

• Threadworm (pinworm) infestation in children can cause severe anal and vulval pruritus. The small worms are seen best at night-time when the itch is worst. Treatment is with piperazine.

• Swimmer's itch, in tropical waters, may be due to the penetration through the skin of the cercariae of human and non-human schistosomes.

• Multiple firm nodules in the skin may be due to the larval stages of the pork tapeworm (cysticercosis).

• Larger fluctuant cysts may be due to hydatid disease.

CHAPTER 17

Skin reactions to light

Ultraviolet radiation (UVR) can be helpful when it is used to treat skin diseases such as psoriasis. It can also be harmful (Fig. 17.1). It is the leading cause of skin cancers, and it causes or worsens certain skin disorders. UVR is non-ionizing but changes the skin chemically by reacting with endogenous light-absorbing chemicals called chromophores.

The UVR spectrum is divided into three parts (Fig. 17.2). The C spectrum does not penetrate the ozone layer of the atmosphere and is therefore irrelevant to skin disease. The B wavelengths (UVB: 290–320 nm) cause sunburn and are effectively screened out by window glass. The A spectrum (UVA) is long-wave ultraviolet light, from 320 nm to the most violet colour perceptible to the eye (about 400 nm). It ages and tans the skin.

Sunburn

Cause

UVB penetrates the epidermis and superficial dermis, stimulating the production and release of prostaglandins, leukotrienes, histamine, IL-1 and TNF-α which cause pain and redness.

Presentation and course

Areas of skin exposed to too much UVB smart and become red several hours later. Severe sunburn is painful and may blister. Redness is maximal after one day and then settles over the next two or three days, leaving a sheet-like desquamation and pigmentation (Figs 17.3 & 17.4).

Differential diagnosis

Phototoxic reactions due to drugs are like an exaggerated sunburn.

Investigations

None are required.

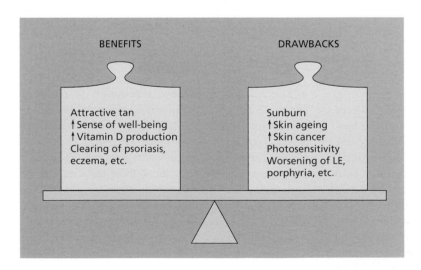

BENEFITS	DRAWBACKS
Attractive tan ↑ Sense of well-being ↑ Vitamin D production Clearing of psoriasis, eczema, etc.	Sunburn ↑ Skin ageing ↑ Skin cancer Photosensitivity Worsening of LE, porphyria, etc.

Fig. 17.1 The balance between the benefits and drawbacks of sun exposure.

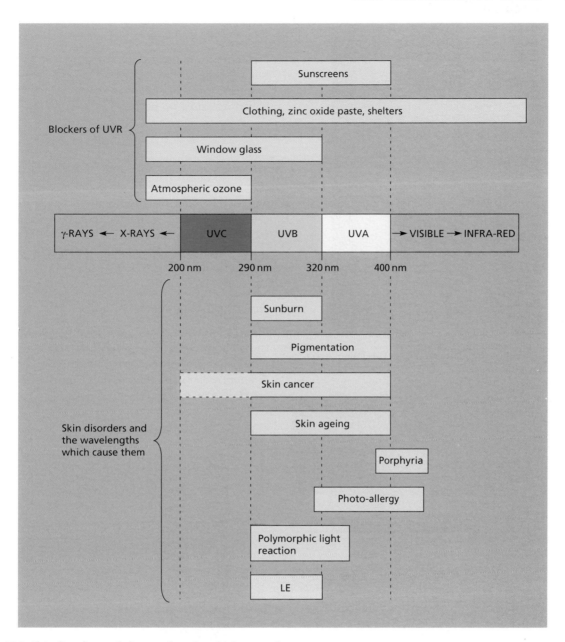

Fig. 17.2 Skin disorders and the wavelengths which cause them.

Treatment

The treatment is symptomatic. Baths may be cooling and oily shake lotions (e.g. oily calamine lotion or oil-in-water lotions and creams) may be comforting. Potent topical corticosteroids (Formulary, p. 290) help if used early and briefly. Oral aspirin (a prostaglandin synthesis inhibitor) relieves the pain.

Phototoxicity

Basic photochemical laws require a drug to absorb UVR to cause such a reaction. Most drugs listed in Table 17.1 absorb UVA as well as UVB, and so window glass, protective against sunburn, will not protect against most phototoxic drug reactions.

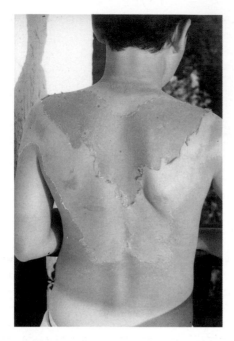

Fig. 17.3 Peeling after acute sunburn. This doctor's son should have known better.

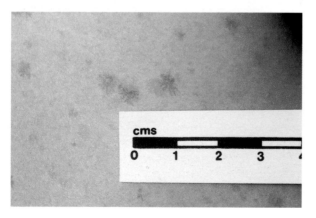

Fig. 17.4 Stellate lentigines — the legacy of sunburn (same patient as in Fig. 17.3).

Table 17.1 Drugs commonly causing photosensitivity

Amiodarone	Psoralens
Chlorpropamide	Quinidine
Nalidixic acid	Sulphonamides
Oral contraceptives	Tetracyclines
Phenothiazines	Thiazides

Presentation and course

Tenderness and redness occur only in areas exposed to sufficient UVR (Fig. 17.5). The signs and symptoms are those of sunburn. The skin may become hyperpigmented on healing.

Cause

These reactions are not immunological. Everyone exposed to enough of the drug and to enough UVR will develop the reaction. Some drugs which can cause phototoxic reactions are listed in Table 17.1. In addition, contact with psoralens in plants can cause localized phototoxic dermatitis termed 'phytophotodermatitis' (Fig. 17.6).

Differential diagnosis

Photo-allergic reactions are difficult to distinguish, the more so as the same drugs can often cause both photo-allergic and phototoxic reactions. The main differences between phototoxicity and photo-allergy are shown in Table 17.2.

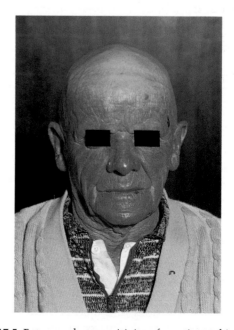

Fig. 17.5 Extreme photosensitivity of a patient taking a thiazide diuretic. Note sparing of the area covered by his cap.

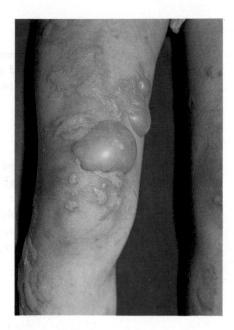

Fig. 17.6 Severe bullous eruption in areas in contact with giant hogweed (contains psoralens) and then exposed to sunlight (phytophotodermatitis).

Table 17.2 Features which distinguish phototoxicity from photo-allergy

Phototoxicity	Photo-allergy
Erythematous	Eczematous
Immediate	Delayed
Hurts	Itches
Photopatch testing negative	Photopatch testing positive

Investigations

None are usually required. Phototesting may be carried out in special centres in difficult cases. The action spectrum (those wavelengths which cause the reaction) may incriminate a particular drug.

Treatment

This is the same as for sunburn. Drugs should be stopped if further exposure to ultraviolet light is likely.

Photo-allergy

Drugs, topical or systemic, and chemicals on the skin can interact with UVR and cause immunological reactions.

Cause

UVR converts an immunologically inactive form of a drug into an antigenic molecule. An immunological reaction, analogous to allergic contact dermatitis, is induced if antigen remains in the skin or is formed there on subsequent exposure to the drug and UVR. Many of the same drugs which cause phototoxic reactions can cause photo-allergic ones.

Presentation

Photo-allergy is often similar to phototoxicity. The areas exposed to UVR become inflamed, but the reaction is more likely to be eczematous. The eruption will be on exposed areas such as the hands, the V of the neck, the nose, the chin, and the forehead. There is also a tendency to spare the upper lip under the nose, the eyelids, and the submental region (Fig. 17.7). Often the eruption does not occur on the first exposure to ultraviolet, but only after a second or further exposures. A lag phase of one or more weeks is necessary for induction of an immune response.

Course

The original lesions are red patches, plaques, vesicles, or bullae, which usually become eczematous. They tend to resolve when either the drug or the exposure to UVR is stopped, but this may take several weeks.

Complications

Some drugs, like the sulphonamides, may cause a persistent light reaction (see below).

Investigations

Photopatch testing can confirm the diagnosis. The chemical is applied for 24 hours and the skin is then irradiated with UVA. An acute photo-allergic contact dermatitis is then elicited. A control patch, not irradiated, rules out ordinary allergic contact dermatitis.

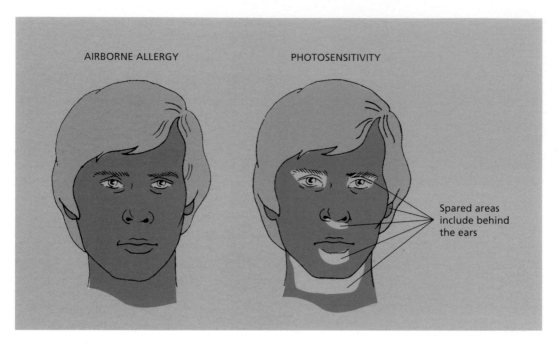

Fig. 17.7 Features distinguishing airborne allergy from photosensitivity.

Treatment

The drug should be stopped and the patient protected from additional UV exposure (avoidance, clothing and sunscreens). Potent topical or a short course of systemic corticosteroid hastens resolution and provides symptomatic relief.

Chronic actinic dermatitis (actinic reticuloid)

Some patients with a photo-allergic reaction never get over it and continue to develop eczematous areas after sun exposure, long after the drug has been stopped.

Cause

This is not clear but some believe minute amounts of the drug persist in the skin indefinitely.

Presentation

This is the same as a photo-allergic reaction to a drug. The patient goes on to develop a chronic dermatitis, with thick plaques, on sun-exposed areas.

Course

These patients may be exquisitely sensitive to UVR. They are usually middle-aged or elderly men who react after the slightest exposure, even through window glass or from fluorescent lights. Affected individuals also become allergic to a range of contact allergens, especially oleoresins in some plants (e.g. chrysanthemums).

Complications

None, but the persistent, severe, pruritic eruption may lead to depression and even suicide.

Differential diagnosis

Airborne allergic contact dermatitis may be confused, but does not require sunlight. Sometimes the diagnosis is difficult as exposure both to sunlight and to the airborne allergen occurs only out of doors. Airborne allergic contact dermatitis also affects sites which sunlight is less likely to reach, such as under the chin (Fig. 17.7). A continuing drug photo-allergy, a polymorphic light eruption (see below), or eczema due to some other cause must also be considered.

Although histology shows a dense, lymphocytic infiltrate and sometimes atypical lymphocytes suggestive of a lymphoma, the disorder seldom becomes malignant.

Investigations

Persistent light reaction can be confirmed experimentally by exposing uninvolved skin to UVA or UVB. Patch tests and photopatch tests help to distinguish between photo-allergy and airborne allergic contact dermatitis, and the action spectrum may point to a certain drug. Testing is difficult, and should be carried out only in specialist centres.

Treatment

These patients need extreme measures to protect their skin from UVR. These include protective clothing, and frequent applications of combined UVA and UVB blocking agents (Formulary, p. 289). Patients must protect themselves from UVR coming through windows or from fluorescent lights. Some can only go out at night. As even the most potent topical steroids are often ineffective, systemic steroids or immunosuppressants (e.g. azathioprine) may be needed for long periods.

Polymorphic light eruption

This is the most frequent cause of 'sun allergy'.

Cause

It is speculated that UVR causes a natural body chemical to change into an allergen. Mechanisms are similar to those in drug photo-allergy.

Presentation

Small itchy, red papulovesicles or eczematous plaques arise from two hours to five days, most commonly at 24 hours, after exposure to UVR. The eruption is itchy and usually confined to sun-exposed areas (Fig. 17.8), remembering that some UVR passes through thin clothing.

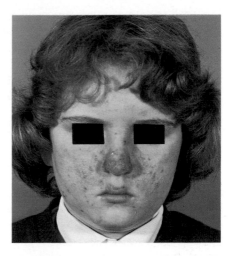

Fig. 17.8 Polymorphic light eruption: excoriated erythematous papules on the face of a young girl. Persists throughout the summer but fades in the winter.

Course

The disorder tends to recur each spring after UVR exposure. Tanning protects some patients so that if the initial exposures are limited, few or no symptoms occur later. Such patients can still enjoy sun exposure and outdoor activities. Others are so sensitive, or their skin pigments so little, that fresh exposures continue to induce reactions throughout the summer. They require photoprotection, and must limit their sun exposure and outdoor activities. The rash disappears during the winter.

Differential diagnosis

Phototoxic reactions, photo-allergic reactions, chronic actinic dermatitis, ordinary eczemas, and airborne allergic contact dermatitis should be considered.

Investigations

It may be possible to reproduce the dermatitis by testing non-sun-exposed skin with UVB or UVA.

Treatment

If normal tanning does not confer protection, sunscreens (Formulary, p. 289) should be used.

Protective clothing, such as wide-brimmed hats, longsleeved shirts, and long trousers is helpful. In some patients, a four-week PUVA course (p. 62) in the late spring can create enough of a tan to confer protection for the rest of the season. Moderately potent topical steroids (Formulary, p. 290) usually improve the eruption.

Actinic prurigo

This is clinically distinct from polymorphic light eruption although the cause may be the same. Papules, crusts, and excoriations arise on sun-exposed areas and sometimes also on other sites: lesions may persist through the winter. It is common among North American Indians and may resemble excoriated acne, bites, eczema, erythropoetic proto-porphyria or neurotic excoriations. It may be associated with atopy.

Solar urticaria

This is discussed in Chapter 10. Wheals occur in the sun-exposed areas within minutes. Some patients have erythropoietic protoporphyria (p. 251) and this should be considered particularly when solar urticaria starts in infancy.

Actinic keratoses

These are discussed in Chapter 19.

Actinic cheilitis

This term describes the inflammation and scaling of the lower lips of those who have led an outdoor life. It can be treated by cryosurgery, laser ablation, excision with lip advancement, or the judicious use of 5-fluorouracil cream (Formulary, p. 296).

Lupus erythematosus

Many patients with lupus erythematosus (p. 124) notice that they get worse after exposure to UVR, especially to UVB. They should be warned about this, and protect themselves from the sun (avoidance, clothing and sunscreens).

Carcinoma

The sun can cause basal cell carcinomas, squamous cell carcinomas, and malignant melanomas. These are discussed in Chapter 19.

Exacerbated diseases

UVR is useful in the treatment of many skin diseases, but it can also make some worse (Table 17.3).

Porphyria cutanea tarda

This condition is described in Chapter 20.

LEARNING POINTS
If the skin reacts badly to light through glass then:
1 *Sunscreens are usually ineffective.*
2 *Think of drugs or porphyria.*

Cutaneous ageing

The trouble with old skin is the way it looks rather than the way it behaves. UVR is the main factor speeding the ageing process in white skin. The bronzed young skins of today will become the wrinkled, spotted, rough prune-like ones of tomorrow.

Wrinkles occur when the dermis loses its elastic recoil, failing to snap back properly into shape. UVR damages elastic tissue and hastens the process. In skin chronically exposed to UVR, the elastic fibres

Table 17.3 The effect of sunlight on some skin diseases

Helps	Worsens
Atopic eczema	Darier's disease
Cutaneous T cell lymphoma	Herpes simplex
Parapsoriasis	Lupus erythematosus
Pityriasis lichenoides	Pellagra
Pityriasis rosea	Photo-allergy/toxicity
Pruritus of renal failure, liver disease	Porphyrias (excluding acute intermittent)
AIDS	Xeroderma pigmentosum
Psoriasis	

are clumped and amorphous, leading clinically to a yellow, pebbly look called *actinic elastosis*.

Although face lifts can smooth wrinkles out, there is no way to reverse this damage fully, although tretinoin cream (Formulary, p. 294) seems to help some patients. Prevention, by reducing exposure to UVR, is better than any cure and it is especially important in sunny climates (Table 17.4).

Skin ages even in sun protected areas, albeit much more slowly. The dermis thins. Skin collagen falls by about 1% per year throughout adult life, and it becomes more stable (less elastic). Fibroblasts become sparser in the dermis, accounting for reduced collagen synthesis and slower wound healing.

Table 17.4 Tips to avoid skin damage for those living in a sunny climate

1 Apply sunscreen daily — rain or shine
2 Reapply sunscreen often when outdoors
3 Use a sunscreen with a protective factor (SPF) of at least 15
4 Wear protective clothing, including wide-brimmed hats
5 Target outdoor activities for early morning or late afternoon
6 Seek shade
7 Avoid tanning salons
8 Do not sunbathe
9 Wear cosmetics, including lipstick
10 Help your children to protect themselves

CHAPTER 18

Disorders of pigmentation

Normal skin colour

It is a mixture of pigments, and not one alone, that gives normal skin its colour. Untanned Caucasoid skin is pink, due to oxyhaemoglobin in the blood within the papillary loops and superficial horizontal plexus (Fig. 2.14). Melanin may blend with this colour, for example after a suntan. Melanin is, of course, responsible too for the shades of brown seen in Negroid skin. Other hues are due to the addition to these pigments of yellow from carotene, found mainly in subcutaneous fat and in the horny layer of the epidermis. There is no natural blue pigment; when blue is seen it is due either to an optical effect from normal pigment (usually melanin) in the dermis or to the presence of an abnormal pigment (see below).

Abnormal skin colours

These may be due to an imbalance of the normal pigments mentioned above (e.g. in cyanosis, chloasma and carotenaemia) or to the presence of abnormal pigments (Table 18.1).

Sometimes it is difficult to distinguish between the colours of these pigments. For example, the gingery brown colour of haemosiderin is readily confused with melanin. Histological stains may be needed to settle the issue.

In practice, apart from tattoos, most pigmentary problems are due to too much, or too little melanin.

Decreased melanin pigmentation

Some conditions in which there is a lack of melanin are listed in Table 18.2. A few of the more important,

Table 18.1 Some abnormal pigments

Endogenous

Haemoglobin-derived
methaemoglobin ⎱	⎰ blue colour in vessels
sulphaemoglobin ⎰	⎱ cyanosis
carboxyhaemoglobin	pink
bilirubin ⎱	
biliverdin ⎰	yellow green
haemosiderin	brown

Drugs
gold	blue-grey (chrysiasis)
silver	blue-grey (agyria)
bismuth	grey
mepacrine	yellow
clofazamine	red
phenothiazines	slate-grey
amiodarone	blue-grey

Diet
carotene	orange

Exogenous

Tattoo pigments
carbon	blue-black
coal dust	blue-black
cobalt	blue
chrome	green
cadmium	yellow
mercury	red
iron	brown

Local medications
silver nitrate	black
magenta paint	magenta
gentian violet	violet
eosin	pink
potassium permanganate	brown
dithranol	purple
tar	brown
iodine	yellow

Table 18.2 Some causes of hypopigmentation

Genetic	Albinism
	Piebaldism
	Phenylketonuria
	Waardenburg's syndrome
	Chediak–Higashi syndrome:
	autosomal recessive
	lysosomal defect
	(susceptible to infections)
	Tuberous sclerosis
Endocrine	Hypopituitarism
Chemical	Substituted phenols (in rubber
	industry)
	Chloroquine and
	hydroxychloroquine
Post-inflammatory	Eczema
	Pityriasis alba
	Psoriasis
	Sarcoidosis
	Lupus erythematosus
	Lichen sclerosus et atrophicus
	Cryotherapy
Infections	Leprosy
	Pityriasis versicolor
	Syphilis, yaws and pinta
Tumours	Halo naevus
	Malignant melanoma
Miscellaneous	Vitiligo
	Idiopathic guttate hypomelanosis

and the mechanisms involved, are summarized in Fig. 18.1.

Oculocutaneous albinism

Little or no melanin is made in the skin and eyes (oculocutaneous albinism) or in the eyes alone (ocular albinism — not discussed further here). The prevalence of albinism of all types ranges from 1 in 20000 in the USA and UK to 5% in some communities.

Cause

The hair bulb test (see Investigations) separates oculocutaneous albinism into two main types: tyrosinase negative and tyrosinase positive. Roughly equal numbers of the two types are found in most communities, both being inherited as autosomal recessives. This explains how children with two albino parents can sometimes themselves be normally pigmented, the genes being complementary in the double heterozygote.

The tyrosinase gene lies on chromosome 11q14-q21. More than 20 allelic variations have been found there in patients with tyrosinase-negative albinism. The gene for tyrosinase positive human albinism has been mapped to chromosome 15q11-q13. It

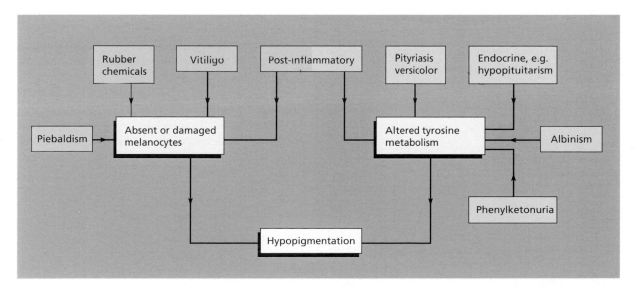

Fig. 18.1 The mechanisms involved in some types of hypopigmentation.

probably encodes for a polypeptide component of the melanosomal membrane involved in the transport of tyrosine.

Presentation and course

The whole skin is white and pigment is also lacking in the hair, iris, and retina (Fig. 18.2). Albinos have poor sight, photophobia, and a rotatory nystagmus. As they grow older tyrosinase-positive albinos gain a little pigment in their skin, iris and hair. Negroid skin becomes yellow-brown and the hair becomes yellow. Albinos may also develop freckles. Sunburn is common on unprotected skin. As melanocytes are present, albinos have non-pigmented melanocytic naevi and may develop amelanotic malignant melanomas.

Complications

In the tropics these unfortunate individuals develop numerous skin tumours even when they are young, confirming the protective role of melanin.

Differential diagnosis

Piebaldism and vitiligo are described below.

Investigations

Prenatal diagnosis of albinism is now possible but may not be justifiable in view of the good prognosis. A biopsy from fetal skin, taken at 20 weeks, is examined by electron microscopy for arrested melanosome development.

The hair bulb test, in which plucked hairs are incubated in dihydroxyphenylalanine, distinguishes tyrosinase-positive from tyrosinase-negative types. Those whose hair bulbs turn black (tyrosine-positive) are less severely affected.

Treatment

Avoidance of sun exposure, and protection with opaque clothing, wide-brimmed hats and sunscreen creams (Formulary, p. 289), are essential and allow albinos in temperate climates to live a relatively normal life. In the tropics the outlook is less good and the termination of affected pregnancies may be considered.

Piebaldism

These patients often have a white forelock of hair and patches of depigmentation lying symmetrically on the limbs, trunk and central part of the face, especially the chin. The condition is present at birth and is inherited as an autosomal dominant trait. A genetic abnormality in mice (dominant white spotting) provided the clue which allowed the human piebaldism gene to be mapped to chromosome 4q12, where the KIT protooncogene lies. This encodes the tyrosine kinase transmembrane cellular receptor on certain stem cells; without this they cannot respond to normal signals for development and migration. Melanocytes are absent from the hypopigmented areas. The depigmentation, often mistaken for vitiligo, may improve with age. There is no effective treatment. The Waardenburg syndrome includes piebaldism, widening of the medial epicanthic folds, prominent inner third of eyebrows, irides of different colour, and deafness.

Phenylketonuria

This rare metabolic cause of hypopigmentation has a prevalence of about 1 : 25 000. It is described in Chapter 20.

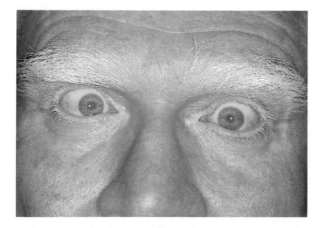

Fig. 18.2 Oculocutaneous albinism in an Asian. The skin and hair are depigmented and the irides translucent. The patient had a rotary nystagmus.

Hypopituitarism

The skin changes here may alert an astute physician to the diagnosis. The complexion has a pale, yellow tinge; there is thinning or loss of the sexual hair; the skin itself is atrophic. The hypopigmentation is due to a decreased production of pituitary melanotrophic hormones (see Chapter 2).

Vitiligo

The word vitiligo comes from the Latin word *'vitellus'*, which means veal, that is pale, pink flesh. It is an acquired circumscribed depigmentation, found in all races; its prevalence may be as high as 0.5–1%; its inheritance is polygenic.

Cause and types

There is a complete loss of melanocytes from affected areas. There are two main patterns; a common generalized one and a rare segmental type. *Generalized vitiligo*, including the acrofacial variant, usually starts after the second decade. There is a family history in 30% of patients and this type is most frequent in those with autoimmune diseases such as diabetes, thyroid disorders and pernicious anaemia. *Segmental vitiligo* is restricted to one part of the body, but not necessarily to a dermatome. It occurs earlier than generalized vitiligo, and is not associated with autoimmune diseases. Trauma and sunburn may precipitate both types.

Clinical course

Generalized type. The sharply defined, white patches are especially common on the backs of the hands (Fig. 18.3), wrists, fronts of knees, neck and around body orifices. The hair of the scalp and beard may depigment too. The surrounding skin in Caucasoids is sometimes hyperpigmented.

The course is unpredictable: lesions may remain static, or spread; occasionally they repigment spontaneously from the hair follicles (Fig. 18.4).

Segmental type. The individual areas look like the generalized type but their segmental distribution is striking (Fig. 18.5). Spontaneous repigmentation

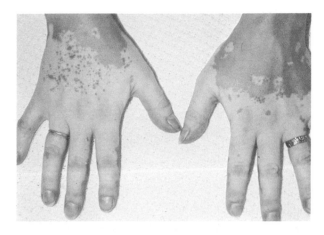

Fig. 18.3 Vitiligo: note the rough symmetry, and the coffee colour of the surrounding skin.

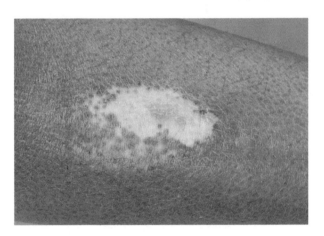

Fig. 18.4 The spottiness of this repigmenting vitiligo is due to the migration of melanocytes from the depths of hair follicles.

occurs more often in this type than in generalized vitiligo.

Differential diagnosis

Contact with depigmenting chemicals, such as hydroquinones and substituted phenols in the rubber industry, should be excluded. Pityriasis versicolor (p. 191) must be considered; its fine scaling and less complete pigment loss separate it from vitiligo. Post-inflammatory depigmentation (see below) may look very like vitiligo but is less white and improves spontaneously. The patches of piebaldism are present

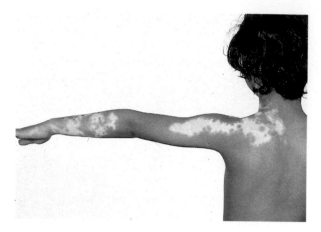

Fig. 18.5 Segmental vitiligo in a young girl. The distribution is not dermatomal.

at birth. Sometimes leprosy must be excluded by sensory testing and a general examination. Other tropical diseases which cause patchy hypopigmentation are leishmaniasis (p. 171), yaws (p. 168) and pinta.

Treatment

Treatment is unsatisfactory. A short course of a potent topical steroid, applied to a few recent patches, occasionally helps. Some patients improve with psoralens (trimethylpsoralen or 8-methoxypsoralen, in a dose of 0.6 mg/kg body weight), taken one to two hours before graduated exposure to natural sunshine or to artificial UVA (PUVA, p. 62). Therapy is needed daily for at least six months: new lesions seem to respond best. Autologous grafts are experimental but interesting. Their use may be limited by cost and the development of vitiligo (Köbner phenomenon) at donor sites. As a general rule established vitiligo is best left untreated in most whites, though advice about suitable preparations (Formulary, p. 289) to cover unsightly patches should be given. Sun avoidance and screening preparations are needed to avoid sunburn of the affected areas (Formulary, p. 289). Patients with extensive vitiligo can be completely and irreversibly depigmented by creams containing the monobenzyl ether by hydroquinone. Carefully considered informed consent is needed before such treatment.

Post-inflammatory depigmentation

This may follow eczema, psoriasis, sarcoidosis, lupus erythematosus and, rarely, lichen planus. It may also result from cryotherapy or a burn. In general, the more severe the inflammation, the more likely pigment is to decrease rather than increase in its wake. These problems are most significant in Negroids or Asians. With time, repigmentation usually occurs.

White hair

Melanocytes in hair bulbs become less active with age (Chapter 2), and white hair (canities) is a universal sign of ageing. Early greying of the hair is seen in the rare premature ageing syndromes, such as Werner's syndrome, and in autoimmune conditions such as pernicious anaemia, thyroid disorders, and Addison's disease.

Disorders with increased pigmentation (hypermelanosis)

Some of these disorders are listed in Table 18.3. The most common will be described below and the mechanisms involved are summarized in Figure 18.6.

Freckles (ephelides)

Freckles are so common that to describe them seems unnecessary. They are most often seen in the red-haired or blond as sharply demarcated light brown-ginger macules, of usually less than 5 mm in diameter (Fig. 18.7). They multiply and become darker with sun exposure.

Increased melanin is seen in the basal layer of the epidermis without any increase in the number of melanocytes, and without elongation of the rete ridges (Fig. 18.8). No treatment is necessary.

Table 18.3 Some causes of hyperpigmentation

Genetic	Freckles
	Lentigines
	Café au lait macules
	Peutz–Jeghers syndrome
	Xeroderma pigmentosum
	Albright's syndrome:
	segmental hyperpigmentation
	fibrous dysplasia of bones
	precocious puberty
Endocrine	Addison's disease
	Cushing's syndrome
	Pregnancy
	Renal failure
Metabolic	Biliary cirrhosis
	Haemochromatosis
	Porphyria
Nutritional	Malabsorption
	Carcinomatosis
	Kwashiorkor
	Pellagra
Drugs	Photosensitizing drugs
	ACTH and synthetic analogues
	Oestrogens and progestogens
	Psoralens
	Arsenic
	Busulphan
	Minocycline
Post-inflammatory	Lichen planus
	Eczema
	Secondary syphilis
	Systemic sclerosis
	Lichen and macular amyloidosis
	Cryotherapy
Poikiloderma	
Tumours	Acanthosis nigricans
	Pigmented naevi
	Malignant melanoma
	Mastocytosis

Lentigo

Simple and senile lentigines look alike. They are light or dark brown macules, ranging from 1 mm to 1 cm across. Although usually discrete, they may have an irregular outline. Simple lentigines arise most often in childhood as a few scattered lesions, often on areas not exposed to sun. Senile or solar lentigines are common after middle age on the backs of the hands ('liver spots') (Fig. 18.9) and on the face (Fig. 18.10). In contrast to freckles, lentigines have increased numbers of melanocytes (Fig. 18.8). They should be distinguished from freckles, from junctional melanocytic naevi (p. 223) and from a lentigo maligna (p. 235). Treatment is usually unnecessary. Ugly lesions may be excised or frozen with liquid nitrogen. Liver spots associated with actinic damage lighten or clear with the daily application of 0.1% tretinoin cream (Formulary, p. 294).

Conditions associated with multiple lentigines

Three rare but striking syndromes feature multiple lentigines:

Peutz–Jeghers syndrome

Profuse lentigines are seen on and around the lips in this autosomal dominant condition (Fig. 18.11). Scattered lentigines also occur on the buccal mucosa, gums, hard palate, hands and feet. The syndrome is important because of its association with polyposis of the small intestine which may lead to recurrent intussusception and, rarely, to malignant transformation of the polyps. Ten per cent of affected women have ovarian tumours.

Cronkhite–Canada syndrome

This consists of multiple lentigines on the backs of the hands and a more diffuse pigmentation of the palms and volar aspects of the fingers. It may also associate with gastrointestinal polyposis. Alopecia and nail abnormalities complete the rare but characteristic clinical picture.

'Leopard' syndrome

This is an acronym for generalized *L*entiginosis associated with cardiac abnormalities demonstrated by *E*CG, *O*cular hypertelorism, *P*ulmonary stenosis, *A*bnormal genitalia, *R*etardation of growth and *D*eafness.

Chloasma

Chloasma is a patterned pigmentation of the face occurring in women during pregnancy or on oral

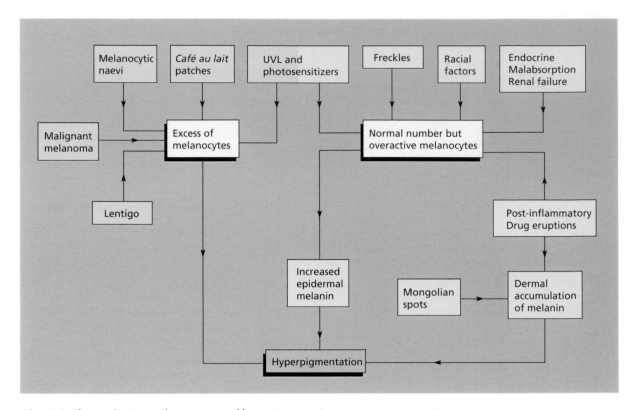

Fig. 18.6 The mechanisms of some types of hyperpigmentation.

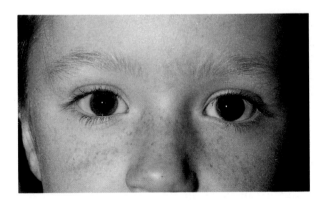

Fig. 18.7 Characteristic freckling in a red-headed boy.

contraceptives. The areas of increased pigmentation are well-defined, symmetrical, and their edge is often scalloped (the mask of pregnancy) (Fig. 18.12). The light brown colour becomes darker after exposure to the sun. The placenta may secrete hormones which stimulate melanocytes. Chloasma should be differentiated from a phototoxic reaction to a scented cosmetic or to a drug. Treatment is unsatisfactory, though some find bleaching agents which contain hydroquinone helpful. A sunscreen will make the pigmentation less obvious during the summer.

Endocrine hyperpigmentation

Addison's disease

Hyperpigmentation due to the overproduction of ACTH is often striking (Fig. 18.13); it may be generalized or limited to the skin folds, creases of the palms, scars and the buccal mucosa.

Cushing's syndrome

Increased ACTH production may cause a picture like that of Addison's disease. The hyperpigmen-

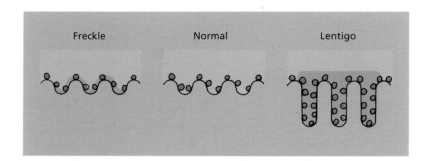

Fig. 18.8 Histology of a freckle and a lentigo.

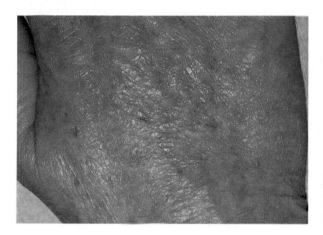

Fig. 18.9 Senile lentigines on the back of an elderly hand ('liver spots'). Note accompanying atrophy.

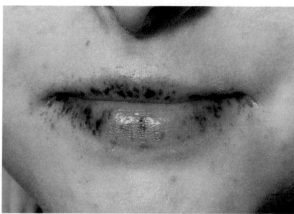

Fig. 18.11 Profuse lentigines on and around the lips in the Peutz–Jeghers syndrome.

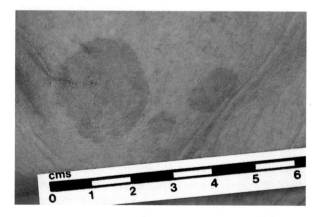

Fig. 18.10 Simple lentigines on the jaw line of an elderly lady. Note the even colour and regular edge.

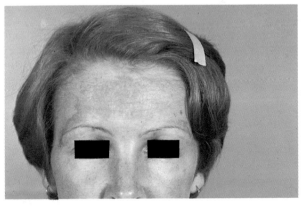

Fig. 18.12 Chloasma which became more obvious after a holiday in the sun.

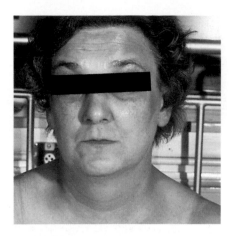

Fig. 18.13 Marked, diffuse facial pigmentation in Addison's disease.

tation may become even more marked after adrenalectomy (Nelson's syndrome).

Pregnancy

There is a generalized increase in pigmentation during pregnancy, especially of the nipples and areolae, and of the linea alba. Chloasma (see above) may also occur. The nipples and areolae remain pigmented after parturition.

Chronic renal failure

The hyperpigmentation of chronic renal failure and of patients on haemodialysis is due to an increase in levels of pituitary melanotrophic peptides, normally cleared by the kidney.

Porphyria

Formed porphyrins, especially uroporphyrins, are produced in excess in cutaneous hepatic porphyria and congenital erythropoietic porphyria (p. 251). These endogenous photosensitizers induce hyperpigmentation on exposed areas; skin fragility, blistering and hypertrichosis are equally important clues to the diagnosis.

Nutritional hyperpigmentation

Any severe wasting disease, such as malabsorption,

AIDS, tuberculosis or cancer, may be accompanied by diffuse hyperpigmentation. Kwashiorkor is a cause of hyperpigmentation in the tropics, and in this condition the hair is red-brown or grey.

Drugs causing hyperpigmentation

Table 17.1 lists drugs that commonly photosensitize. All may cause hyperpigmentation of the exposed skin. Psoralens are used in the photochemotherapy of psoriasis (Chapter 6) and, more rarely, of vitiligo.

The term 'Berloque dermatitis' refers to a 'pendant' of hyperpigmentation, often on the side of the neck, where cosmetics have been applied which contain the photosensitizing 5-methoxypsoralen. Cosmetics for men (pre- and after-shaves, etc.) are a thriving source of these.

Arsenic is seldom used medically nowadays. Once it caused 'raindrop' depigmentation within a diffuse bronzed hyperpigmentation.

Busulphan and bleomycin, used to treat some forms of leukaemia, frequently cause diffuse hyperpigmentation but may cause streaks of brown colour (flagellate hyperpigmentation). Minocycline can leave blue-black drug deposits in inflamed acne spots on the shins or on the mucosae.

Post-inflammatory hyperpigmentation

This is common after lichen planus (p. 67). It is also a feature of systemic sclerosis (p. 131) and some types of cutaneous amyloidosis, and is often an unwelcome sequel of cryotherapy.

Poikiloderma

Poikiloderma is the name given to a triad of signs: reticulate pigmentation, atrophy, and telangiectasia. It is not a disease but a reaction pattern with many causes including X-irradiation, photocontact reactions, and connective tissue and lymphoreticular disorders. Congenital variants (Rothmund–Thomson syndrome, Bloom's syndrome and Cockayne's syndrome) associated with photosensitivity, dwarfism and mental retardation also occur.

CHAPTER 19

Skin tumours

This chapter will deal both with skin tumours arising from the epidermis and its appendages, and with those arising from the dermis (Table 19.1).

Prevention

Actinic keratoses, lentigines, keratoacanthomas, basal cell carcinomas, squamous cell carcinomas, malignant melanomas and, arguably, acquired melanocytic naevi would all become less common if Caucasoids, especially those with a fair skin, protected themselves against exposure to sunlight. Education of those living in sunny climates or holidaying in the sun has already reaped great rewards here. Successful campaigns have focussed on regular self-examination and the ways in which sun exposure can be reduced by avoidance, clothing and sunscreen preparations (Figs 19.1 & 19.2). Public awareness and compliance has been encouraged by imaginative and gimmicky slogans like the Australian 'slip, slap and slop' advice (slip on the shirt, slap on the hat and slop on the sunscreen) and the lovable American creature Joel Mole.

Tumours of the epidermis and its appendages

Benign

Viral warts

These are discussed in Chapter 15, but are mentioned here for two reasons: first, they are sometimes misdiagnosed if solitary on the face or hands of

Table 19.1 Skin tumours

Derived from	Benign	Premalignant	Malignant
Epidermis and appendages	Viral wart Squamous cell papilloma Seborrhoeic keratosis Skin tag Milium Melanocytic naevus Epidermoid/pilar cyst Chondrodermatitis nodularis helicis	Kerato-acanthoma Intra-epidermal carcinoma Actinic keratosis	Basal cell carcinoma Squamous cell carcinoma Malignant melanoma Paget's disease of the nipple
Dermis	Haemangioma Lymphangioma Glomus tumour Pyogenic granuloma Dermatofibroma Keloid Lipoma Lymphocytoma cutis		Kaposi's sarcoma Lymphoma Dermatofibrosarcoma protuberans Secondary deposits

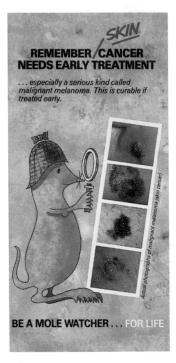

Fig. 19.1 An eye-catching and effective way of teaching the public how to look at their moles. Pamphlet produced by the Cancer Research Campaign in the UK.

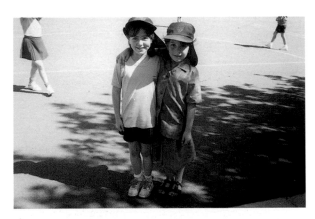

Fig. 19.2 These Australian schoolchildren are wearing legionaire's caps with large peaks and flaps. They are becoming fashionable after several clever campaigns, and the 'no hat — no play' rule has become an accepted way of life.

the elderly; and, second, warts are one of the few tumours in humans which are, without doubt, caused by a virus. Seventy per cent of transplant patients who have been immunosuppressed for over five years have multiple viral warts: there is growing evidence that immunosuppression, viral warts and ultraviolet radiation interact in this setting to cause squamous cell carcinoma (p. 232).

Squamous cell papilloma

This common tumour, arising from keratinocytes, may resemble a viral wart clinically. Sometimes an excessive hyperkeratosis produces a horn-shaped excrescence. Excision, or curettage with cautery to the base, is the treatment of choice. The histology should be checked.

Seborrhoeic keratosis (basal cell papilloma, seborrhoeic wart)

This is a common, benign, epidermal tumour, unrelated to sebaceous glands. The term senile wart should be avoided as it offends many patients.

Cause

Usually unexplained but:
• Multiple lesions may be inherited (autosomal dominant).
• Occasionally follow an inflammatory dermatosis.
• Very rarely the sudden eruption of hundreds of itchy lesions is associated with an internal neoplasm (sign of Leser–Trélat).

Presentation

Seborrhoeic keratoses usually arise after the age of 50, but flat inconspicuous lesions are often visible earlier. They are often multiple (Figs 19.3 & 19.4) but may be single. Lesions are most common on the face and trunk. The sexes are equally affected.
Physical signs:
• A distinctive 'stuck-on' appearance.
• May be flat, raised or pedunculated.
• Colour varies from yellow to dark brown.
• Surface may have greasy scaling and scattered keratin plugs ('currant bun' appearance).

Clinical course

Lesions may multiply with age but remain benign.

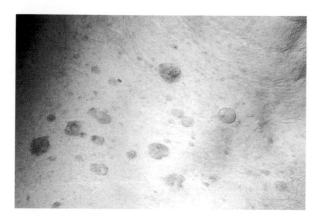

Fig. 19.3 Typical multiple seborrhoeic warts at the base of the neck.

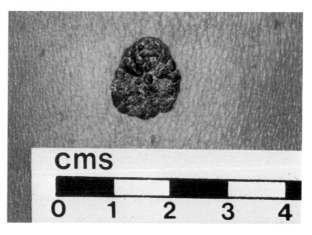

Fig. 19.5 Darkly pigmented seborrhoeic wart needing biopsy to exclude a malignant melanoma.

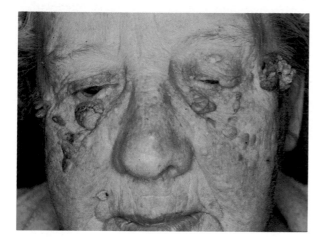

Fig. 19.4 Numerous ugly seborrhoeic warts of the face.

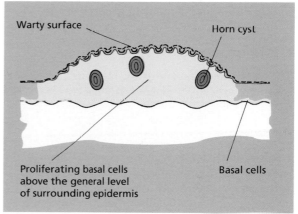

Fig. 19.6 Histology of a seborrhoeic keratosis.

Differential diagnosis

Seborrhoeic keratoses are easily recognized. Occasional confusion arises with a pigmented cellular naevus, a pigmented basal cell carcinoma and, most importantly, with a malignant melanoma (Fig. 19.5).

Investigations

Biopsy is needed only in rare dubious cases. The histology is diagnostic (Fig. 19.6). The lesion lies above the general level of the surrounding epidermis and consists of proliferating basal cells and horn cysts.

Treatment

Seborrhoeic keratoses may be left alone, but ugly or easily traumatized ones can be removed by curetting them off under local anaesthetic (this has the advantage of providing histology), or by cryotherapy.

LEARNING POINT

If you cannot tell most seborrhoeic warts from a melanoma you will send too many old people to the pigmented lesion clinic.

Skin tags (acrochordon)

These common benign outgrowths of skin affect mainly the middle-aged and elderly.

Cause

This is unknown but the trait is sometimes familial. Skin tags are most common in obese women, and rarely are associated with tuberous sclerosis (p. 263), acanthosis nigricans (p. 246) or acromegaly, and diabetes.

Presentation and clinical course

Skin tags occur around the neck and within the major flexures. They look bad and may catch on clothing and jewellery. They are soft, skin-coloured or pigmented, pedunculated papules (Fig. 19.7).

Differential diagnosis

The appearance is unmistakable. Tags are rarely confused with small melanocytic naevi.

Treatment

Small lesions can be snipped off with fine scissors, frozen with liquid nitrogen, or destroyed with a hyfrecator without local anaesthesia. There is no way of preventing new ones from developing.

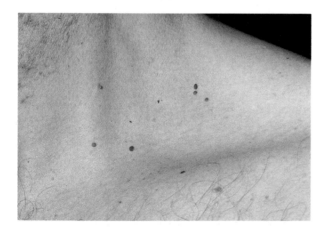

Fig. 19.7 A cluster of pigmented skin tags in the supraclavicular fossa.

Melanocytic naevi

The term 'naevus' refers to a lesion, often present at birth, which has a local excess of one or more normal constituents of the skin. Melanocytic naevi (moles) are localized benign proliferations of melanocytes. Their classification is shown in Table 19.2 and depends on where the aggregations of naevus cells lie (Fig. 19.8).

Cause and evolution

The cause is unknown. A genetic factor is likely in many families, working together with excessive sun exposure during childhood.

With the exception of congenital melanocytic naevi, most appear in early childhood, often with a sharp increase in numbers during adolescence. Further crops may appear during pregnancy, oestrogen therapy, or rarely after cytotoxic chemotherapy and immunosuppression, but new lesions come up less often after the age of 20.

Melanocytic naevi in childhood are usually of the 'junctional' type, with proliferating melanocytes in clumps at the dermo-epidermal junction. Later, the melanocytes round off and 'drop' into the dermis. A 'compound' naevus has both dermal and junctional components. With maturation the junctional component disappears so that the melanocytes in an 'intradermal' naevus are all in the dermis (Fig. 19.8).

Presentation

Congenital melanocytic naevi (Figs 19.9 & 19.10). These are present at birth or appear in the neonatal period and are seldom less than 1 cm in diameter. Their colour varies from brown to black or blue-

Table 19.2 Classification of melanocytic naevi

1 Congenital melanocytic naevi
2 Acquired melanocytic naevi
    Junctional naevus
    Compound naevus
    Intradermal naevus
    Spitz naevus
    Blue naevus
    Dysplastic naevus

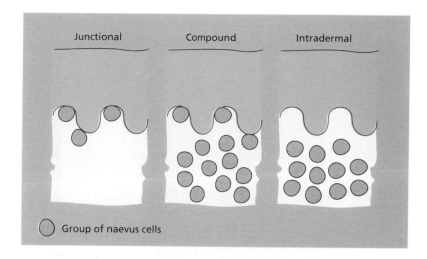

| Junctional | Compound | Intradermal |

◯ Group of naevus cells

Fig. 19.8 Types of acquired melanocytic naevi.

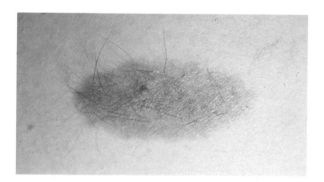

Fig. 19.9 Congenital melanocytic naevus measuring 5 × 2 cm.

black. With maturity some become protruberant and hairy, with a cerebriform surface. Such lesions can be disfiguring, e.g. a 'bathing trunk' naevus, and carry an increased risk of malignant transformation.

Junctional melanocytic naevi (Fig. 19.11). These are roughly circular macules. Their colour ranges from mid to dark brown and may vary even within a single lesion. Most naevi of the palms, soles and genitals are of this type.

Compound melanocytic naevi (Fig. 19.12). These are domed pigmented nodules of up to 1 cm in diameter. They may be light or dark brown but their colour is more even than that of junctional naevi. Most are smooth, but larger ones may be

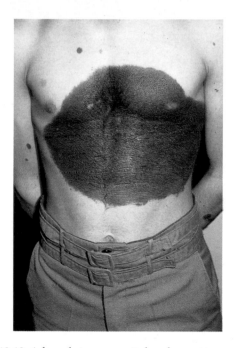

Fig. 19.10 A large hairy congenital melanocytic naevus.

cerebriform, or even hyperkeratotic and papillomatous; many bear hairs.

Intradermal melanocytic naevi (Fig. 19.13). These look like compound naevi but are less pigmented and often skin-coloured.

Spitz naevus (juvenile melanoma) (Fig. 19.14). These are usually found in children. They develop over a

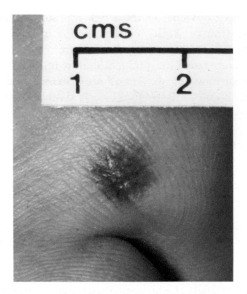

Fig. 19.11 Junctional melanocytic naevus at the base of the little toe.

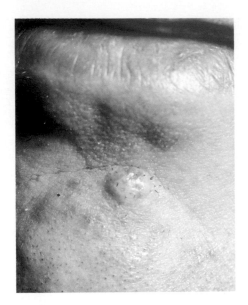

Fig. 19.13 Intradermal melanocytic naevus with numerous shaved hairs.

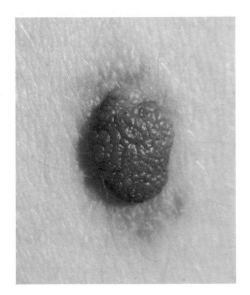

Fig. 19.12 Compound melanocytic naevus. No recent change.

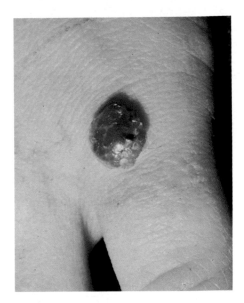

Fig. 19.14 Spitz naevus. Rapid evolution and red colour cause diagnostic confusion.

month or two as solitary pink or red nodules of up to 1 cm in diameter and are most common on the face and legs. Though benign, they are often excised because of their rapid growth.

Blue naevus. So-called because of their striking slate grey-blue colour, blue naevi usually appear in child-

hood and adolescence, on the limbs, buttocks and lower back (Fig. 19.15). They are usually solitary.

Mongolian spots. Pigment in dermal melanocytes is responsible for these bruise-like greyish areas seen on the lumbosacral area of most Down's syndrome

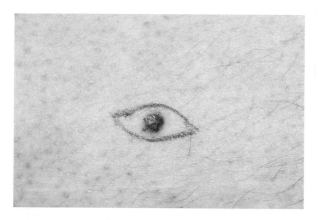

Fig. 19.15 The blue ink matches the blue naevus.

and many Negroid babies. They usually fade during childhood.

Dysplastic naevus syndrome (atypical mole syndrome) (Fig. 19.16). Dysplastic naevi may occur sporadically or run in families as an autosomal dominant trait, with incomplete penetrance, affecting several generations. Some families with dysplastic naevi are melanoma prone. Genes for susceptibility to melanoma have been mapped to chromosomes 1p36 and 9p13 in a few of these families. The many large irregularly pigmented naevi

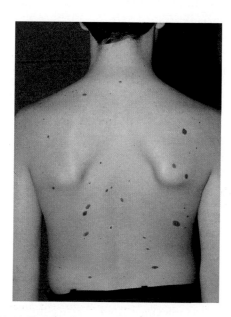

Fig. 19.16 Dysplastic naevus syndrome.

are most obvious on the trunk but some may be present on the scalp. Their edges are irregular and they vary greatly in size; many are over 1 cm in diameter. Some are pinkish and an inflamed halo may surround them. Some have a mamillated surface. Patients with multiple atypical melanocytic or dysplastic naevi with a positive family history of malignant melanoma should be followed up six monthly for life.

Differential diagnosis of melanocytic naevi

• *Malignant melanoma.* Most important in the differential diagnosis. These are very rare before puberty. Melanomas are single and more variably pigmented and irregularly shaped. Other features are listed below under Complications.
• *Seborrhoeic keratoses.* These may cause confusion in adults but they have a stuck-on appearance and are warty. Tell-tale keratin plugs and horny cysts may be seen with the help of a lens.
• *Lentigines.* May be found on any part of the skin and mucous membranes. More profuse than junctional naevi, they are usually grey-brown rather than black, and develop more often after adolescence.
• *Ephelides (freckles).* These are tan macules less than 5 mm in diameter. They are confined to sun-exposed areas, being most common in blonds or redheads.
• *Haemangiomas.* Benign proliferations of blood vessels, including haemangiomas and pyogenic granulomas, may be confused with a vascular Spitz naevus or an amelanotic melanoma.

Histology

Most acquired lesions fit into the scheme given in Fig. 19.8; orderly nests of benign naevus cells are seen in the junctional region, in the dermis, or in both. However, some types of melanocytic naevi have their own distinguishing features. In congenital naevi the naevus cells may extend to the subcutaneous fat, and hyperplasia of other skin components (e.g. hair follicles) may be seen. A Spitz naevus has a worrisome histology similar to melanoma. It shows dermal oedema and dilated capillaries, and is composed of large epithelioid and spindle-shaped naevus cells, some of which may be in mitosis.

In a blue naevus, naevus cells are seen in the mid and deep dermis.

The main features of a dysplastic naevus are lengthening and bridging of rete ridges, and the presence of junctional nests showing melanocytic dysplasia (nuclear pleomorphism and hyperchromatism). Fibrosis of the papillary dermis and a lymphocytic inflammatory response are also seen.

Complications

- *Inflammation.* Pain and swelling are common but are not features of malignant transformation. They are due to trauma, bacterial folliculitis, or a foreign body reaction to hair after shaving or plucking.
- *Depigmented halo* (Fig. 19.17). The so-called 'halo naevus' is uncommon but benign. There may be vitiligo elsewhere. The naevus in the centre often involutes spontaneously before the halo repigments.
- *Malignant change.* This is extremely rare except in congenital melanocytic naevi, where the risk has been estimated at between 3 and 6% depending on their size (Fig. 19.18) and in the dysplastic naevi of melanoma-prone families. It should be considered if the following *changes* occur in a melanocytic naevus:
  - Itch.
  - Enlargement.
  - Increased or decreased pigmentation.
  - Altered shape.

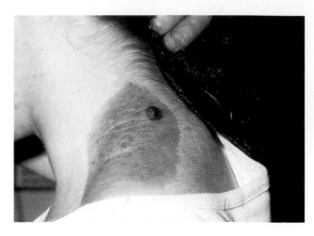

Fig. 19.18 Malignant melanoma developing within a congenital melanocytic naevus.

- Altered contour.
- Inflammation.
- Ulceration.
- Bleeding.

If such changing lesions are examined carefully, remembering the 'A B C D E' features of malignant melanoma (Table 19.3), few malignant melanomas should be missed.

Treatment

Excision is needed when:
1 A naevus is deemed ugly.
2 Malignancy is suspected or is a known risk, e.g. in a large congenital melanocytic naevus.
3 A naevus is repeatedly inflamed or traumatized.

LEARNING POINT
Do not be frightened, even if you think they are harmless, to refer moles which have **changed** *to a dermatologist.*

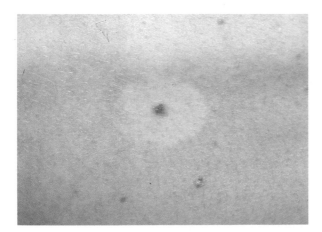

Fig. 19.17 Halo naevus. Involuting melanocytic naevus within area of symmetrical and total depigmentation.

Table 19.3 The A B C D E of malignant melanoma

Asymmetry
Border irregularity
Colour variability
Diameter greater than 0.5 cm
Elevation irregularity

Epidermoid and pilar cysts

Often incorrectly called 'sebaceous cysts', epidermoid cysts are common and occur on the scalp, face, behind the ears, and on the trunk. They often have a central punctum; when they rupture, or are squeezed, foul-smelling cheesy material comes out. Histologically the lining of a cyst resembles normal epidermis (epidermoid cyst) or the outer root sheath of the hair follicle (pilar cyst). Occasionally an adjacent foreign body reaction is noted. Treatment is by excision, or by incision followed by expression of the contents and removal of the cyst wall.

Milium

Milia are small, subepidermal keratin cysts (Fig. 19.19). They are common on the face in all age groups and appear as tiny, white, millet seed-like papules of from 0.5 to 2 mm in diameter. They are occasionally seen at the site of a previous subepidermal blister (e.g. in epidermolysis bullosa and porphyria cutanea tarda). The contents of milia can be picked out with a sterile needle without local anaesthesia.

Chondrodermatitis nodularis helicis
(painful nodule of the ear, ear corn)

This terminological mouthful is, strictly, not a neoplasm, but a chronic inflammation. A painful nodule develops on the helix or antehelix of the ear, most often in men. It looks like a small corn, is tender, and prevents sleep if that side of the head touches the pillow. Histologically, a thickened epidermis overlies inflamed cartilage. Wedge resection under local anaesthetic is effective if cryotherapy or intralesional triamcinolone injection fails.

Premalignant tumours

Kerato-acanthoma

Some argue that this rapidly growing tumour should be classed as benign, but a very few transform into a squamous cell carcinoma.

Cause

Photosensitizing chemicals such as tar and mineral oils may act as co-carcinogens with ultraviolet radiation. They may also follow therapeutic immunosuppression.

Clinical features

They occur mainly on the exposed skin of fair individuals. More than two-thirds are on the face and most of the rest are on the arms. The lesion starts as a pink papule which rapidly enlarges; it may reach a diameter of 1 cm in a month or two. After five or six weeks the centre of the nodule forms either a keratinous plug or a crater (Fig. 19.20). If left, the lesion often resolves spontaneously over 6–12 months but leaves an ugly depressed scar.

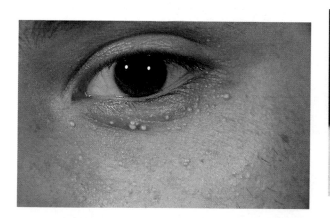

Fig. 19.19 Milia.

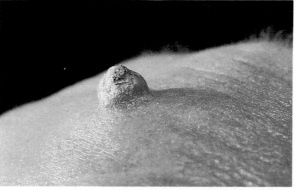

Fig. 19.20 Kerato-acanthoma with its epidermal shoulders and central plug of keratin.

Differential diagnosis

Squamous cell carcinoma is the main tumour to be distinguished from a kerato-acanthoma. However, carcinomas grow more slowly, and usually lack symmetry.

Histology

It is not possible to tell a kerato-acanthoma from a squamous cell carcinoma histologically unless the architecture of the whole lesion can be assessed, including its base (Fig. 19.21). A typical lesion is symmetrical and composed of proliferating fronds of epidermis which show mitotic activity but retain a well-differentiated squamous appearance with the production of much 'glassy' keratin. The centre of the cup-shaped mass is filled with keratin.

Treatment

Excision or curettage and cautery are both effective. Occasionally a further curetting may be needed but this should be done only once; if this is still ineffective, the lesion must be excised.

Intra-epidermal carcinoma (Bowen's disease)

Usually single, these slowly expanding pink, scaly plaques (Fig. 19.22) take years to reach a diameter of a few centimetres. Their border is sharply defined, with reniform projections and notches. These lesions occasionally change into an invasive squamous cell

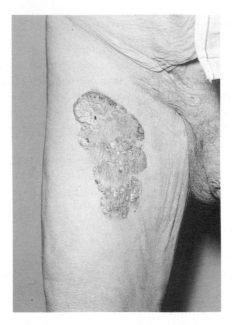

Fig. 19.22 Intra-epidermal carcinoma: a slowly expanding psoriasiform plaque on the thigh. Note the reniform projections and notches so suggestive of an *in situ* malignancy.

carcinoma. The presence of several may be a clue to previous exposure to carcinogens (e.g. arsenic in a tonic when young).

Differential diagnosis

Intra-epidermal carcinoma is often mistaken for psoriasis (Chapter 6), discoid eczema (p. 100) or a superficial basal cell carcinoma (see below).

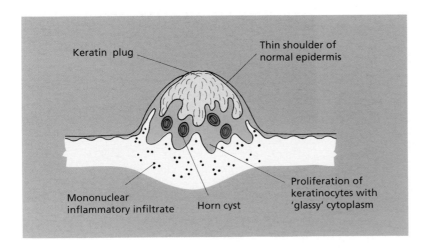

Keratin plug

Thin shoulder of normal epidermis

Mononuclear inflammatory infiltrate

Horn cyst

Proliferation of keratinocytes with 'glassy' cytoplasm

Fig. 19.21 Histology of kerato-acanthoma.

Treatment

These lesions are unaffected by local steroids; excision or cryotherapy is therefore needed, though small lesions may be left under observation in the frail and elderly.

Actinic keratoses

These discrete, rough-surfaced lesions crop up on sun-damaged skin. They are premalignant, although only a few turn into a squamous cell carcinoma.

Cause

The effects of sun exposure are cumulative. Those with fair complexions living near the equator are most at risk and invariably develop these 'sun warts'. Melanin protects, and actinic keratoses are not seen in black skin. Conversely, albinos are especially prone to develop them.

Presentation

They affect the middle-aged and elderly in temperate climates, but younger people in the tropics. The pink or grey, rough, scaling macules or papules seldom exceed 1 cm in diameter. Their rough surface (Fig. 19.23) is sometimes better felt than seen.

Complications

Transition to a squamous cell carcinoma, although rare, should be suspected if a lesion enlarges, ulcerates or bleeds (Fig. 19.24). Luckily such tumours seldom metastasize. A 'cutaneous horn' is a hard keratotic protrusion based on an actinic keratosis or viral wart (Fig. 19.25).

Differential diagnosis

There is usually no difficulty in telling an actinic keratosis from a seborrhoeic wart, a viral wart

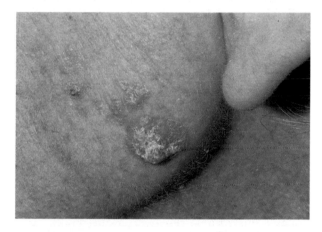

Fig. 19.24 A large neglected actinic keratosis at the angle of the jaw. Already showed transition to a squamous cell carcinoma on biopsy.

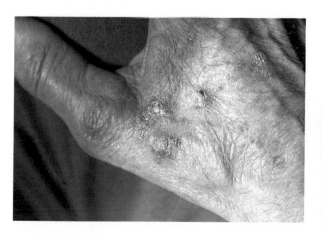

Fig. 19.23 The back of the hand of a farm worker showing numerous typical rough-surfaced actinic keratoses.

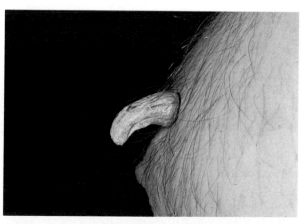

Fig. 19.25 Cutaneous horn with a bulbous fleshy base.

(p. 172), a kerato-acanthoma, an intra-epidermal carcinoma, or a squamous cell carcinoma.

Investigations

A biopsy is needed if there is worry over malignant change.

Histology

Alternating zones of hyper- and parakeratosis overlie a thickened or atrophic epidermis. The normal maturation pattern of the epidermis may be lost and occasional pleomorphic keratinocytes may be seen. Solar elastosis is seen in the superficial dermis.

Treatment

Freezing with liquid nitrogen or carbon dioxide snow is simple and effective. Curettage is best for large lesions and cutaneous horns. Multiple lesions can be treated with 5-fluorouracil cream (Formulary, p. 296) after specialist advice. Lesions which do not respond should be regarded with suspicion, and biopsied.

Malignant epidermal tumours

Basal cell carcinoma (rodent ulcer)

This is the most common form of skin cancer. It crops up most commonly on the faces of the middle-aged or elderly. Lesions invade locally but, for practical purposes, never metastasize.

Cause

Prolonged sun exposure is the most important factor so these tumours are most common in whites living near the equator. They may also occur in scars caused by X-rays, vaccination or trauma. Photosensitizing pitch, tar and oils can act as co-carcinogens with ultraviolet radiation. Previous treatment with arsenic, once present in many 'tonics', predisposes to multiple basal cell carcinomas often after a lag of many years. Multiple basal cell carcinomata are found in the naevoid basal cell carcinoma syndrome (Gorlin's syndrome) where they may be associated with palmoplantar pits, jaw cysts and abnormalities of the skull, vertebrae and ribs.

The syndrome is inherited as an autosomal dominant trait and recent studies indicate that the genetic abnormality lies on chromosome 9q.

Presentation

Nodulo-ulcerative. This is the most common type. An early lesion is a small, glistening, translucent, skin-coloured papule which slowly enlarges. Central necrosis, though not invariable, leaves an ulcer with an adherent crust and a rolled pearly edge (Fig. 19.26). Fine telangiectatic vessels often run across the tumour's surface. Without treatment such lesions may reach 1−2 cm in diameter in 5−10 years.

Cystic. The lesion is at first like the nodular type, but later cystic changes predominate and the nodule becomes tense and more translucent, with marked telangiectasia (Fig. 19.27).

Cicatricial (morphoeic). These are slowly expanding, yellow or white, waxy plaques with an ill-defined edge. Ulceration and crusting, followed by fibrosis, are common, and the lesion may look like an enlarging scar (Fig. 19.28).

Superficial (multicentric). These arise most often on the trunk. Several lesions may be present, each expanding slowly as a pink or brown scaly plaque with a fine 'whipcord' edge (Fig. 19.29). Such lesions can grow to more than 10 cm in diameter.

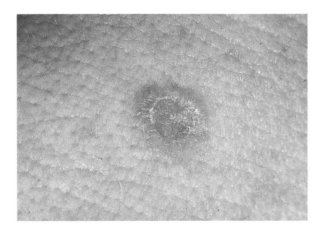

Fig. 19.26 Early basal cell carcinoma with rolled opalescent edge and central crusting.

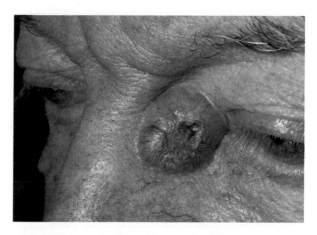

Fig. 19.27 Cystic basal cell carcinoma with marked telangiectasia, on the point of ulcerating.

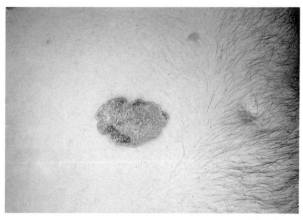

Fig. 19.29 Persistent scaly plaque — the whipcord edge gives away the diagnosis of a superficial basal cell carcinoma.

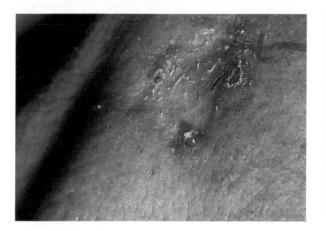

Fig. 19.28 Poorly defined cicatricial basal cell carcinoma.

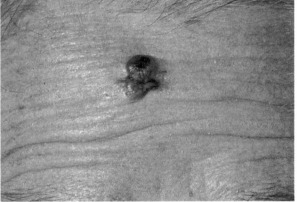

Fig. 19.30 A pigmented tumour on the forehead. The opalescence and telangiectasia point to the diagnosis of a basal cell carcinoma.

Pigmented. Pigment may be present in all types of basal cell carcinoma causing all or part of the tumour to be brown or have specks of brown or black within it (Fig. 19.30).

Clinical course

Slow but relentless growth destroys tissue locally. Untreated, a basal cell carcinoma may invade underlying cartilage or bone (Fig. 19.31) or damage important structures such as the tear ducts.

Histology

Small, darkly blue staining basal cells grow in well-defined aggregates which invade the dermis (Fig. 19.32). Their outer layer of cells is arranged in a palisade. Numerous mitoses and apoptotic bodies are seen. In the cicatricial type the islands of tumour are surrounded by fibrous tissue.

Differential diagnosis

A nodular basal cell carcinoma may be confused with an intradermal melanocytic naevus, a squamous cell carcinoma, a giant molluscum contagiosum (p. 180) or a kerato-acanthoma. Pigmented basal cell carcinomas should be distinguished from

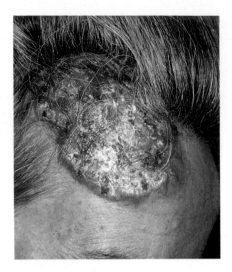

Fig. 19.31 A grossly neglected basal cell carcinoma already invading underlying bone.

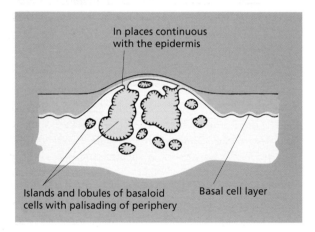

In places continuous with the epidermis

Islands and lobules of basaloid cells with palisading of periphery

Basal cell layer

Fig. 19.32 Histology of nodular basal cell carcinoma.

seborrhoeic warts and malignant melanomas. A cicatricial basal cell carcinoma may mimic morphoea (p. 133) or a scar. A superficial basal cell carcinoma may be confused with an intra-epidermal carcinoma, with psoriasis (Chapter 6) or with nummular eczema (p. 100).

Treatment

Excision, with 0.5 cm of surrounding normal skin, is the treatment of choice for patients under 60. Cicatricial tumours, with their ill-defined edges, and

lesions near vital structures, should be excised by specialist surgeons. Mohs' micrographic surgical technique is highly effective; it includes careful histological checks in all planes of tissue excised during the operation (p. 282). Radiotherapy is also effective; it is seldom used now for biopsy-proven lesions in patients under 70, but it is helpful when surgery is contraindicated. Cryotherapy, or curettage and cautery, is sometimes useful for small superficial lesions (p. 283). The five-year cure rate for all types of basal cell carcinoma is over 95%, but regular follow up is necessary to detect local recurrence.

LEARNING POINTS

1 *Catch lesions early: small ones are easy to get rid of; large ones may eat into cartilage or bone.*
2 *Do not sit and watch doubtful lesions near the eye.*

Squamous cell carcinoma

This is a common tumour in which malignant keratinocytes show a variable capacity to form keratin.

Cause

These tumours often arise in skin damaged by long-term UVR and also by X-rays and infra-red rays. Other carcinogens include pitch, tar, mineral oils and inorganic arsenic (see Basal cell carcinoma). Certain rare genetic disorders, with defective DNA repair mechanisms, such as xeroderma pigmentosum (p. 264), lead to multiple squamous and basal cell carcinomas, and to malignant melanoma; this illustrates the importance of altered DNA in the pathogenesis of malignancy. Multiple self-healing squamous cell carcinomata are found in the autosomal dominant trait described by Ferguson–Smith. The abnormal gene apparently lies on chromosome 9q. The DNA of the human papilloma virus (p. 172) may be integrated into the nuclear DNA of keratinocytes and cause malignant transformation. Immunosuppression and UVR predispose to this.

Clinical presentation and course

Tumours may arise as thickenings in an actinic keratosis, or, *de novo*, as small scaling nodules; rapidly growing anaplastic lesions may start as ulcers with a granulating base and an indurated edge (Fig. 19.33). Squamous cell carcinomas are common on the lower lip (Fig. 19.34) and in the mouth. Those arising in actinic keratoses seldom metastasize, but those arising in scars, ulcers, sinus tracks, X-irradiated skin and on mucous membranes often do. All lesions should be treated without delay.

Histology

Keratinocytes disrupt the dermo-epidermal junction and proliferate irregularly into the dermis. Malignant cells usually retain the capacity to produce keratin (Fig. 19.35).

Treatment

After the diagnosis has been confirmed by biopsy, the tumour should be excised with a 0.5 cm border of normal skin. Radiotherapy is effective but should be reserved for the frail and the elderly.

Malignant melanoma

Malignant melanoma attracts a disproportionate amount of attention because it is so often lethal. The public now knows more about its increasing incidence and dangers.

Incidence

The incidence in whites in the UK and USA is increasing, doubling approximately every 10 years. In Scotland the incidence is now about 10 per 100 000 per year with females affected almost twice as often as males. There is a higher incidence in whites living near the equator than in temperate zones and the female preponderance is lost. The tumour is rare before puberty and in blacks, Asians and Orientals and when it does occur in these races it is most often found on the palms and soles or affecting mucous membranes.

Cause

Genetic. These tumours are most common in whites with blond hair, many freckles and fair skin which tans poorly. Those of Celtic origin are the most susceptible. Melanoma may affect several members of a single family, in association with dysplastic naevi (p. 225).

Sunlight. Both incidence and mortality increase with decreasing latitude. Tumours occur most often, but not exclusively, on exposed skin.

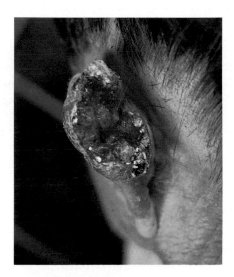

Fig. 19.33 Moderately differentiated squamous cell carcinoma presenting as an ulcerated keratotic nodule on the rim of an ear.

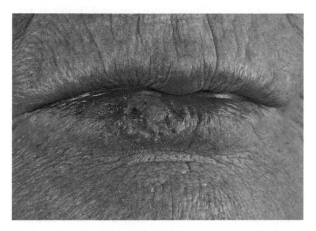

Fig. 19.34 Persistent nodule of the lower lip of a smoker: squamous cell carcinoma until proved otherwise by biopsy.

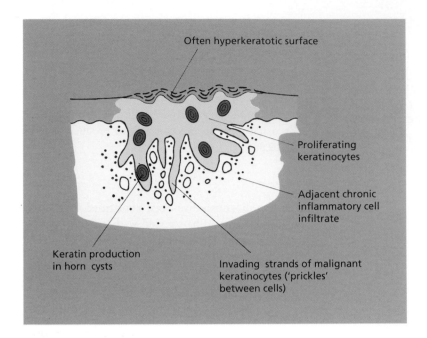

Often hyperkeratotic surface

Proliferating keratinocytes

Adjacent chronic inflammatory cell infiltrate

Keratin production in horn cysts

Invading strands of malignant keratinocytes ('prickles' between cells)

Fig. 19.35 Histology of squamous cell carcinoma.

Pre-existing melanocytic naevi. The risk of developing a malignant melanoma is highest in those with dysplastic naevi, congenital melanocytic naevi or many banal melanocytic naevi. A pre-existing naevus is seen histologically in about 30% of malignant melanomas.

Virus. RNA tumour viruses have occasionally been found in metastatic deposits of human melanoma, and in some animal melanomas.

Clinical features

Eighty per cent of invasive melanomas are preceded by a superficial and radial growth phase, shown clinically as an expanding, irregularly pigmented macule or plaque (Fig. 19.36). Most are multicoloured mixtures of black, brown, blue, tan and pink. Their margins are irregular with reniform projections and notches (see Table 19.3). Malignant cells are at first usually confined to the epidermis and uppermost dermis, but eventually invade deeper and may metastasize.

There are four main types of malignant melanoma:
- *Lentigo maligna melanoma* occurs on the exposed skin of the elderly. An irregularly pigmented, irregularly shaped, macule (lentigo maligna) may have been enlarging slowly for many years as an 'in situ' melanoma before an invasive nodule (lentigo maligna melanoma) appears (Fig. 19.37).
- *Superficial spreading melanoma* is the most common type in Caucasoids. Its radial growth phase shows varied colours and is often palpable (Figs 19.38 & 19.39). A nodule coming up within such a plaque signifies deep dermal invasion and a poor prognosis (Table 19.4).
- *Acral lentiginous melanoma* occurs on the palms and soles and, although rare in Caucasoids, is the most common type in the Chinese and Japanese. The invasive phase is again signalled by a nodule coming up within an irregularly pigmented macule or patch.
- *Nodular melanoma* (Fig. 19.40) appears as a pigmented nodule with no preceding *in situ* phase. It is the most rapidly growing and aggressive type.
- Totally *amelanotic melanomas* (Fig. 19.41) are rare, and flecks of pigment can usually be seen with a lens.
- *Subungual melanomas* are painless areas of pigmentation expanding under the nail and onto the nail fold.
- *Metastatic melanoma* has spread to surrounding skin, regional lymph nodes, or to other organs. At this stage it is only rarely cured.

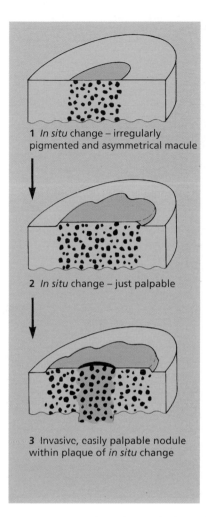

Fig. 19.36 Radial intra-epidermal growth phase of melanoma (1 and 2) precedes vertical and invasive dermal growth phase (3).

Within the illustration:

1 *In situ* change – irregularly pigmented and asymmetrical macule

2 *In situ* change – just palpable

3 Invasive, easily palpable nodule within plaque of *in situ* change

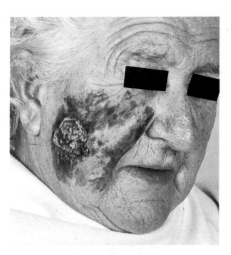

Fig. 19.37 This elderly patient had ignored for too long the slowly spreading macule of a lentigo maligna: now she has a frankly invasive melanoma within it.

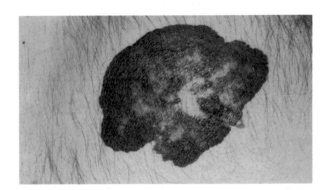

Fig. 19.38 Superficial spreading melanoma, chest wall, 8×6 cm: this lesion has been present for two years and, as yet, has invaded only the superficial dermis. Clearly malignant because of its colour variation, scalloped and notched outline.

Malignant melanoma is staged clinically into:
- Stage I: primary lesion only.
- Stage II: regional nodal disease.
- Stage III: distant disease (visceral or nodes).

Histology (Fig. 19.42)

- *Lentigo maligna*. Numerous atypical melanocytes, many in groups, are seen along the basal layer extending downwards in the walls of hair follicles.
- *Lentigo maligna melanoma*. Dermal invasion occurs, with a breach of the basement membrane region. *In situ* changes are seen in the adjacent epidermis.

- *Superficial spreading melanoma in situ*. Large epithelioid melanoma cells permeate the epidermis.
- *Superficial spreading melanoma*. The dermal nodule may be composed of epithelioid cells, spindle cells or naevus-like cells. *In situ* changes are seen in the adjacent epidermis.
- *Acral lentiginous melanoma in situ*. Atypical melanocytes are seen in the base of the epidermis and permeating the mid-epidermis.
- *Acral lentiginous melanoma*. Melanoma cells invade the dermis. *In situ* changes are seen in the adjacent epidermis.

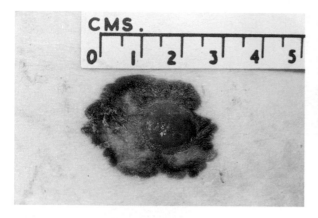

Fig. 19.39 This shows all the hallmarks of a malignant melanoma with its asymmetry, irregular borders and variations in colour. The pink amelanotic nodule signifies deep dermal invasion.

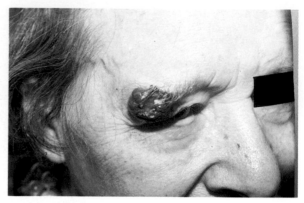

Fig. 19.40 A neglected nodular malignant melanoma: a thick tumour with a poor prognosis.

Table 19.4 Prognostic indicators in malignant melanoma

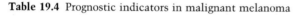

Indicator	Significance
Depth of primary tumour	Breslow <1.5 mm 5-year survival 90% 1.5−3.5 mm 5-year survival 75% >3.5 mm 5-year survival 50%
Sex	Females do better than males
Age	Prognosis worsens after 50 years, especially in males
Site	Poor prognosis with tumours on trunk, upper arms, neck and scalp
Ulceration	Signifies poor prognosis
Clinical stage	Stage I: 5-year survival 75% Stage II: 5-year survival 25% Stage III: 5-year survival 0−5%

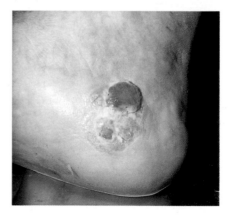

Fig. 19.41 An amelanotic malignant melanoma on the heel of an elderly person. Always obtain histology even if you think it is just a pyogenic granuloma or a wart.

- *Nodular melanoma.* The tumour comprises epithelioid, spindle and naevoid cells and there is no *in situ* melanoma in the adjacent epidermis.

Microstaging

Histology can help to assess prognosis. Breslow's method is to measure, with an ocular micrometer, the vertical distance from the granular cell layer to the deepest part of the tumour. Clark's method is to assess the depth of penetration of the melanoma (Fig. 19.43) in relation to the different layers of the dermis. The thicker and more penetrating a lesion, the worse is its prognosis (see below).

Differential diagnosis

This includes melanocytic naevus, seborrhoeic keratosis, pigmented actinic keratosis, pigmented basal cell carcinoma, and sclerosing haemangioma; all are discussed in this chapter. A malignant melanoma may also be confused with a subungual or peri-ungual haematoma. A history of trauma will help here, as may paring. *'Talon noir'* is a pigmented

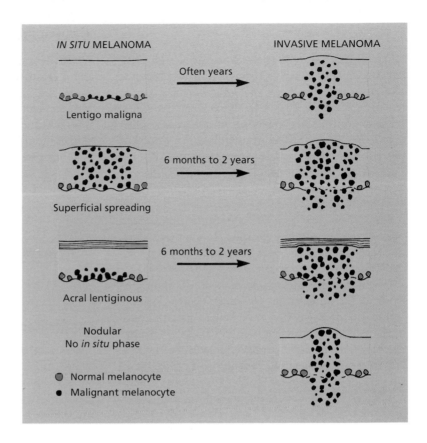

Fig. 19.42 Histology of the different types of melanoma.

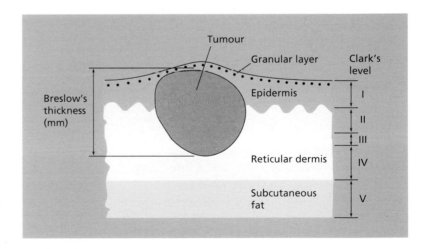

Fig. 19.43 Schematic representation of Breslow's and Clark's methods of microstaging malignant melanoma.

petechial area on the heel following minor trauma from ill-fitting training shoes. An amelanotic melanoma is most often confused with a pyogenic granuloma and with a squamous cell carcinoma.

Prognosis

The prognostic indicators, and their significance, are listed in Table 19.4.

Treatment

Surgical excision, with minimal delay, is indicated. Excision biopsy, with a 2 mm margin of clearance laterally, and down to the subcutaneous fat, is recommended for all suspicious lesions. If the histology confirms the diagnosis of malignant melanoma then wider excision, including the wound of the excision biopsy, should be performed as soon as possible. The extent of the wider excision will depend on the thickness of the tumour; 1 cm clearance of all margins is acceptable for thin (<1.5 mm) tumours but 3 cm is more appropriate for deeper ones. Tissue is removed down to, but not including, the deep fascia. Grafting may be necessary to repair the defect. The prognosis is excellent (90% 5-year survival) for patients with shallow tumours, but worsens in proportion to their depth. Elective regional node dissection may benefit patients with tumours of intermediate thickness (2–3.5 mm). Chemotherapy, rarely curative, is palliative in 25% of patients with stage III melanoma. Campaigns to educate doctors and the public to recognize melanoma early, in its superficial and curable phase, must be worthwhile.

LEARNING POINTS

1 Prevention of malignant melanoma is better than cure; remember avoidance of excessive sun exposure and 'slip, slap and slop' advice to patients.
2 All people, but especially those with many moles, should be encouraged to examine their own skin regularly.
3 Take any change in a mole seriously.
4 Do not forget the A B C D and E rules when querying a melanoma (Table 19.3).
5 Excise all doubtful lesions and check their histology.
6 If excision biopsy shows that a melanoma is less than 1 mm thick, the only question to be asked is whether it has been excised with a 1 cm clearance in all directions.

Paget's disease of the nipple

A well-defined red, scaly plaque spreads slowly over and around the nipple due to the invasion of the epidermis by cells from an underlying intraductal carcinoma of the breast (Paget cells). It is unilateral, whereas eczema usually affects both nipples. A skin biopsy should be carried out first and if the diagnosis is confirmed mastectomy will be necessary. Extra-mammary Paget's disease involves sites bearing apocrine glands (Chapter 2) and is due to an underlying ductal carcinoma of these.

Tumours of the dermis

Benign

Developmental abnormalities of blood vessels

These are either present at birth or appear soon after. They can be classified clinically (Table 19.5) but there is no good clinicohistological correlation. A capillary malformation is composed of a network of capillaries in the upper and mid dermis. A capillary-cavernous haemangioma has multiple ectatic channels of varying calibre distributed throughout the dermis and even the subcutaneous fat.

Table 19.5 Common vascular naevi

Malformations Present at birth. Do not involute ('salmon' patch is exception)	1 Capillary ('salmon' patch and 'port-wine' stain) 2 Arterial 3 Venous 4 Combined
Haemangiomas (sometimes called angiomatous naevi) Usually appear after birth. More common in females, 50–60% on head and neck. Involute by 5–9 years after initial proliferation	1 Superficial (capillary) 2 Deep (cavernous) 3 Mixed

Malformations

'Salmon' patches

These are the commonest malformation, present in about 50% of all babies. They are dull red, often telangiectatic macules, most commonly on the nape of the neck ('erythema nuchae'), the forehead and the upper eyelids. Nuchal lesions may remain unchanged, but patches in other areas usually disappear within a year.

'Port-wine' stains

These are also present at birth. They are pale, pink to purple macules, and vary from the barely noticeable to the grossly disfiguring. Most occur on the face or trunk. They persist, and in middle age may darken and become studded with angiomatous nodules (Fig. 19.44). Occasionally a port-wine stain of the trigeminal area (Fig. 19.45) is associated with a vascular malformation of the leptomeninges on the same side, which may cause epilepsy or hemiparesis (the Sturge−Weber syndrome), or with glaucoma.

Recently, very encouraging results have been obtained with careful (and time-consuming) pulsed tunable dye laser therapy (p. 285). Treatment sessions can begin in babies and anaesthesia is not always necessary. If a trial patch is satisfactory 40−50 pulses

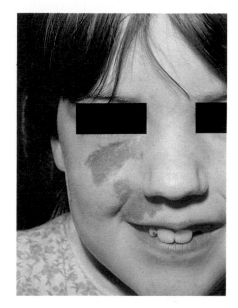

Fig. 19.45 Port-wine stain of the right cheek. No neurological problems in this patient.

can be delivered in a session and the procedure repeated at three monthly intervals. On the other hand, some adults become very adept at using cosmetic camouflage (see Fig. 1.5).

Combined vascular malformations of the limbs

A large port-wine stain of a limb may be associated with overgrowth of all soft tissues of that limb with or without bony hypertrophy. There may be underlying venous malformations (Klippel−Trenaunay syndrome), arterio-venous fistulae (Parkes−Weber) or mixed venous-lymphatic malformations.

Haemangiomas

Capillary-cavernous haemangioma
(strawberry naevus)

Strawberry naevi appear within a few weeks of birth, and grow for a few months, forming a raised, compressible swelling with a bright red surface (Fig. 19.46). Spontaneous regression then follows; the surface whitens centrally (Fig. 19.47) and regression is complete by the age of five in 50% of children and

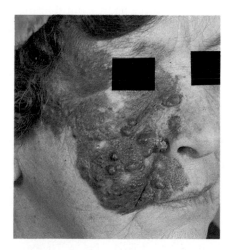

Fig. 19.44 Lifelong capillary malformation of the cheek showing no tendency to resolve. Note port-wine appearance of the upper pole contrasting with the nodular elements elsewhere.

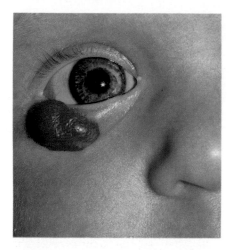

Fig. 19.46 Classic strawberry naevus, occurred and enlarged rapidly shortly after birth.

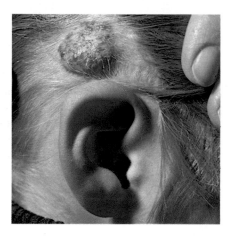

Fig. 19.47 Strawberry naevus above the ear showing the whitening of the surface which is a sign of spontaneous remission.

in 90% by the age of nine, leaving only an area of slight atrophy. Bleeding may follow trauma, and ulceration is common in the napkin (diaper) area.

Strawberry naevi are best treated in infancy by utilizing the pulsed tunable dye laser before they grow large. Small lesions, especially in less obvious sites, can be left untreated. Serial photographs of the way they clear up in other children help parents to accept this. Firm pressure may be needed to stop bleeding. If lesions interfere with feeding, or with vision, or if giant lesions sequestrate platelets (the Kasabach–Merritt syndrome), high doses of sys-

temic steroids should be considered; they are most successful in the proliferative phase. Prednisolone (2–4 mg/kg/day) is given as a single dose in the morning and the dose tapered to zero after one month. Ophthalmological help should be sought for all growing periocular haemangiomas; intralesional steroids have proved effective. Rarely, plastic surgery is necessary.

Campbell de Morgan spots (cherry angiomas)

These benign angiomas are common on the trunks of the middle-aged and elderly. They are small, bright red papules and of no consequence (Fig. 19.48).

Lymphangiomas

The commonest type is lymphangioma circumscriptum which appears as a cluster of vesicles resembling frog spawn. If treatment is needed, excision has to be wide and deep as dilated lymphatic channels and cisterns extend to the subcutaneous tissue.

Glomus tumour

These are derived from the cells surrounding small arteriovenous shunts. Solitary lesions are painful and most common on the extremities and under the nails. Multiple lesions are seldom painful and may affect other parts of the body. Painful lesions can be removed; others may be left.

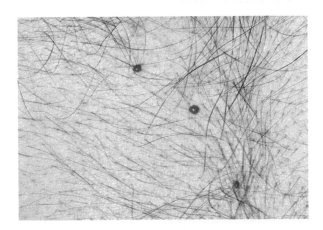

Fig. 19.48 Campbell de Morgan spots (cherry angiomas) of the chest.

Pyogenic granuloma

This badly named lesion is in fact a common benign acquired haemangioma, often seen in children and young adults. It develops at sites of trauma, over the course of a few weeks, as a bright red, raised, sometimes pedunculated and raspberry-like lesion which bleeds easily (Fig. 19.49).

The important differential is from an amelanotic malignant melanoma and, for this reason, the histology should always be checked. It shows leashes of vessels of varying calibre invested by a thin, often ulcerated, epidermis.

Lesions should be removed by curettage under local anaesthetic with cautery to the base. Rarely this is followed by recurrence or an eruption of satellite lesions around the original site.

Other benign dermal tumours

Dermatofibroma (histiocytoma)

These benign tumours are firm, discrete, usually solitary, dermal nodules, often on the extremities of young adults. The lesions have an 'iceberg' effect in that they feel larger than they look. The overlying epidermis is often lightly pigmented and dimples when the nodule is squeezed. Some lesions seem to follow minor trauma or an insect bite. Histologically, the proliferating fibroblasts merge into the sparsely cellular dermis at the margins. A straightforward lesion may be left but, if there is any diagnostic doubt, it should be excised.

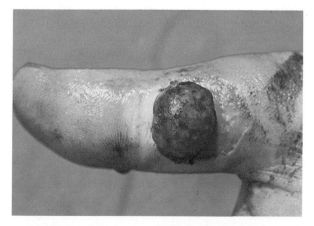

Fig. 19.49 Pyogenic granuloma of the thumb: soggy after elastoplast dressing and bleeding easily.

Keloid

This is an overgrowth of dense fibrous tissue in the skin, arising in response to trauma, however trivial. The tendency to develop keloids is genetically inherited. Keloids are common in Negroids and may be familial. Keloid formation is encouraged by infection, foreign material and by wounds (including surgical ones) especially those not made along the lines of least tension or the skin creases. Even in Caucasoids keloids are seen often enough on the presternal area, the neck, upper back and deltoid region of young adults to make doctors think twice before removing benign lesions there. Intralesional steroid injections are the treatment of choice and are especially helpful if given in early, preferably developing, lesions.

Lipoma

Lipomas are common benign tumours of mature fat cells in the subcutaneous tissue. There may be one or many and lipomas are, rarely, a familial trait. They are most common on the proximal parts of the limbs but may occur at any site. They have an irregular lobular shape and a characteristic soft rubbery consistency. They are rarely painful. They need to be removed only if there is doubt about the diagnosis or if they are painful or ugly.

Malignant

Kaposi's sarcoma

This malignant tumour of proliferating capillaries and lymphatics may be multifocal. There are two types; the classical, and that associated with immunosuppression.

Classical Kaposi's sarcoma is seen most often in Africans and in elderly Jews of European origin. The tumours are usually on the feet and ankles but may be seen on the hands and on parts of the skin which are cold (e.g. ears and nose). Initially they are dark blue to purple macules progressing to tumours (Fig. 19.50) and plaques which ulcerate and fungate. The rate of spread is variable but often slow. Tumours may metastasize to lymph nodes and spread to internal organs; oedema of the legs may be severe.

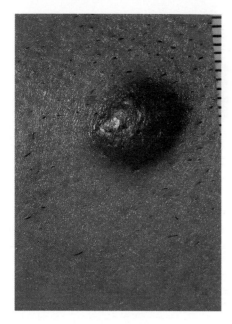

Fig. 19.50 Kaposi's sarcoma (8 mm diameter): classical type of tumour.

The tumours are very sensitive to radiotherapy which is the treatment of choice during the early stages; chemotherapy, with chlorambucil or vinblastine, helps when there is systemic involvement. The life expectancy is five to nine years.

Kaposi's sarcoma and immunosuppression. Smaller and more subtle (e.g. bruise-like) lesions may occur in an immunodeficient host. The tumour has recently become well known because of its association with AIDS (p. 181) due to the human immunodeficiency virus (HIV-1). Lesions of AIDS-related Kaposi's sarcoma may appear anywhere but are most common on the upper trunk and head and neck. The initial bruise-like lesions tend to follow tension lines; they become raised with increasing pigmentation and evolve into nodules and plaques. Lesions frequently arise on mucous membrane in the mouth. Interestingly, HIV-positive intravenous drug abusers do not develop Kaposi's sarcoma as often as do HIV-positive homosexuals. The prognosis of AIDS patients with Kaposi's sarcoma is poor as most will develop opportunistic infections; the life expectancy in this situation is around one year. Single lesions respond to radiotherapy, cryotherapy, or intralesional

vinblastine; systemic treatment with α-interferon has helped some with multiple lesions.

> ## LEARNING POINT
> *Early Kaposi's sarcomas often look trivial but odd in those with immunosuppression. Keep HIV in mind.*

Lymphomas and leukaemias

Skin involvement falls into two broad categories:
1 Disorders which arise in the skin or preferentially involve it. These include:
   • T cell lymphomas (mycosis fungoides).
   • Sézary syndrome.
   • Lymphoma associated with HIV infection.
2 Those arising extracutaneously, which sometimes involve the skin. These include:
   • Hodgkin's disease.
   • B cell lymphomas.
   • Leukaemia.

Cutaneous T cell lymphoma (mycosis fungoides)

This lymphoma of skin-associated helper T lymphocytes usually evolves slowly. There are three clinical phases: the patch, plaque and tumour stages with involvement of lymph nodes and other tissues occurring late in the disease.

The *premycotic plaque phase* may last for years. Most commonly it consists of scattered, barely palpable, erythematous, slightly pigmented, sharply marginated scaly plaques rather like psoriasis or seborrhoeic dermatitis (Fig. 19.51). They often have a bizarre outline (e.g. arciform, or horseshoe shape) and, on close inspection, atrophy with surface wrinkling is usually evident. Less commonly, the premycotic phase is a widespread poikiloderma, with atrophy, pigmentation and telangiectasia (Fig. 19.52). As the lymphoma develops, some plaques become indurated and palpable — *the infiltrated plaque stage.* Some then turn into frank tumours which may ulcerate (Fig. 19.53).

The first two phases of the disease may take as long as 20 years, but the *tumour stage* is often short, with spread and death usually within three years.

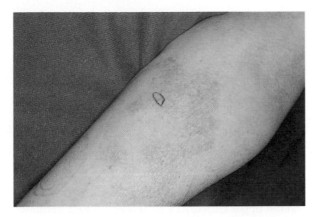

Fig. 19.51 Premycotic stage of mycosis fungoides with scattered, barely palpable, erythematous, atrophic scaly plaques.

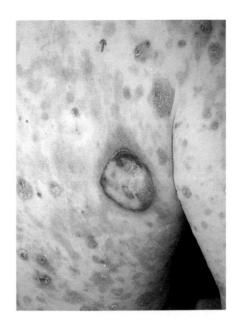

Fig. 19.53 An ulcerated tumour of mycosis fungoides against a background of plaques.

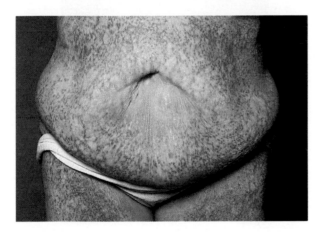

Fig. 19.52 Poikiloderma vasculare atrophicans may be a precursor of mycosis fungoides.

The *Sézary syndrome* is related to mycosis fungoides and is also due to a proliferation of helper T lymphocytes. Generalized erythema and oedema of the skin is associated with pruritus and lymphadenopathy. Abnormal T lymphocytes, with large convoluted nuclei, are found circulating in the blood ('Sézary cells').

Histology

The histological hallmarks of established mycosis fungoides are:
• Intra-epidermal lymphocytic micro-abscesses (Pautrier micro-abscesses).

• A band of lymphoid cells in the upper dermis which infiltrates the epidermis.
• Atypical lymphocytes.

The histology of the premycotic phase poses more problems and may differ little from dermatitis. Many biopsies, over several years, may be needed to prove that a suspicious rash has transformed into mycosis fungoides.

Differential diagnosis

The premycotic patch phase may be mistaken for psoriasis or parapsoriasis (Chapter 6), seborrhoeic dermatitis (p. 98) or tinea corporis (p. 186). However, it responds poorly to treatment for these disorders; the bizarre patterns often raise suspicion. In the early stages skin scrapings may be needed to exclude tinea.

Treatment

Moderately potent or potent local steroids, and UVB treatment, may offer prolonged palliation in the premycotic phase. In the patch phase, PUVA is probably the best treatment choice. As lesions become infiltrated, PUVA or electron beam therapy may be used. Topical nitrogen mustard paint has also been used with success in both patch and plaque stages. Individual tumours respond well to low dose radiotherapy. Systemic chemotherapy for advanced disease is disappointing.

Lymphomas arising extracutaneously

Hodgkin's disease

This is of interest to dermatologists because it may present with severe generalized pruritus (p. 250). Patients with unexplained pruritus must be examined for lymphadenopathy and hepato-splenomegaly. Only rarely does Hodgkin's disease affect the skin directly, as small nodules and ulcers.

Leukaemia

Rarely the first sign of leukaemia is a leukaemic infiltrate in the skin. Clinically, this shows as plum-coloured plaques or nodules or, less often, a thickening and rugosity of the scalp (cutis verticis gyratum) (Fig. 19.54). More often, the rashes associated with leukaemias are non-specific red papules ('leukaemid'). Other non-specific manifestations include pruritus, herpes zoster, acquired ichthyosis and purpura.

B cell lymphomas

B lymphocytic lymphomas presenting with skin lesions are rare. They appear as scattered plum-coloured nodules (Fig. 19.55). Histologically, a B cell lymphoma infiltrates the lower dermis in a nodular or diffuse manner. Immunophenotyping shows a monoclonal expansion of B lymphocytes. Treatment is with radiotherapy and systemic chemotherapy.

Other malignant tumours

Dermatofibrosarcoma protuberans

Dermatofibrosarcoma protuberans is a slowly growing malignant tumour of fibroblasts, arising usually on the upper trunk. At first it seems like a dermatofibroma or keloid but, as it slowly expands, it turns

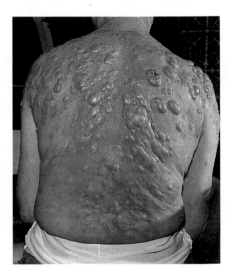

Fig. 19.55 B cell lymphoma of the skin.

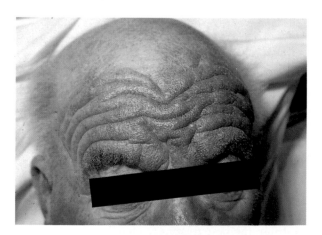

Fig. 19.54 Leukaemic infiltration of the skin.

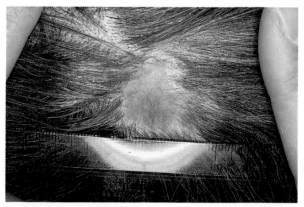

Fig. 19.56 An indurated patch of alopecia due to a solitary metastasis from a breast carcinoma.

into a plaque of red or bluish nodules with an irregular, protuberant surface. It seldom metastasizes. It should be removed with extra wide margins, and even then will sometimes recur.

Cutaneous metastases

About 3% of patients with internal cancers have cutaneous metastases. Usually they arise late and indicate a grave prognosis. Occasionally a solitary cutaneous metastasis is the first sign of the occurrence of a tumour.

The most common cutaneous metastases come from breast cancer. The skin of the breast is also most often involved by the direct extension of a tumour. This may show up as a sharply demarcated and firm area of erythema (carcinoma erysipeloides), firm telangiectatic plaques and papules (carcinoma telangiectoides) or as skin like orange peel (*peau d'orange*) due to blocked and dilated lymphatics. Carcinoma of the breast may also send metastases to the scalp causing patches of alopecia (Fig. 19.56), or to other areas as firm and discrete dermal nodules.

Other common primaries metastasizing to the skin are tumours of the lung, GI tract, uterus, prostate and kidney. The most frequent sites are the umbilicus and the scalp.

CHAPTER 20

The skin in systemic disease

This subject touches on most of general medicine: only selected aspects are covered here.

The skin and internal malignancy

Obvious and easily explicable skin signs may occur when a tumour invades the skin, or sends metastases to it; but there are other, more subtle ways in which tumours can affect the skin. Sometimes tumours act physiologically, causing, for example, acne with some adrenal tumours, flushing in the carcinoid syndrome, or jaundice with a bile duct carcinoma. These cast-iron associations need no further discussion here.

However, the presence of some rare but important conditions should alert the clinician to the possibility of an underlying neoplasm:

1 *Acanthosis nigricans* is a velvety thickening and pigmentation of the major flexures (Figs 20.1–20.3). Setting aside those cases due to obesity, or to diabetes, and characterized by insulin resistance, the chances are high of a tumour being present, usually within the abdominal cavity.

2 *Erythema gyratum repens* is a shifting pattern of waves of erythema covering the skin surface and looking like the grain on wood.

3 *Acquired hypertrichosis lanuginosa* ('malignant down') is an excessive and widespread growth of fine lanugo hair.

4 *Necrolytic migratory erythema* is a figurate erythema with a moving crusted edge. When present, usually with anaemia, stomatitis, weight loss and diabetes, it signals the presence of a glucagon-secreting tumour of the pancreas.

5 *Basex's syndrome* is a papulosquamous eruption of the toes, fingers, ears, and nose, seen with some tumours of the upper respiratory tract.

6 *Dermatomyositis*, other than in childhood (p. 129).

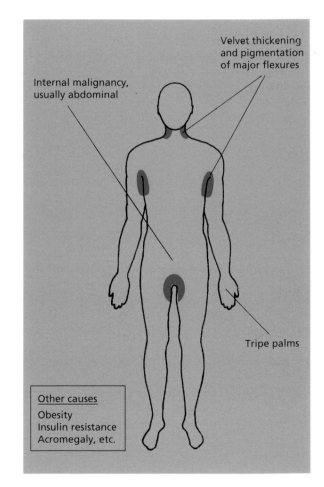

Fig. 20.1 Acanthosis nigricans.

Velvet thickening and pigmentation of major flexures

Internal malignancy, usually abdominal

Tripe palms

Other causes
Obesity
Insulin resistance
Acromegaly, etc.

7 *Generalized pruritus*. One of the long list of causes is an internal malignancy, usually a lymphoma (p. 242).

8 *Superficial thrombophlebitis*. The migratory type has traditionally been associated with carcinomas of the pancreas.

9 *Acquired ichthyosis*. This may result from a

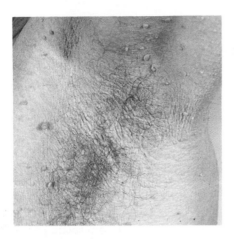

Fig. 20.2 Acanthosis nigricans: velvety thickening of armpit skin associated with skin tags.

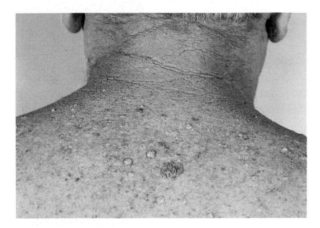

Fig. 20.3 Acanthosis nigricans – pigmentation and thickening of back of the neck. Seborrhoeic wart-like lesions on back.

number of underlying diseases (see p. 46) but it is always important to exclude malignancy, especially lymphomas, as the cause.

The skin and diabetes mellitus

The following are more common in those with diabetes than in others:

1 *Necrobiosis lipoidica*. Less than 1% of diabetics have necrobiosis, but most patients with necrobiosis will have diabetes: the other few should have a glucose tolerance test followed by regular urine tests as some will become diabetic later. The lesions

appear as one or more plaques on the fronts of the shins (Fig. 20.4); they are shiny, atrophic and brown-red or slightly yellow. The underlying blood vessels are easily seen through the atrophic skin (Fig. 20.5) and the margin may be erythematous or violet. Minor knocks may lead to slow-healing ulcers; biopsy may do the same. No treatment is reliably helpful.

2 *Granuloma annulare*. The association with diabetes applies only to a few adults with extensive lesions. Children with standard lesions on the hands need a single urine check for sugar but no more

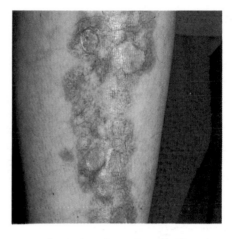

Fig. 20.4 Necrobiosis lipoidica: shiny, yellowish patch with redder edge. Scars have followed indolent ulcers secondary to minor trauma.

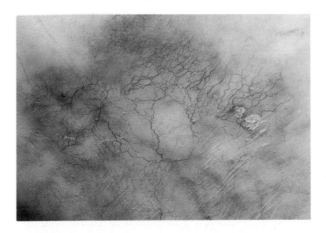

Fig. 20.5 Necrobiosis lipoidica: close-up to show atrophy with telangiectasia.

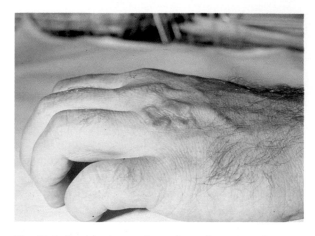

Fig. 20.6 Granuloma annulare: classic lesions on the knuckles.

elaborate tests. The cause is not known. Lesions often lie over the knuckles (Fig. 20.6) and are composed of dermal nodules fused into a rough ring shape. On the hands the lesions are skin-coloured or slightly pink; elsewhere a purple colour may be seen. Although a biopsy is seldom necessary, the histology shows a diagnostic palisading granuloma like that of necrobiosis lipoidica. Lesions tend to go away over the course of a year or two. Stubborn lesions respond to intralesional triamcinolone injections.

3 *Diabetic dermopathy*. In about 50% of diabetics multiple small (0.5−1 cm in diameter), slightly sunken, brownish scars can be found on the limbs, most obviously over the shins.

4 *Candidal infections* (p. 188).

5 *Staphylococcal infections* (p. 161).

6 *Vitiligo* (p. 213).

7 *Eruptive xanthomas* (p. 254).

8 *Tight waxy skin* on the fingers and hands.

9 *Atherosclerosis* with ischaemia or gangrene of feet.

10 *Neuropathic foot ulcers*.

The skin in sarcoidosis

About one-third of patients with systemic sarcoidosis have skin lesions; in addition it is possible to have cutaneous sarcoidosis without systemic abnormalities. The most important skin changes are as follows:

1 *Erythema nodosum* (Fig. 20.7). This occurs in the early stages of sarcoidosis, especially in young women.

2 *Scar sarcoidosis*. Granulomatous lesions arising in long-standing scars should raise suspicions of sarcoidosis.

3 *Lupus pernio*. Dusky infiltrated plaques appear on the nose and fingers, often in association with sarcoidosis of the upper respiratory tract.

4 *Papular, nodular and plaque forms*. These brownish-red, violaceous, or hypopigmented lesions are indolent though often symptom-free. Sometimes they are annular. They vary in number, size and distribution. Chronic lesions respond poorly to any line of treatment short of systemic steroids which are usually best avoided.

The skin in liver disease

Some of the abnormalities are:

1 *Pruritus*. This is related to obstructive jaundice and may precede it (p. 250).

2 *Pigmentation*. With bile pigments and sometimes melanin (Chapter 18).

3 *Spider naevi*. These are often multiple in chronic liver disease (p. 137).

4 *Palmar erythema* (p. 137).

5 *White nails*. These associate with hypo-albuminaemia.

6 *Porphyria cutanea tarda* (p. 251).

7 *Xanthomas*. In primary biliary cirrhosis (p. 254).

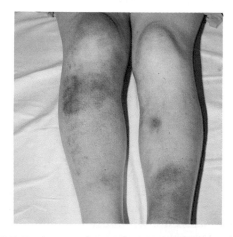

Fig. 20.7 Erythema nodosum: large, painful, dusky plaques on the shins.

8 *Hair loss and generalized asteatotic eczema* may occur in alcoholics with cirrhosis who become zinc deficient.

The skin in renal disease

The main changes are:

1 *Pruritus* and a generally dry skin.

2 *Pigmentation.* A yellowish sallow colour and pallor from anaemia.

3 *Half-and-half nail.* The proximal half is white and the distal half is pink or brownish.

4 *The skin changes of the conditions leading to renal disease.* For example, leucocytoclastic vasculitis (p. 113), connective tissue disorders (Chapter 12), Fabry's disease (p. 255).

Pyoderma gangrenosum

An inflamed nodule or pustule breaks down centrally to form an expanding ulcer with a polycyclic or serpiginous outline, and a characteristic undermined bluish edge (Fig. 20.8). The condition is not bacterial in origin but its pathogenesis, presumably immunological, is not fully understood. It may arise in the absence of any underlying disease, but tends to associate with the following conditions:

1 Ulcerative colitis.

2 Crohn's disease (Fig. 20.9).

3 Conditions causing polyarthritis, including rheumatoid arthritis.

4 Monoclonal gammopathies.

5 Leukaemia (with a bullous form of pyoderma).

Lesions may be single or multiple. If gut disease is present then control of this will help the pyoderma. Otherwise the condition responds to systemic steroids but not to antibiotics, and lesions heal leaving papery scars.

Graft-versus-host (GVH) disease

Marrow grafting is now used for several disorders including aplastic anaemia and leukaemia. Immunologically competent donor lymphocytes, however, may cause problems by reacting against host tissues, especially the skin, liver and gut.

Acute GVH disease appears within four weeks. Fever accompanies malaise and a worsening mor-

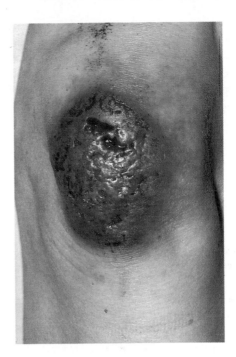

Fig. 20.8 Pyoderma gangrenosum: a plum-coloured lesion with a typical cribriform appearance.

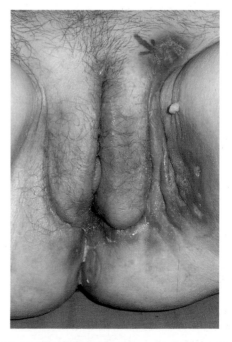

Fig. 20.9 Crohn's disease: grossly oedematous vulva with inter-connecting sinuses. Biopsy at the site arrowed showed a granulomatous histology.

billiform rash which may progress to a generalized desquamation or even toxic epidermal necrolysis. Chronic GVH disease occurs later: its skin changes are variable but may be like those of lichen planus or a pigmented scleroderma. The skin changes may be severe enough to need treatment with systemic prednisolone and azathioprine or cyclosporin A.

Malabsorption and malnutrition

Some of the commonest skin changes are listed in Table 20.1.

Table 20.1 Skin changes in malabsorption and malnutrition

Condition	Skin changes
Malnutrition	Itching Dryness Symmetrical pigmentation Brittle nails and hair
Protein malnutrition (kwashiorkor)	Dry, red-brown hair Pigmented 'cracked skin'
Iron deficiency	Itching Diffuse hair loss Koilonychia Smooth tongue
Vitamin A deficiency	Dry skin Follicular hyperkeratoses Xerophthalmia
Vitamin B_1 (aneurin) deficiency	Beri-beri oedema
Vitamin B_2 (riboflavine) deficiency	Angular stomatitis Smooth purple tongue Seborrhoeic dermatitis-like eruption
Vitamin B_6 (pyridoxine) deficiency	Ill-defined dermatitis
Vitamin B_7 (niacin) deficiency	Pellagra with dermatitis, dementia and diarrhoea Dermatitis on exposed areas, pigmented
Vitamin C deficiency (scurvy)	Skin haemorrhages especially around follicular keratoses containing coiled hairs Bleeding gums Oedematous 'woody' swellings of limbs in elderly

Generalized pruritus

Pruritus is a symptom with many causes, but not a disease in its own right. Itchy patients fall into two groups: those whose pruritus is due simply to surface causes (e.g. eczema, lichen planus, and scabies), which seldom need much investigation; and the others, who may or may not have an internal cause for their itching, such as:

1 *Liver disease.* Itching signals biliary obstruction. It may be an early symptom of primary biliary cirrhosis. Cholestyramine often helps cholestatic pruritus, possibly by promoting the elimination of bile salts.

2 *Chronic renal failure.* Urea itself seems not to be responsible for this symptom which plagues about one-third of patients undergoing renal dialysis.

3 *Iron deficiency.* Treatment with iron may help the itching.

4 *Polycythaemia.* The itching here is usually triggered by a hot bath; it has a curious pricking quality and lasts about an hour.

5 *Thyroid disease.* Itching and urticaria may occur in hyperthyroidism: the dry skin of hypothyroidism may also be itchy.

6 *Diabetes.* Generalized itching may be a rare presentation of diabetes.

7 *Internal malignancy.* The prevalence of itching in Hodgkin's disease may be as high as 30%. It may be unbearable, yet the skin often looks normal. Pruritus may occur long before other manifestations of the disease. Itching is uncommon in carcinomatosis.

8 *Neurological disease.* Paroxysmal pruritus has been recorded in multiple sclerosis and in neurofibromatosis. Brain tumours infiltrating the floor of the fourth ventricle may cause a fierce persistent itching of the nostrils.

9 The skin of the elderly may itch because it is too dry.

The search for a cause has to be tailored to the individual patient, and must start with a thorough history and physical examination. Unless a treatable cause is found, therapy is symptomatic and consists of sedative antihistamines, and the avoidance of rough clothing, overheating and vasodilatation, including that brought on by alcohol. UVB may help the itching associated with chronic renal, and perhaps liver disease. Local applications include calamine and mixtures containing small amounts of menthol or phenol (Formulary, p. 289). Sometimes lubricating the skin with emollients may help.

LEARNING POINTS

1 Learn how to spell pruritus (not pruritis) but do not accept it as a diagnosis in its own right.
2 Ponder underlying causes in those with no primary skin disease.

The porphyrias

An important multistage metabolic pathway leads from glycine and succinyl CoA, through a sequence of porphyrins, to the formation of haem and thence of haemoglobin, myoglobin, cytochromes and various haem-containing enzymes. Each step of the pathway is regulated by enzymes, and deficiencies of these lead to the accumulation of intermediate metabolites, some of which may cause photo-sensitivity to UVR of wavelength 400 nm (capable of penetrating through window glass).

Porphyrias are rare and most types are inherited. They can be separated on clinical grounds, aided by the biochemical investigation of urine, faeces and blood. Only the following five varieties will be mentioned here.

Congenital erythropoietic porphyria

This is very rare and due to mutations in the uropor-phyrinogen synthase gene. Severe photosensitivity is noted soon after birth, and leads to blistering, scarring and mutilation of the exposed parts which become increasingly hairy. The urine is pink, and the teeth are brown, though fluorescing red under Wood's light. A haemolytic anaemia is present. Treatment is unsatisfactory but gene therapy may be possible in the future. The hairy appearance, discoloured teeth, and the tendency to avoid daylight may have given rise to legends about werewolves (Fig. 20.10).

Erythrohepatic protoporphyria
(erythropoietic protoporphyria)

In this commoner, autosomal dominant condition due to mutations in the ferrochelatase gene, a less severe photosensitivity develops during childhood. A burning sensation occurs within minutes of exposure to sunlight. Soon the skin becomes swollen and crusted vesicles sometimes appear, leading to pitted scars. Liver disease and gallstones occur. In addition to sun avoidance and the use of sun-screens (Formulary, p. 289) beta-carotene may be given orally.

Cutaneous hepatic porphyria
(porphyria cutanea tarda)

Perhaps occurring against a background of genetic susceptibility in which mutations in the uropor-phyrinogen decarboxylase gene have been demon-strated, this condition is usually seen in men who have damaged their livers by drinking too much alcohol. Recently it has been shown that some cases are due to previous hepatitis C virus infection. Blisters and milia form on the exposed parts of the face, and on the backs of the hands (Fig. 20.11), in response to sunlight or to minor trauma. These areas become scarred and hairy (Fig. 20.12). The urine is pink and fluoresces a bright coral-pink under Wood's light (p. 39) due to excessive uroporphyrins (Fig. 20.13). Treatment is based on avoiding alcohol and oestrogens, but other measures are usually needed too, including regular venesection or very low-dose hydroxychloroquine therapy (e.g. 100 mg twice weekly) under specialist supervision. Higher doses cause toxic hepatitis in these patients.

Acute intermittent porphyria

This condition, inherited as an autosomal dominant trait due to mutations of the porphobilinogen deaminase gene, is most common in Scandinavia. Skin lesions do not occur. Attacks of abdominal pain, accompanied by neuropsychiatric symptoms and the passage of dark urine, are sometimes trig-gered by drugs (especially barbiturates, griseofulvin, oestrogens and sulphonamides).

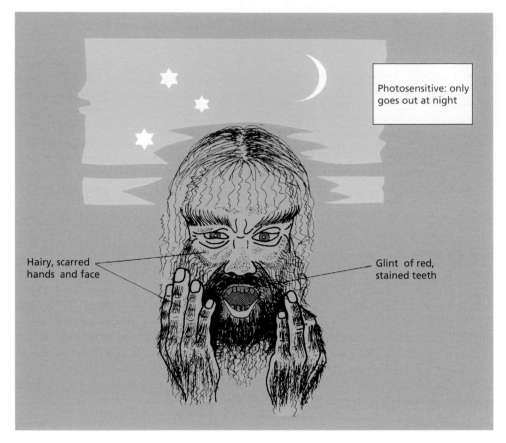

Photosensitive: only
goes out at night

Hairy, scarred
hands and face

Glint of red,
stained teeth

Fig. 20.10 Congenital erythropoietic porphyria — perhaps the origin of the term 'werewolf'.

Variegate porphyria

This disorder, inherited as an autosomal dominant trait, due to mutations of the protoporphyrinogen oxidase gene, is particularly common in South Africa. It shares the skin features of porphyria cutanea tarda and the systemic symptoms and drug provocation of acute intermittent porphyria.

Amyloid

Amyloid is a protein which can be derived from several sources, including immunoglobulin light chains and keratins. It is deposited in the tissues under a variety of circumstances and is then usually in combination with a P component derived from the plasma. Systemic amyloidosis of the type which is secondary to chronic inflammatory disease, such as rheumatoid arthritis or tuberculosis, tends not to affect the skin. In contrast, skin changes are prominent in primary systemic amyloidosis and also in the amyloid associated with multiple myeloma. Skin blood vessels infiltrated with amyloid rupture easily, causing 'pinch purpura' to occur after minor trauma. The waxy deposits of amyloid, often most obvious around the eyes, may also be purpuric. Distinct from the systemic amyloidoses are localized deposits of amyloid. These are uncommon and usually take the form of macular areas of rippled pigmentation or of plaques made up of coalescing papules. Both types are itchy.

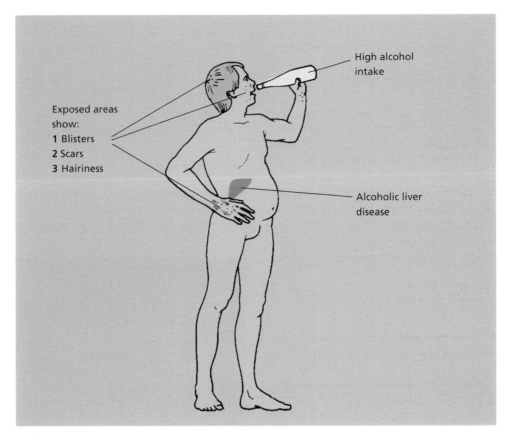

Fig. 20.11 Cutaneous hepatic porphyria (porphyria cutanea tarda).

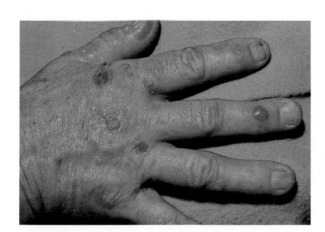

Fig. 20.12 Blisters on the backs of the hands and fingers in a patient with cutaneous hepatic porphyria.

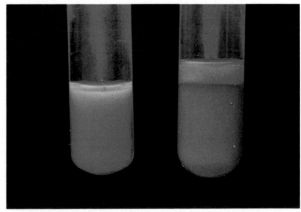

Fig. 20.13 Cutaneous hepatic porphyria. Coral-red fluorescence of urine under Wood's light denoting excessive uroporphyrins.

Mucinoses

The dermis may become infiltrated with mucin in certain disorders:

1 *Myxoedema.* In the puffy hands and face of hypothyroidism.

2 *Pretibial myxoedema.* Pink or flesh coloured mucinous plaques on the lower shins are seen, together with marked exophthalmos, in some patients with hyperthyroidism. They may also occur after the thyroid abnormality has been treated.

3 *Scleromyxoedema.* A diffuse thickening and papulation of the skin may occur in connection with an IgG monoclonal paraproteinaemia.

4 *Follicular mucinosis.* Infiltrated plaques showing loss of hair; some cases are associated with a lymphoma.

Xanthomas

Deposits of fatty material in the skin and subcutaneous tissues (xanthomas) may provide the first clue to important disorders of lipid metabolism.

Primary hyperlipidaemias are usually genetic. They fall into six groups, classified on the basis of an analysis of fasting blood lipids and electrophoresis of plasma lipoproteins. All, save type I, carry an increased risk of atherosclerosis — in this lies their importance and the need for treatment.

Secondary hyperlipidaemia may be found in a variety of diseases including diabetes, primary biliary cirrhosis, the nephrotic syndrome and hypothyroidism.

The clinical patterns of xanthoma correlate well with the underlying cause. The main patterns and their most common associations are shown in Table 20.2.

Phenylketonuria

Phenylketonuria is a rare metabolic cause of hypopigmentation. Its prevalence is about $1:25\,000$. It is inherited as an autosomal recessive trait, the

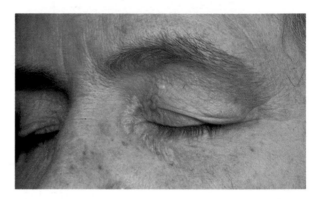

Fig. 20.14 Xanthelasma: flat, yellow lesions on the eyelids; in this patient the blood lipids were normal.

Table 20.2 Xanthomas: clinical appearance and associations

Type	Clinical appearance	Types of hyperlipidaemia and associated metabolic abnormalities
Xanthelasma palpebrarum (Fig. 20.14)	Soft yellowish plaques on the eyelids	None or type II, III or IV
Tuberous xanthomas (Fig. 20.15)	Firm yellow papules and nodules, most often on points of knees and elbows	Types II, III and secondary
Tendinous xanthomas	Subcutaneous swellings on fingers or by Achilles tendon	Types II, III and secondary
Eruptive xanthomas (Fig. 20.16)	Sudden onset, multiple small yellow papules Buttocks and shoulders	Types I, III, IV, V and secondary (usually to diabetes)
Plane xanthomas	Yellow macular areas at any site Yellow palmar creases	Type III and secondary
Generalized plane xanthomas	Yellow macular lesions over wide areas	Myeloma

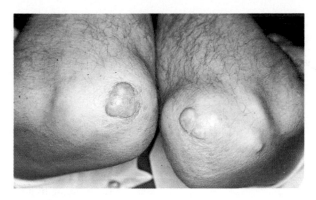

Fig. 20.15 The nodular form of tuberous xanthoma on the points of the elbows.

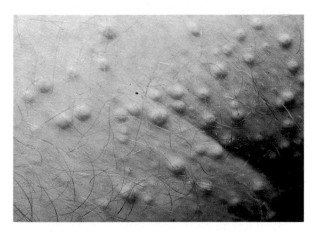

Fig. 20.16 The numerous, small, yellowish papules of eruptive xanthoma. The patient was diabetic.

abnormal gene lying on chromosome region 12q22–q24, and is due to a deficiency of the liver enzyme phenylalanine hydroxylase, which catalyses the hydroxylation of phenylalanine to tyrosine. This leads to the accumulation of phenylalanine, phenylpyruvic acid and their metabolites.

Affected individuals have fair skin and hair. They often develop eczema, usually of atopic type, and may be photosensitive. The accumulation of phenylalanine and its metabolites damages the brain during the phase of rapid development just before and just after birth. Extrapyramidal manifestations such as athetosis and mental retardation may occur.

Oculocutaneous albinism can usually be distinguished by its eye signs. The Guthrie test, which detects raised blood phenylalanine levels, is carried out routinely at birth in most developed countries.

Treatment with a low-phenylalanine diet should be started as soon as possible to prevent further neurological damage.

Alkaptonuria

In this rare, recessively inherited disorder, based on a homogentisic acid oxidase deficiency, dark urine may be seen in childhood, and in adult life pigment may be deposited in various places including the ears and sclera. Arthropathy may occur.

Fabry's disease
(angiokeratoma corporis diffusum)

A deficiency of the enzyme α-galactosidase A is found in this sex-linked disorder (chromosome region Xq21.3–22): abnormal amounts of glycolipid are deposited in many tissues as a result. The skin lesions are grouped, almost black, small telangiectatic papules especially around the umbilicus and pelvis. Progressive renal failure occurs in adult life. Most patients have attacks of excruciating unexplained pain in their hands. Some female carriers have skin changes, though these are usually less obvious than those of affected males. Similar skin lesions may be seen in lysomal storage disorders such as fucosidosis.

CHAPTER 21

The skin and the psyche

Lay people accept, perhaps too easily, that there are strong links between skin disease and the emotions. Dermatologists vary in their ability to see such associations, and only in a few skin disorders, such as dermatitis artefacta, are emotional factors obviously their direct cause.

The relationships between the mind and the skin are usually more subtle and more complex than this. Skin patients do have a higher prevalence of psychiatric abnormalities than the general population, but specific personality profiles and disorders are seldom tied to specific skin diseases. Similarly it is still not clear how, or even how often, psychological factors trigger, worsen or perpetuate such everyday problems as atopic eczema or psoriasis.

Each school of psychiatry has its own theories on the subject, but their explanations do not satisfy everyone. Do people really damage their skin to satisfy guilt feelings? Does their skin 'weep' because they have themselves suppressed weeping? Perhaps, until more is known, it may be better to adopt a simple and more pragmatic approach, in which interactions between the skin and psyche are divided into two broad groups: first, the emotional reactions to the presence of skin disease, real or imagined; and, second, the effects of emotions on skin disease (Fig. 21.1).

Reactions to skin disease

The presence of disfiguring skin lesions may distort the emotional development of a child: some become withdrawn, others become aggressive, but many adjust well. The range of individual reactions to skin disease is, therefore, wide. At one end lies indifference to grossly disfiguring lesions and, at the other, lies an obsession with skin which is quite normal. Between these extremes are reactions ranging from

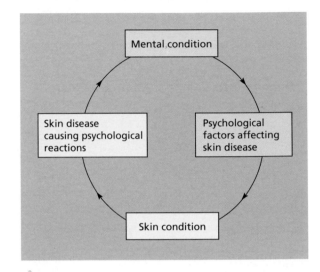

Fig. 21.1 Mind–skin interactions.

natural anxiety over ugly skin lesions to disproportionate worry over minor blemishes. The concept of 'body image' is useful here.

Body image

All of us think we know how we look, but our ideas may not tally with those of others. The nose, face, hair and genitals tend to rank high in a person's 'corporeal awareness', and trivial lesions in those areas may generate much anxiety. For example, the facial lesions of acne, may lead to an excessive loss of self-esteem.

Dysmorphophobia

This is the term applied to distortions of the body image. Minor and inconspicuous lesions are magnified in the mind to grotesque disfiguring images.

Dermatological 'non-disease'

This is a form of dysmorphobia: no skin abnormality can be found by the clinician, but the distress felt by the patient may lead to anxiety, depression, or even suicide. Such patients are not uncommon. They expect dermatological solutions for complaints such as hair loss, or burning, itching and redness of the face or genitals. The dermatologist, who can see nothing wrong, cannot solve matters and no treatment seems to help. Such patients are reluctant to see a psychiatrist though some may suffer from a monosymptomatic hypochondriacal psychosis.

Monosymptomatic hypochondriacal psychosis

Patients may sustain, for long periods, single hypochondriacal delusions in the absence of other recognizable psychiatric disease. Some are eccentric and live in social isolation. In dermatology many of these patients have the delusion that their skin is infested with parasites. Others believe that they have syphilis, AIDS or skin cancer.

Delusions of parasitosis (Fig. 21.2)

This term is better than 'parasitophobia' which implies a fear of becoming infested. Patients with delusions of parasitosis are unshakably convinced that they are already infested. No rational argument can convince them that they are not; their physician then must be wrong. Their symptoms include odd sensations of crawling and biting, and they often bring to the clinic with them, in a box, specimens of the 'parasite' at different stages of its supposed life cycle. These must be examined microscopically but usually turn out to be fragments of skin, hair, clothing, or unclassifiable debris.

Such patients become angry if doubts are cast on their ideas or if they are referred to a psychiatrist. Direct confrontations are best avoided, and much tact is needed to secure any co-operation with treatment.

The delusions of a few of these patients are based on an underlying depression or schizophrenia, and of a further few on organic problems such as vitamin deficiency or cerebrovascular disease. These disorders must be treated on their own merits. Most patients, however, suffer from monosymptomatic hypochondriacal delusions which can often be suppressed by treatment with pimozide, accepting that this will be needed long-term. Otherwise the outlook for resolution is poor. High doses of pimozide carry cardiac risks. An ECG should be done before starting treatment and the drug should not be given to those with a prolonged Q–T interval or with a history of cardiac arrhythmia. In those patients receiving pimozide in excess of 16 mg daily, periodic ECGs should be performed. Tardive dyskinesia may develop and persist despite withdrawal of the drug. Sulpiride is a reasonable alternative.

Their skin changes may include gouge marks and scratches, but it is convenient to consider these patients separately from dermatitis artefacta.

Dermatitis artefacta

Here the skin lesions are caused and kept going by the patient's own actions, but parasites are not held to be to blame. Patients with dermatitis artefacta continue to deny self-trauma but, naturally, if treatment is left to them to carry out, their problems do not improve. Lesions will heal under occlusive dressings, but these do not alter the underlying psychiatric problems, and lesions may recur or crop up outside the bandaged areas. Different types of dermatitis artefacta are listed in Table 21.1.

The lesions (Fig. 21.3) favour accessible areas, and do not fit with known pathological processes. The diagnosis is often difficult to make but an experienced clinician will suspect it because there are no primary lesions and because of the bizarre shape or grouping of the lesions, which may be rectilinear or oddly grouped and are often limited to accessible parts (Fig. 21.4). Areas damaged by burning, corrosive

Table 21.1 Types of dermatitis artefacta

Type	Personality
Minor habits, e.g. excoriated acne	Relatively normal
More obvious lesions	Hysterical or neurotic (secondary gain)
Bizarre	Psychotic
Malingering	Criminal

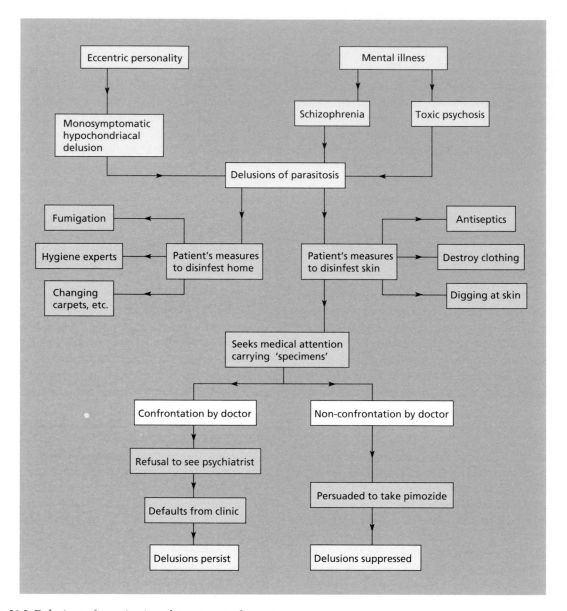

Fig. 21.2 Delusions of parasitosis — the sequence of events.

chemicals, or by digging have their own special appearance.

Apart from frank malingerers, the patients are often young women with some medical knowledge, perhaps a nurse. Some form of 'secondary gain' from having skin lesions may be obvious. The psychological problems may be superficial and easily resolved, but sometimes psychiatric help is needed and the artefacts are part of a prolonged psychiatric illness (Fig. 21.5). Direct confrontation and accu-

LEARNING POINTS
1 Try pimozide for those with delusions of parasitosis (caution; see p. 257).
2 Direct confrontations with patients with dermatitis artefacta or delusions of parasitosis may make you feel better but do little for them.

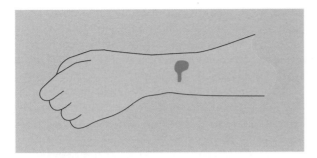

Fig. 21.3 Look for a trickle effect in self-inflicted corrosive injuries.

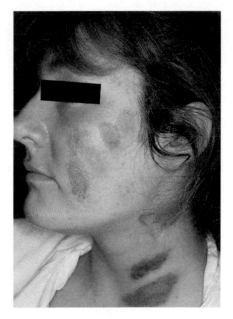

Fig. 21.4 Obvious dermatitis artefacta: back your own judgement against the patient's here.

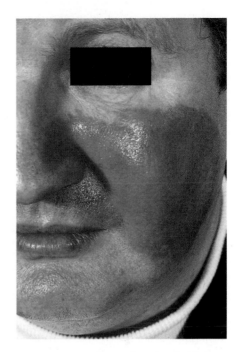

Fig. 21.5 Dermatitis artefacta: denials of self trauma did not convince us that this was due to any other skin disease.

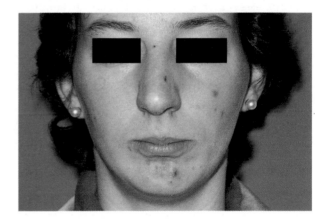

Fig. 21.6 Neurotic excoriations: they do not respond to treatment for acne which she has never had.

sations are usually best avoided, and the condition may last for some years.

Neurotic excoriations

Patients with neurotic excoriations differ from those with other types of dermatitis artefacta in that they admit to picking and digging at their skin. This habit affects women more often than men and is most active at times of stress. The clinical picture is mixed, with crusted excoriations and pale scars, often with a hyperpigmented border, mainly on the face, neck, shoulders and arms (Fig. 21.6). The condition may last for years and psychiatric treatment is seldom successful.

Acne excoriée

Here the self-inflicted damage is based to some extent on the lesions of acne vulgaris which may, in themselves, be mild but become disfiguring when dug and squeezed to excess (Fig. 14.7). The patients are usually young girls who may leave themselves with ugly scars. A psychiatric approach is often unhelpful and a daily ritual of attacking the lesions, helped by a magnifying mirror, may persist for years.

Localized neurodermatitis (lichen simplex)

This term refers to areas of itchy lichenification, perpetuated by bouts of scratching in response to stress. The condition is not uncommon and may occur on any area of skin. In men the lesions are often on the calves; women favour the nape of the neck where the redness and scaling may look like psoriasis. Some examples of persistent itching in the anogenital area are due to lichen simplex there.

Patients with localized neurodermatitis develop conditioned scratch responses to minor itch stimuli more readily than controls. Local therapy does not alter the underlying cause, but topical steroids, sometimes only the most potent ones, may ameliorate the symptoms. Occlusive bandaging of suitable areas may clear the lesions which are covered.

Hair-pulling habit

Trichotillomania is too dramatic a word for what is usually only a minor comfort habit in children, ranking alongside nail-biting and lip-licking. Perhaps it should be dropped now. The matter is usually of little consequence and children who twist and pull their hair, often as they are going to sleep, seldom have major psychiatric disorders. The habit may go away more quickly if it is ignored. However, more severe degrees of hair pulling are sometimes seen in disturbed adolescents and in the mentally deficient. Here the outlook for full regrowth is less good, even with formal psychiatric help.

The diagnosis can usually be made on the history, but some parents do not know what is going on. The areas of hair loss do not show the exclamation mark hairs of alopecia areata, or the scaling and inflammation of scalp ringworm. The patches are irregular in outline and hair loss is never complete. Those hairs that remain tend to be bent or broken, and of variable length.

Dermatoses precipitated or perpetuated by emotional factors

Fancy rather than fact rules here. Popular candidates for inclusion in this group of diseases are psoriasis, urticaria, atopic eczema, pompholyx, discoid eczema, alopecia areata, and lichen planus. Every dermatologist will have seen associations between external stress and exacerbations of most of the conditions listed here, but proof that stress causes the diseases is hard to find. For example, some studies suggest that even hyperhidrosis of the palms and soles, once thought to be an accentuated response to stress, may have no relationship to chronic anxiety at all.

CHAPTER 22

Other genetic disorders

The human genome consists of 23 pairs of chromosomes carrying an estimated 50 000–100 000 genes. The pairs of matching chromosomes as seen at colchicine-arrested metaphase are numbered in accordance with their size. A centromere divides each chromosome into a shorter (p) and a longer (q) arm.

Any individual's chromosomal make-up (karyotype) can be expressed as their total number of chromosomes plus their sex chromosome constitution. A normal male, therefore, is 46XY. A short-hand notation exists for recording other abnormalities such as chromosome translocations and deletions.

The precise location of any gene can be given by naming the chromosome, the arm of the chromosome (p or q), and the numbers of the band and sub-band of the chromosome, as seen with Giemsa staining, on which it lies. One of the genes important for atopy, for instance, lies on chromosome 11q13, i.e. on the long arm of chromosome 11 at band 13.

Several techniques can be used to identify the position of a gene.

1 A clue may be offered by finding that some affected individuals have chromosomal deletions or unbalanced translocations, suggesting that the gene in question lies on the abnormal segments.

2 Linkage analysis. Genes are linked if they lie close together on the same chromosome; they will then be inherited together. The closer together they are, the less is the chance of their being separated by cross overs, one to six of which, depending on length, occur on each chromosome at meiosis.

Each member of an affected family has to be examined both for the presence of the trait to be mapped, and also of a marker, usually a DNA probe, which has already been mapped. If linkage is established then the two loci will be close on the same chromosome.

The probability of the results of such a study representing true linkage can be expressed as a Lod (standing for logarithm of the odds) score. A score of three or more suggests that the linkage is likely to be genuine.

3 Somatic cell hybridization. A hybrid made by fusing a human cell with a mouse cell will at first have two sets of chromosomes. Later human chromosomes are lost randomly until a stable state is reached. Those cells which produce a particular human protein must contain the relevant chromosome. A panel of such hybrid cells can be created which differ in their content of human chromosomes. By comparing these the chromosomal site of the relevant gene can be deduced.

4 *In situ* hybridization. A cloned sequence of DNA, if made single stranded by heat, will anneal to its complementary sequence on a chromosome. Radioactive or fluorescent labelling can be used to indicate its position there.

Non-mendelian genetics

Traditional genetics has also been extended by the introduction of several new non-mendelian concepts of importance in dermatology. These include:

1 *Mosaicism.* A mosaic is a single individual made up of two or more genetically distinct cell lines: the concept is important in several skin disorders including incontinentia pigmenti (p. 265) and segmental neurofibromatosis (p. 263). A mutation of a single cell in a fetus may form a clone of abnormal cells. In the skin these often adopt a bizarre pattern of lines and whorls — Blaschko's lines, named after the dermatologist who recorded them in linear epidermal naevi in 1901.

2 *Contiguous gene deletions.* Complex phenotypes occur when several adjacent genes are lost. In this

way, for example, X-linked ichthyosis may associate with hypogonadism or anosmia.

3 *Genomic imprinting* means that genes may differ in their effect depending on the parent from which they are inherited. Genes from the father seem especially important in psoriasis, and from the mother in atopy (p. 94).

4 *Uniparental disomy* occurs when both pairs of genes are derived from the same parent so that an individual lacks either a maternal or a paternal copy. In this way a disorder usually inherited as a recessive trait can arise even though only one parent is a carrier.

Inheritance is important in many of the conditions discussed in other chapters and this has been highlighted in the sections on aetiology. This chapter includes some genetic disorders not covered elsewhere.

Neurofibromatosis

This relatively common disorder affects about one in 3000 people and is inherited as an autosomal dominant trait. There are two main types: von Recklinghausen's neurofibromatosis (NF1, which accounts for 85% of all cases) and bilateral acoustic neurofibromatosis (NF2); these are phenotypically and genetically distinct.

Cause

The NF1 gene has been localized to chromosome 17q11.1: it is unusually large (300 kb) and several different mutations have now been identified. The inheritance of NF1 is as an autosomal dominant but one-third to one-half of index cases have no preceding family history. New mutations usually arise on the paternally derived chromosome 17. The gene encodes an amino acid important in the inactivation of the ras p21 oncogene, perhaps explaining the susceptibility of NF1 patients to tumours.

The inheritance of NF2 is also autosomal dominant. Mapping to chromosome 22q11.21–13.1 followed the observation of changes in chromosome 22 in meningiomas as these tumours may be seen in NF2.

Clinical features

The physical signs include:

Von Recklinghausen's neurofibromatosis (NF1)
• Six or more *café au lait* patches (light brown oval macules) (Fig. 22.1), developing usually in the first year of life.
• Axillary freckling (Fig. 22.2) in two-thirds of affected individuals.
• Variable numbers of skin neurofibromas, some small and superficial, others larger and deeper, ranging from flesh-coloured to pink, purple or brown (Fig. 22.1). Most are dome-like nodules, but others are irregular raised plaques. Some are firm, some soft and compressible through a deficient dermis ('button-hole' sign); others feel 'knotty' or 'wormy'. Neurofibromas may not appear until puberty and become larger and more numerous with age.
• Small circular pigmented hamartomas of the iris (Lisch nodules), appear in early childhood.

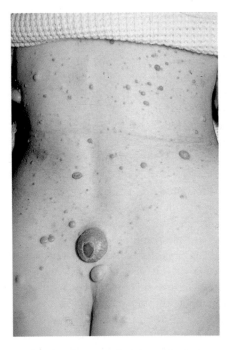

Fig. 22.1 Neurofibromatosis: one large, but benign, neurofibroma has ulcerated over the sacrum. Several *café au lait* patches are visible.

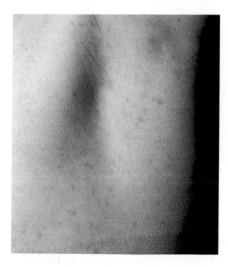

Fig. 22.2 Freckling of the axilla implies that this child has neurofibromatosis though surface nodules have not yet appeared.

Bilateral acoustic neurofibromatosis (NF2).
- Bilateral acoustic neuromas.
- Few, if any, cutaneous manifestations.
- No Lisch nodules.

Diagnosis

The *café au lait* marks, axillary freckling and Lisch nodules should be looked for, as they appear before the skin neurofibromas. Isolated neurofibromas are not uncommon in individuals without neurofibromatosis and are of little consequence unless they are painful.

Complications

Von Recklinghausen's neurofibromatosis. A neurofibroma will occasionally change into a neurofibrosarcoma. Other associated features may include kyphoscoliosis, mental deficiency, epilepsy, renal artery stenosis and an association with phaeochromocytoma. 'Forme-fruste' variants occur, for example segmental neurofibromatosis.

Bilateral acoustic neurofibromatosis. Other tumours of the central nervous system may occur, especially meningiomas and gliomas.

Management

Affected adults may ask about the risk of their children developing the disorder; the chances are one in two. It should soon be possible to devise a prenatal DNA screening test that will show deleted or mutated genes, thereby identifying those at risk. Ugly or painful lesions, and any suspected of undergoing malignant change, should be removed.

Tuberous sclerosis

This uncommon condition, with a prevalence of about 1 in 12 000 in children under ten years old, is also inherited as an autosomal dominant trait, with variable expressivity even within the same family. As fertility is reduced, transmission through more than two generations is rare.

Cause

There is genetic heterogeneity and abnormal genes have already been found on chromosomes 9 and 11. Since several pedigrees have normal genes at these sites, a third and possibly other loci may exist.

Clinical features

The skin changes include:
- *Small oval white patches* ('ash leaf macules') occur in 80% of those affected. These are important as they may be the only manifestation at birth.
- *Adenoma sebaceum* occur in 85% of those affected. They develop at puberty as pink or yellowish acne-like papules on the face, often around the nose (Fig. 22.3).
- *Peri-ungual* fibromas occur in 50% of patients. These develop in adult life as small pink sausage-like lesions emerging from the nail folds (Fig. 22.4).
- *Connective tissue naevi* ('Shagreen patches') are seen in 40% of patients. Cobblestone, somewhat yellow plaques often arise in the skin over the base of the spine.
Other features may include:
- Epilepsy (in 75% of patients).
- Mental retardation (in 50% of patients).
- Ocular signs, including retinal phakomas and pigmentary abnormalities (in 50% of patients).
- Hyperplastic gums.

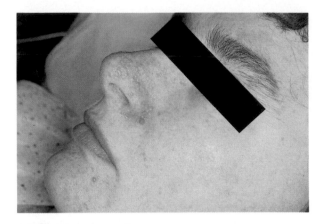

Fig. 22.3 Tuberous sclerosis. Adenoma sebaceum.

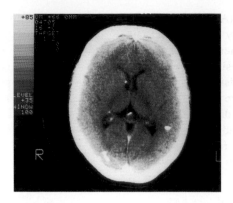

Fig. 22.5 A CT scan of a patient with tuberous sclerosis. Modern imaging techniques can sometimes show cortical tubers (white) even when the skin changes are minimal.

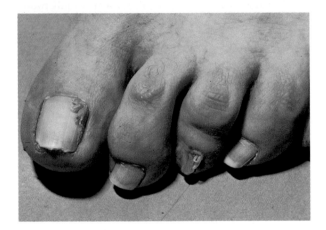

Fig. 22.4 The peri-ungual fibromas of tuberous sclerosis are found in adult patients.

- Gliomas along the lateral walls of the lateral ventricles (80% of cases) and calcification of the basal ganglia.
- Renal and heart tumours.

Diagnosis and differential diagnosis

Any baby with unexplained epilepsy should be examined with a Wood's light (p. 39) to look for ash leaf macules. Skull X-rays and CT scans (Fig. 22.5) help to exclude involvement of the central nervous system and kidneys. The lesions of adenoma sebaceum (a misnomer, as histologically they are angiofibromas) may be mistaken for acne.

Management

Affected families need genetic counselling. Apparently unaffected parents with an affected child will wish to know the chances of further children being affected. Before concluding that an affected child is the result of a new mutation, the parents should be examined with a Wood's light and by an ophthalmologist to help exclude the possibility of genetic transmission from a subtly affected parent. As the gene defects become established prenatal screening of DNA should indicate those at risk.

Adenoma sebaceum improves cosmetically after electrodesiccation, dermabrasion, or destruction by laser but tends to recur.

Xeroderma pigmentosum

Xeroderma pigmentosum is a heterogeneous group of autosomal recessive disorders, characterized by the defective repair of DNA after its damage by ultraviolet radiation. The condition is rare affecting about five per million in Europe.

Cause

Ultraviolet light damages DNA by producing covalent linkages between adjacent pyrimidines. These distort the double helix and inhibit gene expression. Cells from xeroderma pigmentosum patients lack the ability of normal cells to repair this damage.

DNA repair is a complex process using a large family of genes that encode a variety of interacting products which coordinate, locate, and prepare damaged sites for excision and replacement. It is not surprising therefore that many genetic defects can lead to a similar clinical picture. The condition has been divided into several complementation groups by studying the behaviour of cells obtained by fusing those from two patients but this is a research procedure not used clinically.

Clinical features

There are many variants but all follow the same pattern:
- The skin is normal at birth.
- Multiple freckles, roughness and keratoses on exposed skin appear between the ages of six months and two years (Fig. 22.6). Photosensitivity increases thereafter.
- The atrophic facial skin shows telangiectases and small angiomas.
- Many tumours develop on light-damaged skin: these include basal cell carcinomas, squamous cell carcinomas, kerato-acanthomas and malignant melanomas. Many patients die before the age of 20.
- The eyes are affected in most patients. Problems include photophobia, conjunctivitis, and ectropion.
- The condition may be associated with microcephaly, mental deficiency, dwarfism, deafness and ataxia (de Sanctis–Caccione syndrome).

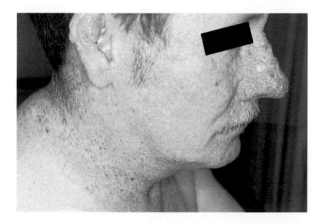

Fig. 22.6 Xeroderma pigmentosum: obvious freckling on neck. Scars on nose mark the spots where tumours have been removed.

Diagnosis

This becomes evident on clinical grounds, though variants with minor signs may cause difficulty. The DNA repair defect can be detected in a few laboratories after the ultraviolet irradiation of cultured fibroblasts or lymphocytes from the patient.

Treatment

Skin cancers can be prevented by strict avoidance of sunlight, protective clothing, wide brimmed hats and the use of reflectant sunscreens and dark glasses. Early and complete removal of all tumours is essential. Radiotherapy should be avoided.

Incontinentia pigmenti

This rare condition is an X-linked dominant disorder, usually lethal before birth in males. The gene for familial cases has been mapped to Xq28 and that for the more severe sporadic cases to Xp11. The bizarre patterning of the skin is due to random X-inactivation (Lyonization). The lines of affected and normal skin represent clones of cells in which either the abnormal or normal X chromosome is active.

Clinical features

There are three stages in the evolution of the skin signs.
- *Vesicular.* Linear groups of blisters occur more on the limbs than trunk.
- *Warty.* After a few weeks the blisters dry up and the predominant lesions are papules with a verrucous hyperkeratotic surface.
- *Pigmented.* A whorled or 'splashed' macular pigmentation, ranging from slate-grey to brown, replaces the warty lesions. Its bizarre patterning is a strong diagnostic pointer.

Occasionally the vesicular and warty stages occur *in utero*; warty or pigmented lesions may therefore be the first signs of the condition. There is also a variant in which pale rather than dark whorls and streaks are seen.

Associated abnormalities are common. A quarter of the patients have defects of their central nervous system, most commonly mental retardation, epilepsy or microcephaly. Skull and palatal abnormalities may also be found. Delayed dentition, and even a total absence of teeth, are recognized features. The incisors may be cone- or peg-shaped. Ocular defects occur in a third of patients, the most common being strabismus, cataract and optic atrophy.

Differential diagnosis

Diagnosis is usually made in infancy when bullous lesions predominate so the differential diagnosis includes bullous impetigo (p. 161), candidiasis (p. 188), and the rarer linear IgA bullous disease of childhood (p. 121) and epidermolysis bullosa (see below).

Investigations

There is frequently an eosinophilia in the blood. Biopsy of an intact blister reveals an intra-epidermal vesicle filled with eosinophils.

Management

This is symptomatic and includes measures to combat bacterial and candidal infection during the vesicular phase. Family counselling should be offered.

Epidermolysis bullosa

There are several types of epidermolysis bullosa; the five main ones are listed in Table 22.1. All are characterized by an inherited tendency to develop blisters, though at different levels in the skin, after minimal trauma (Fig. 22.7). Acquired epidermolysis bullosa is not inherited and is discussed on p. 123.

Table 22.1 Simplified classification of epidermolysis bullosa

Type	Mode of inheritance
Simple epidermolysis bullosa	Autosomal dominant
Junctional epidermolysis bullosa (epidermolysis bullosa letalis)	Autosomal recessive
Dystrophic epidermolysis bullosa	Autosomal dominant
Dystrophic epidermolysis bullosa	Autosomal recessive
Acquired epidermolysis bullosa	Not inherited

Simple epidermolysis bullosa

Several subtypes are recognized, most being inherited as autosomal dominant conditions with abnormalities in genes responsible for keratin production.

The paired keratins expressed in the basal keratinocytes are K5 and K14. Linkage studies show that the genetic defect for the commonest types of simple epidermolysis bullosa maps to loci for types I and II keratin and is found on chromosomes 17 and 12.

Blisters form within or just above the basal cell layers of the epidermis and so tend to heal without scarring. Nails and mucosae are not involved. The problems are made worse by sweating and ill-fitting shoes. Blistering can be minimized by avoiding trauma, wearing soft, well-fitting shoes, and using foot powder. Large blisters should be pricked with a sterile needle and dressed. Their roofs should not be removed. Local antibiotics may be needed.

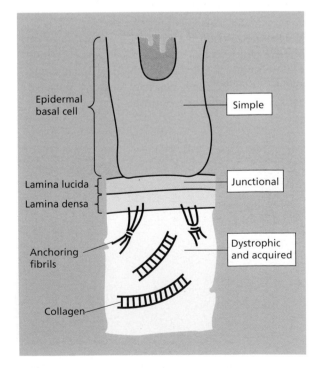

Fig. 22.7 Level of blister in epidermolysis bullosa at the epidermal–dermal junction.

Junctional epidermolysis bullosa

Due to an abnormality in the basal lamina involving loss of anchoring filaments and defective nicein (p. 17; Fig. 2.14). This rare and often lethal form is evident at birth. The newborn child shows large raw areas and flaccid blisters which are slow to heal (Fig. 22.8). The peri-oral and peri-anal skin is usually involved, as are the nails and oral mucous membrane. There is no effective treatment though systemic steroids and phenytoin are often tried.

Dystrophic epidermolysis bullosa

All types probably result from abnormalities of collagen VII, the major structural component of anchoring fibrils. Close linkage has already been found between the dominantly inherited type and the gene for the alpha-1 chain of type VII collagen on chromosome 3p21.

Autosomal dominant dystrophic epidermolysis bullosa

Blisters in this type appear in late infancy. They are most common on friction sites, e.g. knees, elbows and fingers. They heal with scarring, and with milia formation. The nails may be deformed or even lost. The mouth is not affected. The only treatment is to avoid trauma and to dress the blistered areas.

Autosomal recessive dystrophic epidermolysis bullosa

Due to loss of anchoring fibrils (Type VII collagen). In this tragic form of epidermolysis bullosa, blisters start in infancy. They are subepidermal, and may be filled with blood. They heal with scarring which may be so severe that the nails are lost and webs form between the digits (Fig. 22.9). The hands and feet may become useless balls which have lost all of the fingers and toes. The teeth, mouth and upper part of the oesophagus are all affected; oesophageal strictures may form. Treatment is unsatisfactory but phenytoin, which reduces the raised dermal collagenase levels found in this variant, sometimes helps. Systemic steroids are disappointing. It is especially important to minimize trauma, to prevent contractures and web formation between the digits, and to combat secondary infection. Referral to centres with expertise in management of these patients is strongly recommended.

Ehlers–Danlos syndrome

Eleven types are now recognized and this complicated subject has earned its own scientific group which continuously updates its classification and molecular biology.

Cause

All types of Ehlers–Danlos syndrome are likely to

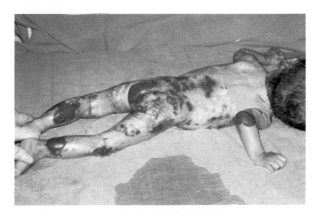

Fig. 22.8 Junctional epidermolysis bullosa; a baby with numerous large raw areas. The condition was fatal.

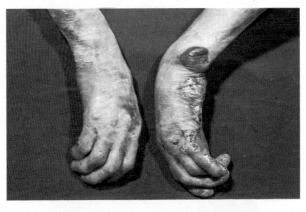

Fig. 22.9 Autosomal recessive dystrophic epidermolysis bullosa: note large blood-filled blister. Scarring has led to fixed deformity of the fingers and loss of nails.

be based on mutations in genes important in the formation or modification of collagen and the extracellular matrix. The first to be detected was the lysyl hydroxylase deficiency found in some type VI patients, and this enzyme is also important in type IX. In type IV Ehlers–Danlos syndrome mutations are found in one of the type III collagen genes on chromosome 2q31. Structural defects in type I collagen occur in type VII Ehlers–Danlos syndrome. The detailed pathogenesis of some of the other types has still to be elucidated.

Clinical features

- Elasticity of the skin.
- Hyperextensibility of the joints (Fig. 22.10).
- Fragility of skin and blood vessels.
- Easy bruising.
- Ugly ('papyraceous') scars.

Complications

These depend on the type. They include subluxation of joints, varicose veins in early life, an increased liability to develop hernias, kyphoscoliosis, aortic aneurysms and ruptured large arteries, and intra-

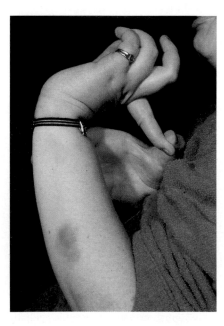

Fig. 22.10 Ehlers–Danlos syndrome: showing hyperextensible joints and easy bruising.

ocular haemorrhage. Affected individuals may be born prematurely as a result of the early rupture of fragile fetal membranes.

Diagnosis and treatment

The diagnosis is made on the clinical features and family history. The frequent skin lacerations and prominent scars may suggest child abuse. The diagnosis and type can sometimes be confirmed by enzyme studies on isolated fibroblasts. There is no effective treatment but genetic counselling is needed.

Pseudo-xanthoma elasticum

Various defects in elastin, and probably collagen, are responsible for this condition of which at least four types are known.

Cause and pathology

Inheritance may be dominant or recessive. As yet no specific enzyme defects have been detected. The elastic fibres in the mid-dermis become swollen and fragmented; their calcification is probably a secondary feature. The connective tissue protein, fibrillin, contains several calcium binding domains and abnormalities in one of the several fibrillin genes may be important in this condition. The elastic tissue of blood vessels and of the retina may also be affected.

Clinical features

The skin of the neck and axillae, and occasionally of other body folds, is loose and wrinkled. Groups of small yellow papules give these areas a 'plucked chicken' appearance. Breaks in the retina show as angioid streaks, which are grey, poorly defined areas radiating from the optic nerve head. Arterial involvement may lead to peripheral, coronary, or cerebral arterial insufficiency.

Complications

The most important are hypertension, recurrent gut haemorrhages, ischaemic heart disease and cerebral haemorrhage.

Diagnosis and treatment

The diagnosis is made clinically and confirmed by the histology. There is no effective treatment.

LEARNING POINTS
The decision to have children, or not to do so, must lie with the family concerned. Make sure they have all the facts before them.

CHAPTER 23

Drug eruptions

Almost any drug can cause a cutaneous reaction, and many inflammatory skin conditions can be caused or exacerbated by drugs. A drug reaction can reasonably be included in the differential diagnosis of most skin diseases.

Mechanisms (Table 23.1)

Non-allergic drug reactions

Not all drug reactions are allergic. Some are due to overdosage, others to the accumulation of drugs, or to unwanted pharmacological effects, e.g. stretch marks from systemic steroids (Fig. 23.1). Other reactions are idiosyncratic (i.e. an odd reaction peculiar to one individual), or due to alterations of ecological balance (see below).

Cutaneous reactions can be expected from the very nature of some drugs. These are normal but unwanted responses. Patients show them when a drug is given in a high dose or even in a therapeutic dose. For example, mouth ulcers frequently occur as a result of the cytotoxicity of methotrexate. Silver-based preparations, given for prolonged periods, can lead to a slate-grey colour of the skin (argyria). Acute

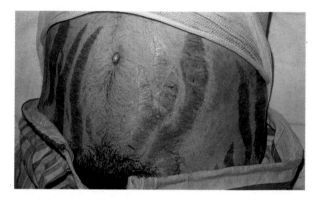

Fig. 23.1 Gross striae due to systemic steroids.

vaginal candidiasis occurs when antibiotics remove the normal resident bacteria from the female genital tract and foster colonization by yeasts. Dapsone or rifampicin, given to patients with lepromatous leprosy, may cause erythema nodosum leprosum as the immune response to the bacillus is re-established.

Non-allergic reactions are often predictable. They affect many, or even all, patients taking the drug at a sufficient dose for a sufficient time. Careful studies before marketing should indicate the types of reaction that can be anticipated.

Allergic drug reactions

Allergic drug reactions are less predictable. They occur in only a minority of patients receiving a drug and can do so even with low doses. Allergic reactions are not a normal biological effect of the drug and usually appear after the latent period required for an immune response. Chemically related drugs may cross-react.

Fortunately allergic drug reactions take up only a limited number of forms, namely urticaria and angioedema, vasculitis, erythema multiforme, or

Table 23.1 Some mechanisms involved in drug reactions

Pharmacological
Due to overdosage or failure to excrete or metabolize
Cumulative effects
Altered skin ecology.
Allergic
  IgE mediated
  Cytotoxic
  Immune complex mediated
  Cell mediated
Idiosyncratic
Exacerbation of pre-existing skin conditions

a morbilliform erythema. Rarer allergic reactions include bullae, erythroderma, pruritus, and toxic epidermal necrolysis.

Presentation

Some drugs and the reactions they can cause

Antibiotics

Penicillins and sulphonamides are among the most common drugs causing allergic reactions. These are often morbilliform (Fig. 23.2), but urticaria and erythema multiforme are common too. Viral infections are often associated with exanthems, and many rashes are incorrectly blamed on an antibiotic when, in fact, a virus was responsible. Most patients with infectious mononucleosis develop a morbilliform rash if ampicillin is administered. Penicillin is a common cause of severe anaphylactic reactions which may be life-threatening. Minocycline can accumulate in the tissues and produce a brown or grey colour in the mucosa, sun-exposed areas, or at sites of inflammation, as in the lesions of acne.

Penicillamine

Like penicillin itself, this can cause morbilliform eruptions or urticaria, but the drug has also been incriminated as a cause of haemorrhagic bullae at sites of trauma, of the extrusion of elastic tissue through the skin, and of pemphigus.

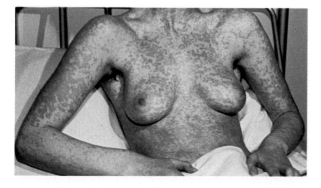

Fig. 23.2 Symmetrical erythematous maculopapular rash due to ampicillin.

Oral contraceptives

The frequency of reactions to these is less now that their hormonal content is small. The hair fall which may follow stopping the drug is like that seen after pregnancy (telogen effluvium) (p. 77). Hirsutism, erythema nodosum, acne, chloasma, and photosensitivity are other reactions.

Gold

This frequently causes rashes. Its side effects range from pruritus to morbilliform eruptions, to curious papulosquamous eruptions like pityriasis rosea or lichen planus. Erythroderma, erythema nodosum, hair fall, and stomatitis may also be provoked by gold.

Steroids

Cutaneous side effects from systemic steroids include a ruddy face, cutaneous atrophy, striae (Fig. 23.1), hirsutism, steroid acne and a susceptibility to cutaneous infections, which may be atypical.

Some common reaction patterns and drugs which can cause them

Toxic (reactive) erythema

This vague term describes the most common type of drug eruption, sometimes looking like measles or scarlet fever, and sometimes with prominent urticarial (Fig. 23.3) or erythema multiforme-like elements. Itching and fever may accompany the rash. Culprits include antibiotics (especially ampicillin), sulphonamides and related compounds (diuretics and hypoglycaemics), barbiturates, phenylbutazone, and PAS.

Urticaria (Chapter 10)

Many drugs may cause this: salicylates are the most common, often working non-immunologically as histamine releasers. Antibiotics are also often to blame. Insect repellants and nitrogen mustards can cause urticaria on contact. Urticaria may be part of a severe and generalized reaction (anaphylaxis) which includes bronchospasm and collapse (Fig. 23.4).

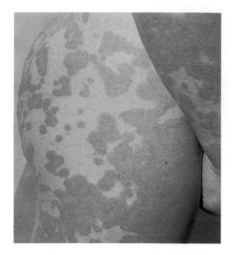

Fig. 23.3 Toxic erythema with urticarial features.

Allergic vasculitis (Chapter 10)

The clinical changes range from urticarial papules, through palpable purpura, to necrotic ulcers. Erythema nodosum may occur. Sulphonamides, phenylbutazone, indomethacin, phenytoin and oral contraceptives are among possible causes.

Erythema multiforme (Chapter 10)

Target-like lesions appear mainly on the extensor aspects of the limbs, and bullae may form. In the Stevens—Johnson syndrome the patients are often ill and the mucous membranes are severely affected. Sulphonamides, barbiturates, and phenylbutazone are known offenders.

Purpura

Clinical features are seldom distinctive apart from the itchy, brown petechial rash on dependent areas that was characteristic of carbromal reactions. Thrombocytopenia and coagulation defects should be excluded (Chapter 13). Thiazides, sulphonamides, phenylbutazone, sulphonylureas, barbiturates and quinine are among the drugs reported to cause purpura.

Bullous eruptions

Some of the reactions noted above may become

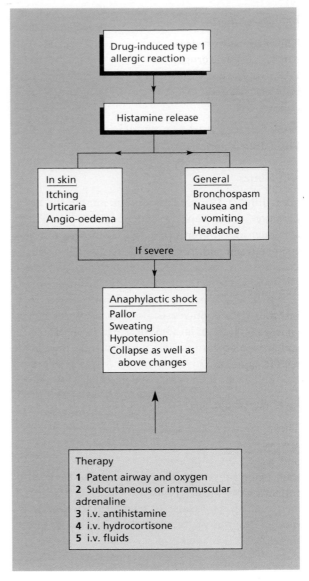

Fig. 23.4 The cause, clinical features and treatment of anaphylaxis.

bullous. Bullae may also develop at pressure sites in drug-induced coma.

Eczema

This is not a common pattern and occurs mainly when patients sensitized by topical application are given the drug systemically. Penicillin, sulphonamides, neomycin, phenothiazines, and local anaesthetics should be considered.

Exfoliative dermatitis

The entire skin surface becomes red and scaly. This can be caused by drugs (particularly phenylbutazone, PAS, isoniazid and gold), but can also be due to a widespread attack of skin diseases such as psoriasis and eczema.

Fixed drug eruptions

Round, erythematous or purple and sometimes bullous plaques recur at the same site each time the drug is taken (Fig. 23.5). Phenolphthalein (in some purgatives), barbiturates, sulphonamides, quinine or tetracycline may be responsible. Pigmentation persists between acute episodes.

Acneiform eruptions

Lithium, iodides, bromides, oral contraceptives, androgens or glucocorticosteroids, antituberculosis and anticonvulsant therapy may cause an acneiform rash (Chapter 14).

Lichenoid eruptions

These resemble lichen planus (Chapter 7), but not always very closely, as mouth lesions are uncommon and as scaling and eczematous elements may be seen. Consider antimalarials, non-steroidal anti-inflammatory drugs, gold, phenothiazines, and PAS.

Toxic epidermal necrolysis (p. 122)

In adults this 'scalded skin' appearance is usually drug-induced (e.g. barbiturates, phenylbutazone, oxyphenbutazone, phenytoin, or penicillin).

Hair loss

This is a predictable side effect of etretinate and cytotoxic agents, an unpredictable response to some anticoagulants, and sometimes seen with antithyroid drugs. Diffuse hair loss may occur during, or just after, the use of an oral contraceptive.

Hypertrichosis

This is a dose-dependent effect of diazoxide, minoxidil, and cyclosporin A.

Pigmentation (see also p. 218)

Chloasma (p. 216) may follow an oral contraceptive plus sun exposure. Large doses of phenothiazines impart a blue-grey colour to exposed areas (Fig. 23.6); heavy metals can cause a generalized browning; clofazamine makes the skin red; and mepacrine turns the skin yellow.

Photosensitivity

This is dealt with in Chapter 17. Always exclude the common drug causes (thiazides, tetracyclines,

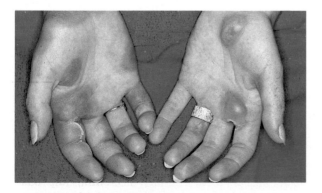

Fig. 23.5 Fixed drug eruption due to barbiturates; unusually severe bullous reaction.

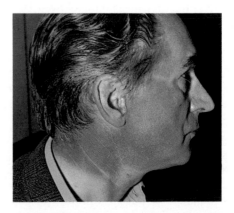

Fig. 23.6 Note sparing of skin creases and area shielded by spectacle frames in this patient with photo-related hyperpigmentation from a phenothiazine drug.

phenothiazines, sulphonamides, psoralens, or nali-
dixic acid).

Xerosis

The skin can become rough and scaly in patients
receiving oral retinoids, nicotinic acid or lithium.

Exacerbation of pre-existing skin conditions

Psoriasis and acne are good examples of this. Psoriasis may be made worse by giving beta-blockers,
anti-malarials, or lithium. Acne may be exacerbated
by androgens, anticonvulsants, and lithium.

Course

The different types of reaction vary so much that a
brief summary is not possible. In previously exposed
patients the common toxic erythema reaction may
start two to three days after the administration of
the drug. If such a reaction occurs during the first
course of treatment, the eruption characteristically
begins later, often coming up at about the ninth day
or even after the drug has been stopped. The speed
with which a drug eruption clears depends on the
type of reaction and the rapidity with which the
drug is eliminated.

Differential diagnosis

The differential diagnosis ranges over the whole
subject of dermatology depending on which disease
is mimicked. For instance, toxic erythema reactions
can look very like measles, pityriasis rosea, or even
secondary syphilis. The general rule is never to forget
the possibility of a drug eruption when an atypical
rash is seen. Six vital questions should be asked
(Table 23.2).

Treatment

The first approach is to withdraw the suspected
drug, accepting that several drugs may need to be
stopped at the same time. This is not always easy.
Sometimes a drug is necessary and there is no

Table 23.2 The six vital questions to be asked when a drug
eruption is suspected

1 Can you exclude a simple dermatosis (such as scabies or
psoriasis) and known skin manifestations of an underlying
disorder (e.g. systemic lupus erythematosus)?
2 Does the rash itself suggest a drug eruption (e.g.
urticaria, erythema multiforme)?
3 Does a past history of drug reactions correlate with
current prescriptions?
4 Was any drug introduced a few days before the eruption
appeared?
5 Which of the current drugs most commonly cause drug
eruptions, e.g. penicillins, sulphonamides, thiazides,
allopurinol, phenylbutazone, etc?
6 Does the eruption fit with a well-recognized pattern
caused by one of the current drugs (e.g. acne from lithium)?

alternative available. At other times the patient may
be taking many drugs and it is difficult to know
which one to stop. The decision to stop or continue
a drug depends upon the nature of the drug, the
necessity of using the drug for treatment, the availability of chemically unrelated alternatives, the
severity of the reaction, its potential reversibility,
and the probability that the drug is actually causing
the reaction.

Assessment depends upon clinical detective work
(Table 23.2). Judgements must be based on prob-
abilities and common sense. Every effort must
be made to correlate the onset of the rash with
prescription records. Often, but not always, the latest
drug to be introduced is the most likely culprit.
Prick tests and *in vitro* tests for allergy are still too
unreliable to be of value. Re-administration, as a
diagnostic test, is usually unwise except when no
suitable alternative drug exists.

Non-specific therapy depends upon the type of
eruption. In urticaria, antihistamines are helpful. In
some reactions, topical or systemic corticosteroids
can be used, and applications of calamine lotion may
be soothing.

Anaphylactic reactions require special treatment
(Fig. 23.4) to ensure that the airway is not compro-
mised (e.g. oxygen, assisted respiration or even
emergency tracheostomy). One or more injections of
adrenaline (epinephrine) (1 : 1000) 0.3–0.5 ml should
be given subcutaneously or intramuscularly in adults
before the slow (over 1 minute) intravenous injection
of chlorpheniramine maleate (10–20 mg diluted in
syringe with 5–10 ml of blood). Although the action

of intravenous hydrocortisone (100 mg) is delayed for several hours it should be given to prevent further deterioration in severely affected patients. Patients should be observed for six hours after their condition is stable, as late deterioration may occur. If an anaphylactic reaction is anticipated, patients should be taught how to self-inject adrenaline, and may be given an adrenaline inhaler to use at the first sign of the reaction.

To re-emphasize, the most important treatment is to stop the responsible drug.

LEARNING POINTS

1 This whole chapter is a warning against polypharmacy. Do your patients really need all the drugs they are taking?

2 Avoid provocation tests unless there are very strong indications for them.

CHAPTER 24

Dermatological therapy

An accurate diagnosis, based on a proper history and examination (Chapter 4), must come before rational treatment can be chosen; and even when a firm diagnosis has been reached, each patient must be treated as an individual. For some, no treatment may even be the best treatment especially when the disorder is cosmetic or if the treatment is worse than the condition. A patient with minimal psoriasis, for example, may be helped more by careful explanation and reassurance than by prescriptions.

If a diagnosis cannot be reached, the doctor has to decide whether a specialist opinion is needed, or whether it is best to observe the rash for a while and treat it perhaps with a bland application. In either case, the indiscriminate use of topical steroids or other medications, in the absence of a working diagnosis, often confuses the picture and may render the future diagnosis more difficult.

Usually, however, a firm diagnosis can be made; and a sensible course of treatment can be planned; but even then results are often better when patients understand their disease and the reason behind their treatment. The cause and nature of their disease should be explained carefully, in language which they can understand, and they must be told what can realistically be expected of their treatment. False optimism or undue pessimism, by patients or doctors, leads only to an unsound relationship. Too often patients become discontented, not because they do not know the correct diagnosis but because they have not been told enough about its cause or prognosis. Even worse, they may have little idea of how to use the treatment and what to expect of it; poor compliance often follows poor instruction. As treatment may be complex, instruction sheets are helpful; they reinforce the spoken word and answer unasked questions.

The principal steps in diagnosis and management are:

- History.
- Examination.
- Investigations.
- Diagnosis.
- Explanation of condition, its cause and prognosis.
- Choice of treatment and instructions about it.
- Discussion of expectations.
- Follow-up, if necessary.

LEARNING POINT
One correct diagnosis is worth a hundred therapeutic trials.

Therapeutic options

Some of the treatments used in dermatology are listed in Table 24.1.

Topical versus systemic therapy

The great advantage of topical therapy is that drugs are delivered directly where they are needed at an

Table 24.1 Therapeutic options in dermatology

Drugs	Topical
	Systemic
Physical	Surgical
	excision
	curettage
	Electrodesiccation
	Cryotherapy
	Radiotherapy
	Phototherapy
	Laser therapy

optimum concentration to the target organ. Systemic side effects from absorption are less than those expected from the same drug given systemically: with topical treatment vital organs such as the marrow, liver and kidneys are exposed to lower drug concentrations than is the skin. However, topical treatment is often messy, time-consuming and incomplete, and takes time to apply whereas systemic treatment is clean and quick and its effect is uniform over the entire skin surface. Cost must also be considered.

Some drugs can only be used topically (e.g. gamma-benzene hexachloride for scabies and mupirocin for bacterial infections), while others work only systemically (e.g. dapsone for dermatitis herpetiformis and griseofulvin for fungal infections).

When a choice exists, and both possibilities are equally effective, then local treatment is usually preferred. Most cases of mild pityriasis versicolor, for example, respond to topical antifungals alone so systemic itraconazole is not the first treatment of choice.

Topical treatment

Percutaneous absorption

Drugs used on the skin must be dissolved or suspended in bases (vehicles). The choice of drug and of the base are both important and depend on the diagnosis and the state of the skin. For a drug to be effective topically it must pass the barrier to diffusion presented by the horny layer (Chapter 2). This requires the drug to be transferred from its base to the horny layer, from which it will diffuse through the epidermis into the papillary dermis. Passage through the horny layer is the rate-limiting step.

The transfer of a drug from its base to the horny layer depends on its relative solubility in each (measured as the 'partition coefficient'). Movement across the horny layer depends upon both the concentration gradient and on restricting forces (its 'diffusion constant'). In general, non-polar substances penetrate more rapidly than polar ones. A rise in skin temperture and in hydration, both achieved by covering a treated area with polyethylene occlusion, encourages penetration.

Some areas of skin present less of a barrier than do others. Two extreme examples are palmar skin, with its impermeable, thick horny layer, and scrotal skin, which is thin and highly permeable. The skin of the face is more permeable than the skin of the body. Body fold skin is more permeable than nearby unoccluded skin. In humans, absorption through the hair follicles and sweat ducts is of little significance and the amount of hair on the treated site is no guide to its permeability.

In many skin diseases the horny layer becomes abnormal, and loses some of its barrier function. The abnormal nucleated (parakeratotic) horny layer of psoriasis and chronic eczema, though thicker than normal, has lost much of its protective qualities. Water loss is increased and therapeutic agents penetrate more readily. Similarly, breakdown of the horny layer by chemicals (e.g. soaps and detergents), and by physical injury, will allow the more rapid penetration of drugs.

In summary, the penetration of a drug through the skin depends on the following factors:

- Its concentration.
- The base.
- Its partition coefficient.
- Its diffusion constant.
- The thickness of the horny layer.
- The state, including hydration, of the horny layer.
- Temperature.

Active ingredients

These include corticosteroids, tar, dithranol, antibiotics, antifungal and antiviral agents, benzoyl peroxide, retinoic acid and many others (Formulary, pp. 287–296). The choice depends on the action required, and the prescriber should know how each works. As topical steroids are the mainstay of much local dermatological therapy their pharmacology is summarized in Table 24.2.

Bases (vehicles)

Most bases are a mixture of powders, water and greases (usually obtained from petroleum). Figure 24.1 shows that blending these bases together produces preparations which retain the characteristics of each of their components.

A base should maximize the delivery of topical drugs but it may also have useful properties in its

Table 24.2 The pharmacology of topical steroid applications

Active constituents	Include hydrocortisone and synthetic halogenated derivatives Halogenation increases activity
Bases	Available as lotions, creams, ointments, sprays and tapes
Penetration	Readily penetrate via the horny layer and appendages Form a reservoir in the horny layer Polyethylene occlusion and high concentrations increase penetration
Metabolism	Some minor metabolism in epidermis and dermis (e.g. hydrocortisone converts to cortisone and other metabolites) Leave skin via dermal vascular plexus and enter general metabolic pool of steroids Further metabolism in liver
Excretion	As sulphate esters and glucuronides
Actions	Anti-inflammatory 1 Vasoconstrict 2 Decrease permeability of dermal vessels 3 Decrease phagocytic migration and activity 4 Decrease fibrin formation 5 Decrease kinin formation 6 Inhibit phospholipase A_2 activity and decrease products of arachidonic acid metabolism 7 Depress fibroblastic activity 8 Stabilize lysosomal membranes Immunosuppressive Antigen–antibody interaction unaffected but inflammatory consequences lessened by above mechanisms and by inhibiting cytokines (e.g. IFNγ, GM-CSF, IL-1,2,3 and TNFα) Lympholytic Decrease epidermal proliferation
Side effects	1 Thinning of epidermis 2 Thinning of dermis 3 Telangiectasia and striae (due to **1** and **2**) 4 Bruising (due to **2** and vessel wall fragility) 5 Hirsutism 6 Folliculitis and acneiform eruptions 7 May worsen or disguise infections (bacterial, viral and fungal) 8 Systemic absorption (rare but may be important in infants, when applied in large quantities under polyethylene pants) 9 Tachyphylaxis — lessening of clinical effect with the same preparation 10 Rebound — worsening, sometimes dramatic on withdrawing treatment
Uses	Eczema, psoriasis in some instances (facial, flexural, and palms/soles) Many non-infective pruritic dermatoses

own right. Used carelessly bases may even do harm. Suggested indications are shown in Table 24.3. The choice of base depends upon the action desired, availability, messiness, ease of application, and cost.

Individual bases

Dusting powders are used in the folds to lessen friction between opposing surfaces. They may repel water (for example, talc) or absorb it (for example,

Table 24.3 Bases and their properties

Base	Used on	Effect	Points of note
Dusting powders	Flexures (may be slightly moist)	Lessen friction	If too wet clump and irritate
Alcohol-based applications	Scalp	Clean vehicle for steroid application	Cosmetically elegant, does not gum up hair May sting raw areas
Watery and shake lotions	Acutely inflamed skin (wet and oozing)	Drying, soothing and cooling	Tedious to apply Frequent changes (lessened by polyethylene occlusion) Powder in shake lotions may clump
Creams	Both moist and dry skin	Cooling, emollient and moisturizing	Short shelf life Fungal and bacterial growth in base Sensitivities to preservatives and emulsifying agents
Ointments	Dry and scaly skin	Occlusive and emollient	Messy to apply, soils clothing Removed with an oil
Pastes	Dry, lichenified and scaly skin	Protective and emollient	Messy and tedious to apply (linen or calico needed) Most protective if applied properly
Sprays	Weeping, acutely inflamed skin Scalp	Drying, non-occlusive	Vehicle evaporates rapidly No need to touch skin to treat it
Gels	Face and scalp	Vehicle for steroids, salicylic acid and tretinoin	May sting when applied to inflamed skin Can be covered by make-up

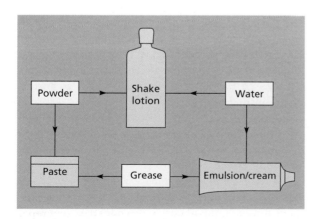

Fig. 24.1 The derivation of bases.

starch); zinc oxide powder has an absorptive power midway between these extremes. Powders ought not be used in moist areas where they tend to cake and abrade.

Watery lotions evaporate and cool inflamed areas. This effect is hastened by adding an alcohol, but glycerol or arachis oil slow evaporation and retain skin moisture. Substances which precipitate protein (astringents), for example silver nitrate, lessen exudation.

Shake lotions are watery lotions to which powder has been added so that the area for evaporation is increased. These lotions dry wet, weeping skin. When water has evaporated from the skin, the powder particles clump together and may become abrasive. This is less likely if an oil such as glycerol has been added.

Creams are used for their cooling, moisturizing, and emollient effects. They are either oil-in-water emulsions (e.g. aqueous cream [UK], acid mantle cream [USA]) or water-in-oil emulsions (e.g. oily cream [UK], cold cream [USA]). Emulsifying agents are added to increase the surface area of the dispersed phase and that of any therapeutic agent in it.

Ointments are used for their occlusive and emollient properties. They allow the skin to remain supple by preventing the evaporation of water from the horny layer. There are three main types: those which are water-soluble (macrogols, polyethylene glycols); those which emulsify with water; and those which repel water (mineral oils, and animal and vegetable fats).

Pastes are used for their protective and emollient properties and usually are made of powder added to a mineral oil or grease. The powder lessens the oil's occlusive effect.

Variations on these themes have led to the numerous topical preparations available today. Rather than use them all, and risk confusion, doctors should limit their choice to one or two from each category; Table 24.3 summarizes the properties and uses of some common preparations.

Methods of application

Ointments and creams are usually applied sparingly twice daily, but the frequency of application will depend on many factors including the nature, severity and duration of the rash, the sites involved, convenience, the preparation (some new local steroids need only be applied once daily; Formulary, p. 290) and, most important, common sense.

Three techniques of application are more specialized: immersion therapy by bathing, wet dressings (compresses) and occlusive therapy.

Baths. Once-daily bathing helps to remove crusts, scales and medications. After soaking for about ten minutes, the skin should be rubbed gently with a sponge, flannel or soft cloth; cleaning may be made easier by soaps, oils, or colloidal oatmeal.

Medicated baths are occasionally helpful, the most common ingredients added to the bath water being bath oils, antiseptics, and solutions of coal tar.

After cleaning, the most important function of a bath is hydration. The skin absorbs water and this can be held in the skin for some time if an occlusive ointment is applied after bathing.

Older patients may need help to get into a bath and should be warned about falling if the bath contains an oil or another slippery substance.

Wet dressings (compresses). These are used to clean the skin or to deliver a topical medication. They are especially helpful for weeping, crusting, and purulent conditions. Five or six layers of soft cloth (e.g. cotton gauze) are soaked in the solution to be used; this may be tap water, saline, an astringent or antiseptic solution, and the compress is then applied to the skin. Open dressings allow the water to evaporate and the skin to cool. They should be changed frequently, for example every 15 minutes for an hour.

Closed dressings are covered with a plastic (usually polyethylene) sheet; they do not dry out so quickly and are usually changed twice daily. They are especially helpful for debriding adherent crusts and for draining exudative and purulent ulcers.

Occlusive therapy. Sometimes steroid-sensitive dermatoses will respond to a steroid only when it is applied under a plastic sheet to encourage penetration. This technique is best reserved for the short-term treatment of stubborn, localized rashes. The drawback of this treatment is that the side effects of topical steroid treatment (Table 24.2) are highly likely to occur. The most important is systemic absorption if a large surface area of skin, relative to body weight, is treated (e.g. when steroids are applied under polyethylene pants to infants).

Monitoring local treatment

One common fault is to underestimate the amount required. The guidelines given in Table 24.4 and Fig. 24.2 are based on twice daily applications. Lotions go further than creams, which go further than ointments and pastes.

Pump dispensers have recently become available for some topical steroids (e.g. Betnovate; Glaxo Laboratories Ltd, UK) which allow measured amounts to be applied. Alternatively, 'finger tip units' (Fig. 24.3) can increase the accuracy of prescribing. As a guide one finger tip unit in an adult male from a standard nozzle provides 0.5 g ointment.

Table 24.4 Minimum amount of cream (g) required for twice-daily application for one week

Age	Whole body	Trunk	Both arms and legs
6 months	35	15	20
4 years	60	20	35
8 years	90	35	50
12 years	120	45	65
Adult (70 kg male)	170	60	90

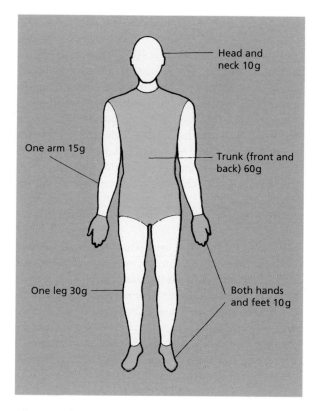

Fig. 24.2 The minimum amount of a cream required in one week by an adult applying it twice daily.

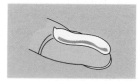

Fig. 24.3 A finger tip measures about 0.5 g ointment.

Systemic therapy

Systemic treatment is needed if a skin condition is associated with systemic disease, or if the medicament of choice is inactive topically (for example, griseofulvin). The principles of systemic therapy in dermatology are no different from those in other branches of medicine. Some drugs act specifically; others non-specifically. For example, antihistamines (H1 blockers) act specifically in urticaria, and non-specifically, by a sedative effect, on the most common skin symptom — itch.

Systemic disease co-exists with skin disease in several ways (Chapter 20). Sometimes a systemic disease such as systemic lupus erythematosus may cause a rash; at other times, a skin disease causes a systemic upset. Examples of this are the depression which occurs in some patients affected with severe rashes, and high-output cardiac failure, which may occur in exfoliative dermatitis from the shunting of blood through the skin. A systemic upset due to skin disease can be treated with drugs designed for such problems while the skin is being treated in other ways.

Physical forms of therapy

The skin is also accessible to treatment by surgery, freezing, burning, ultraviolet radiation, and lasers. As the population grows older, and more concerned about appearances, requests for minor surgery become more common. Some broad principles will be discussed here.

Surgical

The indications for biopsy, and the techniques employed, are described in Chapter 4.

Shave excision

Many small lesions are removed by shaving them off at their bases with a scalpel under local anaesthesia. Although simple, the procedure may leave some cells at the base and these, in the case of tumours, may lead to recurrence.

Excision

Excision under local anaesthetic, using an aseptic technique, is another way to remove small tumours (Figs 24.4 & 24.5). The lesion must be examined carefully and important underlying structures (e.g.

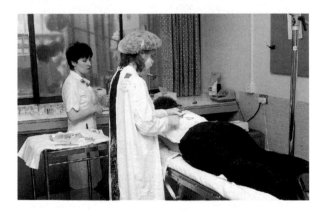

Fig. 24.4 No surgery is minor. Always use an aseptic technique, in proper surroundings, with appropriate help.

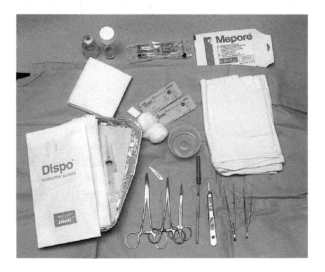

Fig. 24.5 Our standard pack is suitable for most skin surgery.

the temporal artery) noted. If possible the incision should run along the line of a skin crease, especially on the face. If necessary, charts or pictures of standard skin creases should be consulted (Fig. 24.6). After injection of the local anaesthetic (usually 1 or 2% lignocaine [lidocaine, USA] with or without 1 in 200 000 adrenaline [epinephrine]), the lesion is excised as an ellipse with a margin of normal skin which varies with the nature of the lesion and the site (Fig. 24.7). The scalpel should be held perpendicular to the skin surface and the incision should reach the subcutaneous fat. The ellipse of skin is carefully removed with the help of a skin hook (Fig. 24.8) or fine-toothed forceps. Larger wounds, and those where the scar is likely to stretch (e.g. on the back), are closed in layers with absorbable sutures (e.g. dexon) before apposing the skin edges with non-absorbable interrupted or continuous subcuticular sutures such as nylon or prolene. Stitches are removed from the face in 4–5 days and from the trunk and limbs in 7–14 days. Artificial sutures (e.g. Steristrip) may be used to take the tension off the wound edges after the stitches have been taken out.

Curettage

Curettage under local anaesthetic is used to treat benign exophytic lesions (e.g. seborrhoeic keratoses) and, combined with electrodesiccation (see below), to treat some basal cell carcinomas (Fig. 24.9). Its main advantage over purely destructive treatment is that histological examination can be carried out on the curettings. A sharp curette is used to scrape off the lesion and haemostasis is achieved by electrocautery or electrodesiccation. The wound heals by secondary intention over two to three weeks, with good cosmetic results in most cases.

When a basal cell carcinoma is treated, the curette is scraped carefully and firmly along the sides and bottom of the tumour (the surrounding dermis is tougher and more resistant to curettage than the carcinoma) and the bleeding wound bed is then electrodesiccated aggressively. The process is repeated once or twice at the same session to ensure that all of the tumour has been removed or destroyed. With experience and regular follow up the cure rate is good.

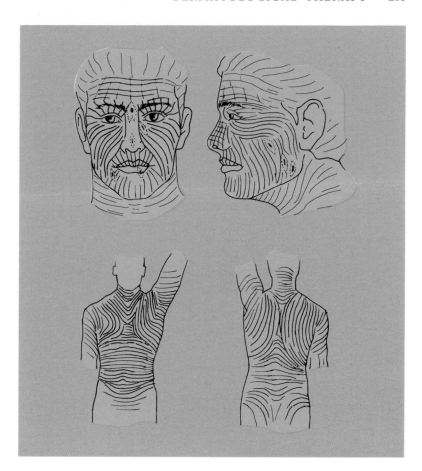

Fig. 24.6 Skin wrinkle figures are helpful in deciding the direction of wounds following skin surgery. Those performing dermatological surgery should have ready access to them.

Microscopically controlled excision
(Mohs' technique)

This is useful to treat:
- A basal cell carcinoma with a poorly defined edge.
- A recurrent basal cell carcinoma.
- A basal cell carcinoma lying where excessive margins of skin cannot be sacrificed to achieve complete removal of the tumour (e.g. one near the eye).
- Basal cell carcinomas in areas with a high incidence of recurrence such as the nose, glabella, or nasolabial folds.
- Occasional tumours other than basal cell carcinomas.

This form of surgery is time-consuming and expensive, but the probability of cure is greater than with excision or curettage. First the tumour is removed with a narrow margin. The excised specimen is then marked at the edges, mapped, and, after rapid histological processing, is immediately examined in horizontal and vertical section. If the tumour extends to any margin, further tissue is removed from the appropriate place, based on the markings and mappings, and again checked histologically. This process is repeated until clearance has been proved histologically at all margins. The resulting wound may then be closed directly, covered with a split skin graft or allowed to heal by secondary intention.

Electrosurgery

This is often combined with curettage, under local anaesthesia, to treat skin tumours. The main types are shown in Figure 24.10.

Cryotherapy

Liquid nitrogen (−196°C) is now used more often than carbon dioxide snow ('dry ice', −79°C). It is

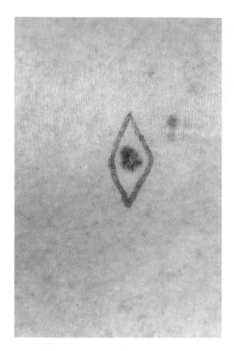

Fig. 24.7 Suspicious pigmented lesions should be removed with a 2 mm margin marked out in advance.

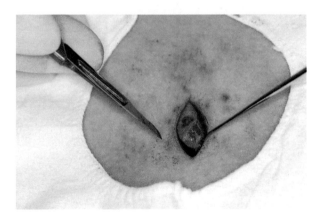

Fig. 24.8 A Gillies hook helps to remove an elliptical biopsy without damaging it.

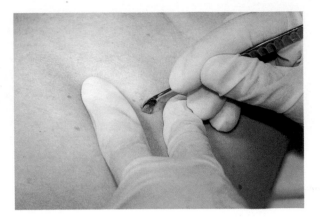

Fig. 24.9 Curettage beats excision if a seborrhoeic wart has to be removed. Stretching the skin helps to hold the lesion steady.

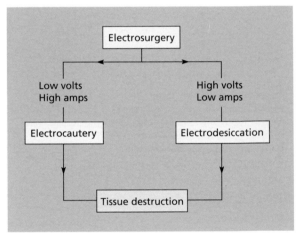

Fig. 24.10 Types of electrosurgery.

effective for viral warts, seborrhoeic keratoses, actinic keratoses and some superficial skin tumours (e.g. intra-epidermal carcinoma and lentigo maligna). It is applied either on a cotton bud or with a special spray gun (Fig. 24.11). The lesion is frozen until it turns white, with a 1–2 mm halo of freezing around. Two freeze–thaw cycles kill tissue more effectively than one but are usually unnecessary for warts and keratoses. Standard freeze–thaw times have been established for superficial tumours but temperature probes in and around deep tumours are needed to gauge the degree of freezing for their effective treatment. A single application of a very potent local steroid, after thawing, may lessen post-treatment pain and prevent blistering. A crust, including the necrotic tumour, should slough off after about two weeks.

Radiotherapy

Superficial radiation therapy (50–100 kV) is often used to treat biopsy-proven skin cancers in those over 60 years old or who are too frail to tolerate

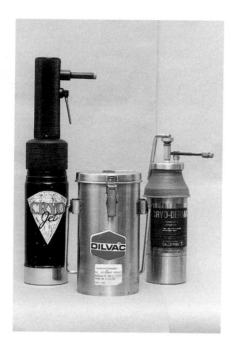

Fig. 24.11 Liquid nitrogen can be applied through a spray, or with a cotton wool bud direct from a vacuum flask (centre).

Phototherapy

UVR helps some conditions, for example psoriasis, parapsoriasis, pityriasis lichenoides, pityriasis rosea, mycosis fungoides, and acne (Table 17.3). For psoriasis, UVB may be given up to three times weekly, for three to eight weeks, on its own or combined with tar (Goeckerman) treatment or dithranol (anthralin) (Ingram) treatment (Chapter 6). After tests to establish a starting dose, irradiance is increased by small increments, aiming to produce minimal erythema only after 24 hours. UVA is combined with psoralens in PUVA treatment (p. 62). Close supervision is needed to avoid side effects such as severe erythema. A careful record should be kept of the cumulative UVR dose.

Laser therapy

Lasers, *L*ight *A*mplification by the *S*timulated *E*mission of *R*adiation, are now being used to treat many skin lesions including capillary haemangiomas, tattoos, epidermal naevi, seborrhoeic keratoses, warts, and tumours.

Since 1960, when T.H. Maiman won the Nobel Prize for inventing the first laser, technology has advanced rapidly and many types of laser are now available for clinical use. Port-wine stains can be treated successfully in children as well as in adults using the flashlamp pulsed dye laser (585 nm); the

surgery (Fig. 24.12). The usual dose is 3000 cGy, given in fractions over five to ten days. The scars from radiotherapy worsen with time, in contrast to surgical scars which improve. Nowadays radiotherapy is seldom used for inflammatory conditions.

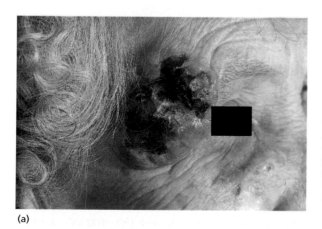

(a)

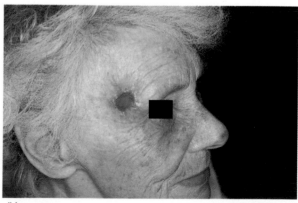

(b)

Fig. 24.12 A 90 year old, unfit for surgery, did well with radiotherapy for this massive basal carcinoma (a). The reaction was healing well after a few weeks (b).

results are better than those using the continuous wave argon laser (488 nm, 514 nm) which may cause hypertrophic scarring and pigmentary changes, especially in children. Most tattoos can be removed by treatment with a q-switched ruby laser (694 nm), a flashlamp pumped pulsed tunable dye laser (510 nm) or an alexandrite laser (760 nm). Scarring should not be a problem. Benign but unsightly pig-mented lesions such as *café au lait* marks, melasma, the naevus of Ota and senile lentigines have been greatly improved by treatment with the flashlamp pumped pulsed tunable dye laser (510 nm) and the q-switched frequency doubled neodymium YAG laser (532 nm). All laser treatments should be carried out by appropriately trained specialists.

Topical treatments

Our selection has been determined by personal preferences and we accept that we have left out many effective remedies. However, the preparations listed here are those which we use most often. As a result some appear only in the UK column but not in the USA one, and vice versa.

Type of preparation and general comments	UK preparations	USA preparations
Emollients These are used to make dry scaly skin smoother. Most are best applied after a shower or bath	Soft white paraffin Emulsifying ointment Aqueous cream — can be used as a soap substitute Diprobase (Schering-Plough) E45 cream (Crookes Products) — contains hypoallergenic lanolin Oilatum cream (Stiefel) Unguentum Merck (E. Merck) — a useful diluent: contains propylene glycol and sorbic acid, which may sensitize Neutrogena dermatological cream — Norwegian formula (Neutrogena) Aquadrate cream (Procter & Gamble Pharm.) — contains urea Calmurid cream (Galderma) — contains urea	Petrolatum alba (USP) Aquaphor (Beiersdorf) Eucerin (Beiersdorf) Lubriderm (Warner-Lambert) Cold Cream (USP) Complex 15 (Baker/Cummins) Carmol range (Syntex) — contains urea Nutraplus (Owen) — contains urea Lacticare (Stiefel) — contains lactic acid LacHydrin lotion (Westwood) — contains ammonium lactate Curel (S.C. Johnson) Moisturel (Westwood) Neutrogena range (Neutrogena)
Bath additives/shower gels These are a useful way of ensuring application to the whole skin. Most contain emollients which help dry itchy skin. Others contain tar (see section on psoriasis) or antibacterials	Balneum range (E. Merck) Emulsiderm (Dermal) — contains benzalkonium chloride Oilatum range (Stiefel) Ster-Zac bath concentrate (Hough) — contains antibacterial triclosan	Alpha Keri (Westwood) Lobana (Ulmer) Oilated Aveeno (Rydelle) — contains colloidal oatmeal, mineral oil Robathol (PharmSpec) — contains cottonseed oil
Shampoos All contain detergents which help to remove debris and scales; some have added ingredients to combat psoriasis, seborrhoeic eczema and bacterial infections. Most work best if their lather is left on the scalp for five minutes before being rinsed off	*Containing tar* Alphosyl shampoo (Stafford-Miller) Polytar range (Stiefel) T-Gel shampoo (Neutrogena) Capasal (Dermal) — also contains salicyclic acid	*Containing tar* Pentrax (GenDerm) Sebutone (Westwood) T-Gel (Neutrogena) Denorex (Whitehall) Ionil-T (Owen)

Continued on p. 288

Type of preparation and general comments	UK preparations	USA preparations
Shampoos (continued)	*Others* Betadine shampoo solution (Seton) – contains antibacterial povidone iodine Ceanel concentrate shampoo (Quinoderm) – contains cetrimide, undecenoic acid Selsun shampoo (Abbott) – contains selenium sulphide and can be used to treat pityriasis versicolor (p. 191) Nizoral shampoo (Janssen) – contains ketoconazole and is useful for seborrhoeic dermatitis and pityriasis versicolor	*Others* Capitrol (Westwood) – contains chloroxine (may stain hair yellow) Ionil Plus (Owen) – contains salicylic acid Head and Shoulders (Procter & Gamble) – contains zinc pyrithione Selsun shampoo (Abbott) – contains selenium sulphide Nizoral (Janssen) – contains ketoconazole
Cleansing agents These are used to remove debris and to combat infection. Some are astringents which precipitate protein and in doing so help to seal the moist surface of a weeping eczema or a stasis ulcer	Normasol (Seton) – 0.9% solution of sodium chloride used to clean wounds and ulcers Permitabs (Bioglan) – one tablet in four litres water makes 0.01% solution of potassium permanganate (will stain clothing and skin) Aluminium acetate lotion – use at 0.65% in water. Mildly astringent and used as wet dressing Silver nitrate – use at 0.5% in water. Astringent. Stains skin brown Cetavlon solution (Zeneca) – contains 40% cetrimide (detergent/antibacterial) and has to be diluted to 1% Hibitane 5% concentrate (Zeneca) – use diluted to one in 100, i.e. a 0.05% solution of chlorhexidine in water for skin disinfection Roccal (Sterling-Winthrop) – contains 1% benzalkonium chloride. Use diluted one in 10 or one in 100	Normal saline Cetaphil lotion (Owen) – a non-lipid soap substitute Domeboro tablets or powder (Miles) – contains aluminium sulphate, calcium acetate Acetic acid – 0.125–0.25% or one part white vinegar to 20 parts water Sodium hypochlorite – 0.25% in water (Dakin's solution)
Barrier preparations These are used to protect the skin from irritants and are of value in the napkin (diaper) area and around stomas. Many contain the silicone, dimethicone. The choice of barrier creams for use at work depends upon individual circumstances: recommendations are not given here	Dimethicone cream Zinc and castor oil ointment Conotrane cream (Yamanuchi: Pharma Ltd) – contains dimethicone, benzalkonium Siopel cream (Zeneca) – contains dimethicone and cetrimide Timodine cream (R & C) – contains dimethicone, hydrocortisone, nystatin, benzalkonium Vasogen cream (Pharmax) – contains dimethicone, calamine, zinc oxide	Zinc oxide paste (USP) Kerodex range (Ayerst) pH Stabil (Hermal) Desitin ointment (Leeming) – contains zinc oxide, vitamins A and D, cod liver oil

Type of preparation and general comments	UK preparations	USA preparations
Depigmenting agents These contain hydroquinone. The use of agents containing monobenzone causes permanent complete depigmentation	None in BNF but some preparations available without prescription from chemists/cosmetic counters	Melanex (Neutrogena) Solaquin (Elder) — also contains sunscreen
Camouflaging preparations Blemishes which cannot be removed can often be made less obvious by covering them: expert cosmetic advice may be needed to obtain the best colour match	Boots Covering cream (Boots) Covermark range of products (Cupharma) Dermablend (Baker Norton) Keromask masking creams and finishing powder (Network Management)	Covermark range (O'Leary) Dermablend (Dermablend Cosmetics) Liquimat acne coverup (Owen/Allercreme) Vitadye (Elder) — vitiligo stain

Sunscreens and sunblocks
These help the light-sensitive but are not a substitute for sun avoidance and sensible protective clothing. The sun protection factor (SPF) is a measure of their effectiveness, which is greater against UVB than UVA
 	
Allergic contact dermatitis from the sunscreen ingredients (usually PABA esters) may be missed and the rash put down to a deterioration of the original photosensitivity
	Contains PABA or PABA ester:
	  Spectraban 15 lotion (Stiefel)
	Contains cinnamate and oxybenzone:
	  RoC Total Sunblock cream
	  Uvistat range (Windsor)
	Contains titanium dioxide:
	  Sun E45 range (Crookes)
		Contain PABA or PABA ester:
		  PreSun (Westwood)
		  Sundown (Johnson & Johnson)
		  Supershade (Plough)
		  Eclipse (Dorsey)
		Contains benzophenone:
		  Solbar (Person & Covey)
		Contains PABA and BMD:
		  Supershade UVA block (Plough)
		Sunblock creams:
		  RVPaque (Elder)
		  Zinc oxide paste
		Lip sunscreens:
		  Chapstick Sunblock (Robins)
		  PreSun Stick (Westwood)

Antipruritics Remember that these are of limited value: try to make a firm diagnosis which will lead to an effective line of treatment	Calamine lotion Calamine lotion, oily — contains arachis oil Menthol (0.5%) or phenol (1.0%) in aqueous cream Eurax cream and lotion (Zyma) — contains crotamiton; also used to treat scabies	Calamine lotion Prax (Ferndale) — contains pramoxine Sarna lotion (Stiefel) — contains menthol, phenol, camphor Tucks (Parke-Davis) — contains glycerin, witch hazel Eurax cream and lotion (Westwood) — contains crotamiton
Antiperspirants The most effective preparations for excessive sweating in the armpits are those which contain aluminium chloride hexahydrate in an alcohol base. They also help palmar sweating but to a lesser extent	Anhydrol forte solution (Dermal) — contains 20% aluminium chloride hexahydrate Driclor solution (Stiefel) — contains 20% aluminium chloride hexahydrate	Xerac AC (Person & Covey) — contains 6.5% aluminium chloride hexahydrate Drysol (Person & Covey) — contains 20% aluminium chloride hexahydrate

Continued on p. 290

Type of preparation and general comments	UK preparations	USA preparations
Keratolytics These are used to counter an excessive production of keratin. Salicylic acid preparations should be used for limited areas only and not above 6%, as absorption and toxicity may follow their prolonged and extensive application, especially in infants	Salicylic acid, 2–4% in emulsifying ointment or soft white paraffin Urea preparations (*see* Emollients)	Salicylic acid, 2–4% in petrolatum alba (USP) Keralyt gel (Westwood) Urea preparations (*see* Emollients)
Depilatories These are used to remove unwanted facial hairs. All are irritating	None in BNF but freely available	Magic shaving powder — contains sulphides Nair (Carter) — contains thioglycollates Neet (Reckit) — contains thioglycollates
Steroids Our selection here has had to be ruthless as so many brands and mixtures are now on the market. Conventionally, they are classified according to their potency; your aim should be to use the least potent preparation which will cope with the skin disorder being treated. Side effects and dangers are listed in Table 24.2 (p. 278) Nothing stronger than 1% hydrocortisone should be used on the face (except in special circumstances, e.g. discoid LE) or in infancy. Be reluctant to prescribe more than 200 g of a mildly potent, 50 g of a moderately potent, or 30 g of a potent preparation per week for any adult for more than a month Most of the preparations listed are available as lotions, creams, oily creams, and ointments; your choice of vehicle will depend upon the condition under treatment (p. 277). Use twice daily except for Cutivate and Elocon which are just as effective if used once a day	*Mildly potent* Hydrocortisone 0.5%, 1.0%, 2.5% (numerous manufacturers) Mildison Lipocream (Brocades) Synalar. One in ten dilution (Zeneca) *Moderately potent* Eumovate (Glaxo) Modrasone (Schering-Plough) Stiedex L.P. (Stiefel) Ultradil (Schering Health) *Potent* Betnovate (Glaxo) Cutivate (Glaxo) Elocon (Schering-Plough) Locoid (Brocades) Synalar (Zeneca) *Very potent* Dermovate (Glaxo) Halciderm (Squibb) Nerisone Forte (Schering Health)	*Mildly potent* Hydrocortisone 0.5%, 1.0%, 2.5% (numerous manufacturers) Tridesilon (Miles) Desowen (Owen) Aclovate (Glaxo) *Moderately potent* Kenalog (Squibb) Aristocort (Lederle) Valisone (Schering) Westcort (Westwood) *Potent* Lidex (Syntex) Cutivate (Glaxo) Halog (Princeton) Diprosone (Schering) *Very potent* Diprolene (Schering) Temovate (Glaxo) Psorcon (Dermik) Ultravate (Westwood)

Steroid combinations

With clioquinol (antiseptic)	*Mildly potent* Vioform hydrocortisone (Zyma) *Potent* Betnovate-C (Glaxo) Locoid-C (Brocades) Synalar-C (Zeneca)	*Mildly potent* Vioform-HC (Ciba)

Continued

Type of preparation and general comments	UK preparations	USA preparations
With antibiotics	*Mildly potent* Terra-Cortril (Pfizer) — with oxytetracycline	*Mildly potent* Neo-Cort-Dome (Miles) — with neomycin, hydrocortisone
	Moderately potent and potent Betnovate-N (Glaxo) — with neomycin Adcortyl with graneodin (Squibb) Synalar-N (Zeneca) — with neomycin	*Moderately potent and potent* Neo-Synalar (Syntex) — with neomycin Cordran-N (Dista) — with neomycin
With antifungals	*Very potent* Dermovate NN — with nystatin and neomycin	
	Mildly potent Canestan HC (Baypharm) Daktacort (Janssen) Econacort (Squibb)	
		Moderately potent and potent Lotrisone (Schering)
With antibacterials and antifungals	*Mildly potent* Nystaform HC (Baypharm) Terra-Cortril Nystatin (Pfizer) Timodine (R & C)	No USA equivalents
	Moderately potent Trimovate (Glaxo)	*Moderately potent* Mycolog II (Squibb)
With tar	*Mildly potent only* Alphosyl HC (Stafford-Miller) Tarcortin (Stafford-Miller)	No USA equivalents
With salicylic acid	*Potent only* Diprosalic (Schering-Plough)	No USA equivalents

Preparations for use in the mouth

Useful mouth washes	Difflam oral rinse (3M) — an analgesic for painful inflammation in the mouth Corsodyl mouth wash (Zeneca) — contains chlorhexidine	Diphenhydramine elixir (Roxane) — anaesthetic Chloraseptic (Richardson-Vicks) — contains phenol Amosan (Oral B) — liberates oxygen upon contact with mouth fluids or blood
Topical steroids	Adcortyl in orabase paste (Squibb) — adheres to mucous membranes Corlan pellets (Evans) — dissolve slowly in mouth near lesion	Kenalog in Orabase (Squibb) — adheres to mucous membranes Lidex gel (Syntex)

Continued on p. 292

Type of preparation and general comments	UK preparations	USA preparations
Preparations for use in the mouth (continued)		
For yeast infections	Daktarin oral gel (Janssen) — contains miconazole Fungilin lozenges (Squibb) — contain amphotericin Nystatin oral suspension (Squibb)	Mycelex troche (Miles) — contains clotrimazole Mycostatin pastilles (Squibb) — contain nystatin Nystatin oral suspension (numerous manufacturers)
Preparations for otitis externa Otitis externa, essentially an eczema, is often complicated by bacterial or yeast overgrowth — hence the combinations listed here	Aluminium acetate ear drops 8% — an effective astringent for the weeping phase: best applied on ribbon gauze Otosporin drops (Wellcome) — hydrocortisone with neomycin and polymyxin Terracortril drops (Pfizer) — hydrocortisone with oxytetracycline and polymyxin Canesten solution (Baypharm) — contains clotrimazole	Otic Domeboro solution (Miles) — contains aluminium sulphate, acetic acid Corticosporin otic suspension (Burroughs Wellcome) — contains polymixin B, neomycin, hydrocortisone Otic-HC ear drops (Hauck) — contains chloroxylenol, hydrocortisone, pramoxine, acetic acid Vo-Sol-HC (Wallace) — contains acetic acid, hydrocortisone
Antibacterial preparations The ideal preparation should have high antibacterial activity, low allergenicity, and the drug should not be available for systemic use; this combination is hard to find. Some compromises are given here	Bactroban ointment (Beecham) — contains mupirocin Fucidin ointment, cream or gel (Leo) — contains fusidic acid Graneodin ointment (Squibb) — contains neomycin (a sensitizer), gramicidin To eliminate nasal carriage of staphylococci: Bactroban-N cream (Beecham) Naseptin cream (Zeneca) — contains neomycin	Polysporin ointment, powder, or spray (Burroughs Wellcome) — contains polymixin B, bacitracin Bacitracin ointment (Fougera) Bactroban ointment (Beecham) — contains mupirocin Betadine ointment (Purdue-Fredrick) — contains povidone iodine
Antifungal preparations In our view imidazole, terbinafine and amorolfine creams have now supplanted their messier, more irritant, and less effective rivals, e.g. Whitfield's ointment. They have the added advantage of combating yeasts as well as dermatophytes Systemic therapy will be needed for tinea of the scalp, of the nails, and of widespread or chronic skin infections which prove resistant to topical treatment	Canesten cream (Baypharm) — contains clotrimiazole Daktarin cream (Janssen) — contains miconazole Ecostatin cream (Squibb) — contains econazole Lamisil cream (Sandoz) — contains terbinafine Loceryl cream and nail lacquer (Roche) — contains amorolfine Trosyl nail solution (Pfizer) — contains tioconazole. Applied locally it may increase the success rate of griseofulvin. Used by itself it may also cure or improve some nails	Naftin cream (Herbert Laboratories) — contains naftifine, not an imidazole Lotrimin cream and solution (Schering) — contains clotrimazole Monistat-derm cream (Ortho) — contains miconazole Oxistat cream (Glaxo) — contains oxiconazole Spectazole cream (Ortho) — contains econazole Nizoral cream (Janssen) — contains ketoconazole Loprox cream (Hoechst) — contains ciclopirox, not an imidazole

Type of preparation and general comments	UK preparations	USA preparations
Antiviral preparations These have little part to play in the management of herpes zoster. However, if used early and frequently, they may help with recurrent herpes simplex infections	Zovirax cream (Wellcome) — contains acyclovir Herpid application (Yamanuchi Pharma Ltd) — contains idoxuridine in dimethyl sulphoxide. Absorption of dimethyl sulphoxide may cause a garlic taste	Zovirax cream (Burroughs Wellcome) — contains acyclovir
Wart treatments		
Palmoplantar warts	Salactol paint (Dermal) Glutarol solution (Dermal) Cuplex gel (S & N Pharm) Occlusal (Euroderma) Veracur gel (Typharm)	Duofilm paint (Stiefel) Occlusal range (GenDerm) Transplantar Pads (Msummura) (in Karaya gum) Duoplant gel (Scholl)
Anoqenital warts	Podophyllin paint compound — contains 15% podophyllin resin (use with care, p. 175)	Podophyllin, 15% in tincture of benzoin (use with care, p. 175) Condylox (Oclassen) — contains podofilox
Preparations for treatment of scabies Poor results follow inefficient usage rather than ineffective preparations. We prefer Lyclear or precipitated sulphur in young children, and pregnant and lactating women. Written instructions are helpful (p. 200)	Lyclear Dermal Cream (Wellcome) — contains permethrin Benzyl Benzoate Application (BP) Ascabiol application (M & B) — contains benzyl benzoate Eurax Cream (Zyma) — contains crotamiton Quellada lotion (Stafford-Miller) — contains lindane (gamma benzene hexachloride) Precipitated sulphur 6% in soft white paraffin Derbac-M liquid (Napp) — contains malathion	Elimite (Herbert) — contains pyrethrin Kwell lotion and cream (Reed & Carnrick) — contains lindane Scabene lotion (Stiefel) — contains lindane Eurax lotion and cream (Westwood) — contains crotamiton Precipitated sulphur 6% in petrolatum alba
Preparations for treatment of pediculosis Resistance to lindane has limited its usefulness for scalp lice. Lotions left on for a minimum of 12 hours are perhaps more effective, though less convenient than shampoos	Prioderm lotion and cream shampoo (Napp) — contains malathion Derbac-M lotion and shampoo (International Labs) — contains carbaryl Quellada lotion (see above) Lyclear Cream Rinse (Wellcome) — contains permethrin	Nix cream rinse (Burroughs Wellcome) — contains pyrethrin R & C spray (Reed & Carnrick) — contains pyrethroids RID lotion (Leeming) — contains pyrethrin Kwell shampoo (Reed & Carnrick) — contains lindane
Preparations for acne Active ingredient:		
Benzoyl peroxide (an antibacterial agent)	Panoxyl and Acetoxyl ranges (Stiefel) 2.5%, 5%, 10%	PanOxyl range (Stiefel) Desquam X range (Westwood) —

Continued on p. 294

Type of preparation and general comments	UK preparations	USA preparations
Preparations for acne (continued) Induces dryness during the first few weeks; this usually settles even with continued use	Quinoderm cream (Quinoderm) — contains potassium hydroxyquinolone	contains laureth-4 Sulfoxyl 5%, 10% (Dermik) — contains 2% sulphur
Retinoids	Isotrex (Stiefel) — contains isotretinoin (avoid during pregnancy/lactation) Retin-A preparations (Ortho-Cilag) — contain tretinoin	Retin-A gel, cream, and solution (Ortho)
Antibiotics	Dalacin-T solution (Upjohn) — contains clindamycin Zineryt (Yamanuchi Pharma Ltd) — contains erythromycin and zinc acetate Stiemycin solution (Stiefel) — contains erythromycin Topicycline solution (Procter & Gamble Pharm.) — contains tetracycline. May stain yellow and fluoresce at discos	Cleocin-T (Upjohn) — contains clindamycin EryDerm (Abbott) — contains erythromycin Topicycline (Norwich Eaton) — contains tetracycline Metrogel (Curatek) — contains metronidazole
Abrasives	Brasivol paste Nos 1 & 2 (Stiefel) Ionax scrub (Galderma)	Bravisol (Stiefel) Ionax scrub (Owen)
Sulphur	2–10% sulphur in calamine lotion	Liquimat (Owen-Allercreme) Rezamid (Dermik) — contains resorcin
Azelaic acid	Skinoren (Schering Health)	
Preparations for rosacea	Metrogel (Sandoz) — contains metronidazole	Metrogel (Curatek) — contains metronidazole
Preparations for psoriasis		
Tar These clean refined tar preparations are suitable for home use. Messier, though more effective, formulations exist but are best used in treatment centres		
Bath additives	Polytar emollient (Stiefel) Psoriderm bath emulsion (Dermal)	Polytar (Stiefel) Balnatar (Westwood)
Applications	Alphosyl cream (Stafford Miller) Carbo-Dome cream (Lagap) Psoriderm cream (Dermal)	Estar gel (Westwood) Psongel (Owen)
Scalp applications	Alphosyl lotion (Stafford-Miller)	
Dithranol/anthralin Stains normal skin and clothing. May be irritant, therefore start with low concentration. For 30-minute regimen *see* p. 61	Anthranol ointment range (Stiefel) Dithrocream range (Dermal) Psoradrate cream range (Procter & Gamble Pharm.) — contains urea	Dithrocreme (American Dermal) Lasan cream and ointment (Stiefel)

Continued

Type of preparation and general comments	UK preparations	USA preparations
Calcipotriol (Calcipotriene, USA) A vitamin D derivative. May irritate initially. Should not exceed 100 g weekly	Dovonex cream and ointment (Leo)	Dovonex (Westwood Squibb Pharmaceuticals Inc.)
Steroids Routine long-term treatment with potent or very potent steroids is not recommended. For indications *see* p. 61		
Scalp applications	Betnovate scalp application (Glaxo) Synalar gel (Zeneca) Diprosalic scalp lotion (Kirby-Warrick) — also contains salicylic acid	Diprolene lotion (Schering) Lidex gel solution (Syntex) Valisone lotion (Schering) Synalar solution (Syntex)
For use elsewhere Tar–steroid combinations are helpful	*See* section on topical steroids above	*See* section on topical steroids above
Salicylic acid Used mostly for scalp psoriasis	*See* Keratolytics	*See* Keratolytics
Tar–salicylic acid combinations	Pragmatar cream (Bioglan) — also contains sulphur Gelcosal (Quinoderm)	T-gel scalp solution (Neutrogena) P & S plus gel (Baker Cummins) Pragmatar ointment (Smith Kline) — also contains sulphur

Preparations for venous ulcers

Regardless of topical applications, venous ulcers will heal only if local oedema is eliminated. Remember that the surrounding skin is easily sensitized. To choose treatment for an individual ulcer *see* p. 146

For cleansing	Saline, potassium permanganate, *see* Cleaning agents Hydrogen peroxide solution (3%)	Prolonged soaks in tap water or saline Hydrogen peroxide solution (3%) Acetic acid aqueous solution (0.25%)
Antibacterial gauze dressings	Bactigras tulle dressing (S & N) Softratulle (Roussel) Fucidin Intertulle (Leo)	
Other applications	Variclene gel (Dermal) — contains brilliant green Flamazine cream (S & N Pharm) — contains silver sulphadiazine active against *Pseudomonas* Silver nitrate aqueous solution (0.5%) Iodosorb (Perstorp) — contains cadexomer iodine	Debrisan (Johnson) a copolymer starch Silver nitrate aqueous solution (0.5%)
Medicated bandages Beware of allergic contact reactions to parabens preservatives which are in most bandages	Calaband (Seton) Ichthopaste (S & N) Viscopaste PB7 (S & N)	

Continued on p. 296

Type of preparation and general comments	UK preparations	USA preparations
Preparations for venous ulcers (continued)		
Other dressings	Granuflex (Convatec) — a hydrocolloid Kaltostat (BritCair) — contains calcium alginate Tielle (T & T) — a hydrogel	Duoderm (Squibb) — a hydrocolloid Vigilon (Bard) — a hydrocolloid Tegaderm (3M) — a film Opsite (American Hospital Co.) — a film Debrisan (Johnson) — a copolymer starch

Miscellaneous

5-flourouracil
The treatment of individual lesions in patients with multiple actinic keratoses is tedious or impossible. For such cases 1—5% cream containing 5-fluorouracil is useful. It should be applied twice daily for two weeks. Patients should be warned about the inevitable inflammation and soreness which appears after a few days. Lesions on the scalp and face do better than those on the arms and hands

Efudix cream (Roche)

Efudex cream and solution (Roche)
Fluoroplex cream and solution (Herbert)

Minoxidil
May be used as a possible treatment for early male-pattern alopecia. The response is slow, and only a small minority of patients will obtain a dense regrowth even after 12 months. Hair regained will fall out when treatment stops — warn patients about this

Regaine topical solution (Upjohn) — only private prescription

Rogaine (Upjohn)

Capsaicin
A topical analgesic useful for the treatment of post-herpetic neuralgia. Apply up to 3—4 times daily after lesions have healed. May take 2—4 weeks to relieve pain

Axsain cream (0.075%) (Euroderma)

Zostrix cream (0.025%)
Zostrix HP cream (0.075%) (Genderm Pharmaceuticals)

Lithium succinate
A topical anti-inflammatory used in seborrhoeic dermatitis

Efalith ointment (Searle) contains 8% lithium succinate and 0.05% zinc sulphate

Lignocaine/prilocaine
A local anaesthetic for topical use. Applied on skin as a thick layer of cream under an occlusive dressing or on adult genital mucosa with no occlusive dressing. Read manufacturer's instructions for times of application

Emla cream (Searle) contains 2.5% lignocaine and 2.5% prilocaine

Systemic medication

We list here only preparations we use commonly for our patients with skin disease. **The doses given are the usual oral doses for adults**. We occasionally use some of these drugs for uses not approved by federal regulatory agencies. We have included some, but not all, of the side effects and interactions; these are more fully covered in the *British National Formulary* (UK) and *Physician's Desk Reference* (USA). Physicians prescribing these drugs should read about them in more detail before treating their patients. If possible, systemic medication should be avoided in pregnant women.

Main dermatological uses and usual adult dosage	Adverse effects	Interactions	Cautions
Antibacterials			
Cefuroxime A cephalosporin not inactivated by penicillinase. For gram-positive and -negative infections resistant to penicillin and erythromycin (250 mg twice daily)	Gut upsets Candidiasis Rarely E. multiforme or toxic epidermal necrolysis Transient hepatotoxicity Rarely nephrotoxic	Probenecid reduces excretion	Not usually indicated as first line or blind therapy. Ten per cent of penicillin allergic patients will react to this
Ciprofloxacin A 4-quinolone used for gram-negative infections, especially pseudomonas, and gram-positive infections. First choice for skin infections in the immunosuppressed if the causative organism is not yet known (500 mg twice daily)	Gut upsets Occasionally hepatotoxic and nephrotoxic Haemolysis in those deficient in glucose-6-phosphate dyhydrogenase	Antacids reduce absorption. Enhances effects of warfarin and theophylline.	Crystalluria if fluid intake is inadequate. Care if renal impairment. Avoid in pregnancy, breast feeding, children and epileptics
Co-amoxyclav A broad spectrum penicillin combined with clavulanic acid: use if organisms resistant to both erythromycin and flucloxacillin. Also for gram-negative folliculitis (375 mg three times daily)	Gut upsets Candidiasis Rashes, especially in infectious mononucleosis	As for other penicillins	Use with care in hepatic or renal failure, pregnancy, and breast feeding. Avoid in those allergic to penicillin

Continued on p. 298

Main dermatological uses and usual adult dosage	Adverse effects	Interactions	Cautions

Antibacterials (continued)

Erythromycin
1 Acne vulgaris (250–500 mg twice daily)
2 Gram-positive infections, particularly staphylococcal and streptococcal. Useful with penicillin allergy (250–500 mg four times daily)

Gut upsets
Rashes
Cholestatic hepatitis if treatment prolonged (reversible and most common with estolate salt)

Increased risk of toxicity if given with theophylline or carbamezapine
Potentiates effects of warfarin, ergotamine, cyclosporin A, disopyramide, carbamezapine, terfenadine, astemizole, theophylline and digoxin

Avoid estolate in liver disease
Care when hepatic dysfunction
Excreted in human milk

Flucloxacillin
Dicloxacillin
Cloxacillin
Penicillins used for infections with penicillinase-forming staphylococci (250 mg four times daily)

Gut upsets
Morbilliform eruptions
Arthralgia
Anaphylaxis

Probenecid increases blood level
Reduces excretion of methotrexate

Accumulate in renal failure
Atopics may be at increased risk of hypersensitivity reactions

Metronidazole
1 Anaerobic infections (200–400 mg three times daily)
2 Stubborn rosacea (200 mg twice daily)
3 Trichomoniasis (200 mg three times daily for seven days)

Gut upsets
Metallic taste
Candidiasis
Ataxia and sensory neuropathy

Potentiates effects of warfarin, phenytoin and lithium
Drugs that induce liver enzymes (e.g. rifampicin, barbiturates, griseofulvin, phenytoin, carbamezapine, and smoking), increase destruction of metronidazole in liver and necessitate higher dosage
May have disulfiram-like effect with alcohol (headaches, flushing, vomiting, abdominal pain)

Use lower dose in presence of liver disease
Neurotoxicity more likely if CNS disease

Minocycline
A tetracycline used for acne and rosacea (50 mg daily or twice daily, or 100 mg daily in a modified release preparation)

Gut upsets
Dizziness and vertigo
Candidiasis
Deposition in bones and teeth of fetus and children
Deposition in skin causes blue-grey pigmentation
Benign intracranial hypertension

May impair absorption of oral contraceptives
May potentiate effect of warfarin

Avoid in pregnancy and in children under 12 years

Continued

Main dermatological uses and usual adult dosage	Adverse effects	Interactions	Cautions
Tetracycline and oxytetracycline Acne and rosacea (250–500 mg twice daily)	Gut upsets Candidiasis Rashes Deposition in bones and teeth of fetus and children Rare phototoxic reactions Benign intracranial hypertension	Absorption impaired when taken with food, antacids, and iron Many impair absorption of oral contraceptives May potentiate effect of warfarin	Avoid in pregnancy and in children under 12 years Should not be used if renal insufficiency
Penicillin V (phenoxymethylpenicillin) **1** For infections with gram-positive cocci (250–500 mg four times daily) **2** Prophylaxis of erysipelas (250 mg daily)	Gut upsets Morbilliform rashes Urticaria Arthralgia Anaphylaxis	Blood level increased by probenecid Reduces excretion of methotrexate	Accumulates in renal failure Atopics at increased risk of hypersensitivity reactions

Antifungals

Terbinafine (not available in USA) Dermatophyte infections when systemic treatment appropriate (due to site, severity or extent) Where available has replaced griseofulvin as first choice systemic antifungal agent. Unlike itraconazole and fluconazole its action does not involve cytochrome p450 dependent enzymes in the liver 250 mg daily Tinea pedis: 2–6 weeks Tinea corporis: 4 weeks Tinea unguium: 12 weeks	Gut upsets Headache Rashes Taste disturbance Rarely liver toxicity	Plasma concentration reduced by rifampicin Plasma concentration increased by cimetidine	Avoid in hepatic and renal impairment and when breast feeding. Not for use in pregnancy Not yet recommended for children
Griseofulvin Dermatophyte infections of skin, nails, and hair. Not for *Candida* or pityriasis versicolor (500 mg microsize daily)	Gut upsets Headaches, rashes, photosensitivity	Induces microsomal liver enzymes and so may increase elimination of drugs such as warfarin and phenobarbitone	Not for use in pregnancy, liver failure, porphyria or systemic LE Absorbed better when taken with fatty foods

Continued on p. 300

Main dermatological uses and usual adult dosage	Adverse effects	Interactions	Cautions

Antifungals *(continued)*

Fluconazole

1 Candidiasis *Acute/ recurrent vaginal* (Single dose of 150 mg) *Mucosal (not vaginal) conditions* (50 mg daily) Oropharyngeal: 7–14 days Oesophagus: 14–30 days *Systemic candidiasis* – see manufacturer's instructions **2** Second line treatment in some systemic mycoses e.g. cryptococcal infections **3** Dermatophyte infections (except of nails) (50 mg daily for 2–6 weeks) **4** Pityriasis versicolor (50 mg daily for 1 week)	Gut upsets Rarely rashes Angioedema/anaphylaxis Liver toxicity May be worse in AIDS patients	Hydrochlorothiazide increases plasma concentration Rifampicin reduces plasma concentration Potentiates effects of warfarin, cyclosporin A and phenytoin May potentiate effects of sulphonylureas leading to hypoglycaemia May inhibit metabolism of terfenadine and astemizole causing serious arrhythmias	Avoid in pregnancy Hepatic and renal impairment Use in children only if imperative and no alternative Avoid in children under one year and when breast feeding

Itraconazole

1 Candidiasis *Vulvovaginal* (200 mg twice daily) one day *Oropharyngeal* (100 mg daily) 15 days **2** Pityriasis versicolor (200 mg daily) – seven days **3** Dermatophyte infections (100 mg daily) Tinea pedis and manuum – 30 days Tinea corporis 15 days Tinea of nails – recently an intermittent regimen has been suggested (200 mg twice daily for one week per month, continued for three or four cycles)	Gut upsets Headache	Antacids reduce absorption Rifampicin and phenytoin reduce plasma concentration May potentiate effects of warfarin May increase plasma levels of digoxin and cyclosporin Inhibits metabolism of terfenadine and astemizole: this may lead to serious arrhythmias	Avoid in hepatic impairment Avoid in children, in pregnancy and when breast feeding

Ketoconazole

Dermatophyte infections of skin and pityriasis versicolor (200 mg daily for 14 days)	Same as fluconazole but greater incidence of liver toxicity	Same as fluconazole	Seldom used in UK. Monitor liver function continually if used for longer than 14 days and chosen because of its cheapness

Nystatin

1 Recurrent vulval and perineal candidiasis **2** Persistant GI candidiasis in immunosuppressed patients (500 000 units three times daily)	Unpleasant taste Gut upsets		Not absorbed and when given by mouth acts only on bowel yeasts

Main dermatological uses and usual adult dosage	Adverse effects	Interactions	Cautions

Antivirals

Acyclovir
1 Severe herpes simplex infections — primary or recurrent (200 mg five times daily for five days)
2 Severe herpes zoster infections (800 mg five times daily for seven days)
3 Prophylaxis for recurrent herpes simplex especially in the immunocompromised, to treat eczema herpeticum and to treat chicken pox in the immunocompromised (for dosages see specialist literature)

	Rapid gut upsets, transient rise in urea and creatinine in 10% of patients after intravenous use Raised liver enzymes Reversible neurological reactions Decreases in haematological indices	Excretion may be delayed by probenicid Lethargy when i.v. acylclovir given with zidovudine	Adequate hydration of patient should be maintained Risk in pregnancy unknown Reduce dose in renal impairment No effect on virus in latent phase Must be given early in acute infections

Famciclovir (not available in USA)
Herpes zoster, pain relief reputed to be quicker than with acyclovir (250 mg three times daily)

	Headache Rashes	See acyclovir	See acyclovir

Antihistamines
All those listed here are H$_1$-blockers though some dermatologists combine these with H$_2$-blockers in recalcitrant urticaria

Non-sedative
Used for urticaria and type I hypersensitivity reactions

Astemizole
Long acting (10 mg once a day; dose must not be exceeded)

	Weight gain Ventricular arrhythmias after excessive dosage	Increased blood concentrations with antifungal imidazoles or erythromycin may lead to serious arrhythmias	Do not exceed recommended dose Never prescribe with erythromycin or antifungal imidazoles Avoid in pregnancy and lactation

Loratadine
(10 mg daily)

		Not reported	Avoid in pregnancy and lactation

Cetirizine
(5 mg twice daily or 10 mg once daily)

	Rarely sedates	Not reported	Use half the usual dose when renal impairment

Continued on p. 302

Main dermatological uses and usual adult dosage	Adverse effects	Interactions	Cautions

Antihistamines (continued)

Terfenadine
(60 mg twice daily or 120 mg once daily in the morning)

	Adverse effects	Interactions	Cautions
	Hair loss Ventricular arrhythmias after excessive dosage	Increased blood concentrations with antifungal imidazoles or erythromycin May lead to serious arrhythmias	Do not exceed recommended dose Never prescribe with erythromycin or antifungal imidazoles

Sedative

Urticaria, type I hypersensitivity including intravenous use in, anaphylaxis (p. 274). Also used as antipruritic agents in e.g. atopic eczema, lichen planus	Sedation (promethazine > trimeprazine > hydroxyzine > chlorpheniramine = diphenhydramine = cyproheptadine) Anticholinergic effects: • dry mouth • blurred vision • urinary retention • tachycardia	Potentiate effect of alcohol and CNS depressants Potentiate effect of other anticholinergic drugs	Increased rate of elimination in children Sedation may be useful in an excited, itchy patient Warn of risk of drowsiness when driving or operating dangerous machinery

Chlorpheniramine
(4 mg three or four times daily)

Diphenhydramine
(25–30 mg four times daily)

Hydroxyzine
(10–50 mg four times daily)

Cyproheptadine
(4 mg four times daily)

Promethazine
(10–25 mg daily to three times daily)

Trimeprazine
(2.5–10 mg once or twice daily)

Anti-androgens

Cyproterone acetate and ethinyl oestradiol
(UK: Dianette; USA: not available)
1 Acne vulgaris, in women only, unresponsive to systemic antibiotics
2 Idiopathic hirsutism
One tablet (cyproterone

	Adverse effects	Interactions	Cautions
	As for combined oral contraceptives	Should not be given with other oral contraceptives	Contra-indicated in pregnancy. Cyproterone acetate is an anti-androgen and if given to pregnant women may feminize a male fetus. For women of childbearing age,

Continued

Main dermatological uses and usual adult dosage	Adverse effects	Interactions	Cautions
acetate 2 mg, ethinyl oestradiol 35 µg) daily for 21 days, starting on fifth day of menstrual cycle and repeated after a seven-day interval. Treat for six months at least			therefore, it must be given combined with a contraceptive (the ethinyl oestradiol component) Also contra-indicated in liver disease, disorders of lipid metabolism, and with past or present endometrial carcinomas Not for use in males or children

Immunosuppressants

Azathioprine

For auto-immune conditions, e.g. systemic LE, pemphigus, and bullous pemphigoid — often used to spare dose of systemic steroids (1–2.5 mg/kg daily)	Gut upsets Bone marrow suppression, usually leucopenia or thrombocytopenia Hepatotoxicity Predisposes to infections, including warts	Increased toxicity if given with allopurinol	Weekly blood checks are necessary for the first eight weeks of treatment and thereafter at intervals of not longer than three months Reduce dose if severe renal impairment Avoid in pregnancy

Cyclosporin

1 Severe psoriasis when conventional treatment is ineffective or inappropriate 2 Short-term (max. eight weeks) treatment of severe atopic dermatitis when conventional treatment ineffective or inappropriate (2.5 mg/kg daily in two divided doses). See p. 64 for guidance in use	Hepatic and renal impairment Gut upset Hypertrichosis Gum hyperplasia Tremor Hyperkalaemia Occasionally facial oedema, hypertension, fluid retention and convulsions	(See BNF and PDR for fuller details) 1 Drugs that may increase nephrotoxicity • Antibiotics (aminoglycosides, cotrimoxazole) • Non-steroidal anti-inflammatory drugs • Melphalan 2 Drugs that may increase cyclosporin blood level (by cytochrome p450 inhibition) • Antibiotics (erythromycin, amphotericin B, cephalosporins, doxycycline, acyclovir) • Hormones (corticosteroids, sex hormones) • Diuretics (frusemide/ furosamide thiazides) • Other (warfarin, H_2 antihistamines, calcium channel blockers) 3 Drugs that may decrease cyclosporin levels (by cytochrome p450 induction)	Contra-indicated if abnormal renal function, hypertension not under control and concomitant premalignant or malignant conditions. Monitor renal function and blood pressure as indicated on p. 64

Continued on p. 304

Main dermatological uses and usual adult dosage	Adverse effects	Interactions	Cautions
Immunosuppressants *(continued)*		• Anticonvulsants (phenytoin, phenobarbitone, carbamezapine, sodium valproate) • Antibiotics (isoniazide, rifampicin)	
Methotrexate Severe psoriasis unresponsive to local treatment (initially, 2.5 mg test dose and observe for one week, then 5–15 mg once every *week* orally or intramuscularly)	Gut upsets Stomatitis Bone marrow depression Liver or kidney dysfunction	Aspirin, probenecid, thiazide diuretics and some non-steroidal anti-inflammatory drugs delay excretion and increase toxicity Anti-epileptics, co-trimoxazole, and pyrimethamine increase antifolate effect Toxicity increased by cyclosporin and acitretin	Regular (weekly for the first six weeks) blood checks are necessary throughout treatment Avoid in pregnancy Reduce dose if renal or hepatic impairment Folinic acid given concomitantly prevents bone marrow depression Many insist on a liver biopsy before treatment and periodically thereafter as this is the best way of detecting hepatic fibrosis Elderly may be more sensitive to the drug

Corticosteroids

Prednisone and prednisolone Acute and severe allergic reactions, severe erythema multiforme, connective tissue disorders, pemphigus, pemphigoid and vasculitis (5–80 mg daily or on alternate days)	Impaired glucose tolerance Redistribution of fat (centripetal) Muscle wasting, proximal myopathy Osteoporosis and vertebral collapse Aseptic necrosis of head of femur Growth retardation in children Peptic ulceration Euphoria, psychosis or depression Cataract formation Precipitation of glaucoma Increase in blood pressure Sodium and water retention Potassium loss	Liver enzyme inducers (e.g. phenytoin, griseofulvin, rifampicin) reduce effect of corticosteroids Carbenoxolone and most diuretics increase potassium loss due to corticosteroids Corticosteroids reduce effect of many antihypertensive agents Corticosteroids will interact with drugs that affect glucose metabolism	**1** Before long-term treatment screen: • Chest X-ray • Blood pressure • Weight • Glycosuria • Electrolytes • Tuberculin skin test (USA) • Past history of peptic ulcer, cataracts/glaucoma, and affective psychosis **2** During treatment check BP, weight, glycosuria, and electrolytes regularly. Patients should carry a steroid treatment card or wear a labelled bracelet. Always bear in mind the

Continued

Main dermatological uses and usual adult dosage	Adverse effects	Interactions	Cautions
	Skin atrophy and capillary fragility Spread of infection Iatrogenic Cushing's syndrome		possibility of masked infections and perforations **3** Long-term treatment has to be tapered off slowly to avoid adrenal insufficiency **4** Do not use for psoriasis or long-term for atopic eczema

Retinoids

Acitretin (Etrerinate in USA)

Severe psoriasis, resistant to other forms of treatment (may be used with PUVA, p. 62), palmoplantar pustulosis, severe ichthyoses, Darier's disease, pityriasis rubra pilaris (0.2–1.0 mg/kg daily)	**1** *Mucocutaneous* (common) Rough, scaly, dry-appearing skin and mucous membranes Chafing Atrophy of skin and nails Diffuse thinning of scalp and body hair Curly hair Exuberant granulation tissue (especially toe nail folds) Disease flare-up Photosensitivity **2** *Systemic* Teratogenesis Diffuse interstitial skeletal hyperostosis Arthralgia, myalgia, and headache Benign intracranial hypertension **3** *Laboratory abnormalities* Haematology: ↓ WBC ↑ ESR Liver function tests: ↓ Bilirubin ↑ AST/ALT ↑ Alkaline phosphatase (abnormal in 20% of patients) Serum lipids: ↑ Cholesterol ↑ Triglycerides ↓ High-density lipoprotein (abnormal in 50% of patients)	Avoid concomitant high doses of vitamin A Possible antagonism to anticoagulant effect of warfarin Increases plasma concentration of methotrexate Increases hepatotoxicity of methotrexate	All women of childbearing age must use effective oral contraception for one month before treatment, during treatment and for at least two years after treatment. They should sign a consent form indicating that they know about the danger of teratogenicity Should not donate blood during or for 1 year after stopping the treatment (teratogenic risk) Regular screening should be carried out to exclude: **1** Abnormalities of liver function **2** Hyperlipidaemia **3** Disseminated interstitial skeletal hyperostosis Avoid if renal or hepatic impairment

Continued on p. 306

Main dermatological uses and usual adult dosage	Adverse effects	Interactions	Cautions
Retinoids (continued)			
Isotretinoin (13 *cis*-retinoic acid)			
Severe acne vulgaris, unresponsive to systemic antibiotics (0.5–1.0 mg/kg daily for 16 weeks)	*See* Acitretin	*See* Acitretin	Females of childbearing age must take effective contraception for one month before treatment is started, during treatment, and for three months after treatment is stopped; check a pregnancy test before starting treatment and monthly. Females should sign a consent form which states the dangers of teratogenicity Avoid in renal or hepatic impairment Blood tests as for acitretin
Drugs acting on the CNS			
Amitriptyline			
1 Depression secondary to skin disease 2 Post-herpetic neuralgia (50–100 mg at night; start with 10–25 mg in the elderly)	Sedation Anticholinergic effects Cardiac arrhythmias Confusion in the elderly Postural hypertension Jaundice Neutropenia May precipitate seizures in epileptics	Potentially lethal CNS stimulation with monoamine oxidase inhibitors Increases effects of other CNS depressants and anticholinergics Metabolism may be inhibited by cimetidine	Avoid in the presence of heart disease or hypertension Use small doses at first to avoid confusion in the elderly Warn about effects on skills such as driving
Diazepam			
Anxiety — often associated with skin disease (2 mg three times daily)	Sedation Impaired skills (e.g. driving) or ataxia Dependence (withdrawal may lead to sleeplessness, anxiety, tremors)	Potentiates effects of other CNS depressants including alcohol Breakdown inhibited by cimetidine and propranolol Liver enzyme inducers (e.g. phenytoin, griseofulvin, rifampicin) increase elimination	Use for short spells only (to avoid addiction) Avoid in pregnancy and breast feeding Use with care in presence of liver, kidney, or respiratory diseases, and in the elderly
Miscellaneous			
Adrenaline (epinephrine) injection			
Emergency treatment for acute anaphylaxis 0.5 mg (0.5 ml of one in 1000 solution given as a slow subcutaneous or rarely intramuscular injection. May be repeated after 10 minutes if necessary)	Tachycardia Cardiac arrhythmias Anxiety Tremor Headache Hypertension Hyperglycaemia Hypokalaemia	If given with some beta-blockers may lead to severe hypertension	Do not confuse the different strengths Give *slowly*, subcutaneously or intramuscularly, but *not* intravenously, except in cardiac arrest

Continued

Main dermatological uses and usual adult dosage	Adverse effects	Interactions	Cautions
Dapsone Leprosy, dermatitis herpetiformis, vasculitis, pyoderma gangrenosum (50–150 mg daily)	Haemolytic anaemia Methaemoglobinaemia Headaches Lethargy Hepatitis Peripheral neuropathy Exfoliative dermatitis Toxic epidermal necrolysis Agranulocytosis Aplastic anaemia Hypoalbuminaemia	Reduced excretion and increased side effects if given with probenecid	Regular blood checks necessary (weekly for first month, then every two weeks until three months, then monthly until six months and then six-monthly) Not felt to be teratogenic, but should not be given during pregnancy and lactation if possible. For dermatitis herpetiformis, a gluten-free diet is preferable at these times Avoid in patients with glucose 6-phosphate dehydrogenase deficiency (screen for this, especially in USA)
Hydroxychloroquine Systemic and discoid LE, porphyria cutanea tarda, polymorphic light eruption, LE: 200–400 mg daily, maintaining level at lowest effective dose. Must not exceed 6.5 mg/kg body weight/day (based on the ideal/lean body weight and not on the actual weight of the patient) Porphyria cutanea tarda: 50–100 mg twice *weekly*	Retinopathy which may cause permanent blindness Corneal deposits Headaches Gut upsets, pruritus and rashes Worsening of psoriasis	Should not be taken at the same time as other antimalarial drugs May raise plasma digoxin levels Potential neuromuscular toxicity if taken with gentamycin, kanamycin, or tobramycin Bioavailability decreased if given with antacids	All patients must have an ophthalmic examination (acuity, ophthalmoscopy, visual fields with red target) before treatment and every six months thereafter whilst on it. Patients should be asked to test themselves with an Amsler grid every two weeks looking for 'faded' squares. Discontinue drug if any change occurs Reduce dose with poor renal or liver function Best avoided in the elderly and children Do not give automatic repeat prescriptions Prefer intermittent short courses to continuous treatment if possible Use minute doses to treat porphyria cutanea tarda; ordinary doses cause toxic reactions

Continued on p. 308

Main dermatological uses and usual adult dosage	Adverse effects	Interactions	Cautions

Miscellaneous (continued)

8-methoxypsoralen (methoxsalen)

Used usually with UVA as PUVA therapy (p. 62) Severe psoriasis, vitiligo, localized pustular psoriasis, cutaneous T cell lymphoma; rarely, lichen planus, atopic dermatitis Tablets: 0.6−0.8 mg/kg body weight taken as a single dose 1−2 hours before exposure to UVA Liquid (Ultra Capsules) (USA): 0.3 mg/kg body weight taken one hour before exposure to UVA	Nausea Itching Photoxicity Cataracts Lentigines Ageing changes of skin Hyperpigmentation Cutaneous neoplasms	Avoid other photosensitizers (Chapter 17)	The following should checked before treatment: • Skin. Examine for premalignant lesions and skin cancer • Eyes. Check for cataracts. Fundoscopic examination of retina. Visual acuity • Blood. Full blood count, liver and renal function tests and antinuclear factor test • Urine analysis Eyes should be protected with polarizing lenses for 24 hours after taking the drug Protective goggles must be worn during radiation If feasible, shield face and genitalia during treatment Patients must protect skin against additional sun exposure after ingestion Monitor eyes for development of cataracts Try to avoid maintenance treatment and a cumulative dose of 1500 joules/cm^2 (skin cancer risk)

Gamolenic acid
(not available in USA)

As adjunctive treatment in atopic eczema. (320−480 mg daily) in two divided doses	Occasional gut upset Headache		Care if history of epilepsy or concomitant treatment with epileptogenic drugs (e.g. phenothiazines)

Index